M.A. Reymond · H.J. Bonjer · F. Köckerling (Eds.)
Port-Site and Wound Recurrences in Cancer Surgery

Springer-Verlag Berlin Heidelberg GmbH

M.A. Reymond · H.J. Bonjer · F. Köckerling (Eds.)

Port-Site and Wound Recurrences in Cancer Surgery

Incidence – Pathogenesis – Prevention

Foreword by Sir Alfred Cuschieri

With 60 Figures and 20 Tables

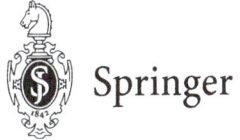

Springer

Marc A. Reymond, M.D., Associate Professor of Surgery,
Department of Surgery, University Hospital of Magdeburg, Leipziger Strasse 44
39120 Magdeburg, Germany

H. Jaap Bonjer, M.D., Ph.D., Head of Laparoscopic Surgery and
Acting Head of Endocrine Surgery, University Hospital Rotterdam
Dijkzigt Hospital, PO Box 2040, 3000 CA, Rotterdam, The Netherlands

Ferdinand Köckerling, M.D., Professor of Surgery and Head Department of Surgery
and Center for Minimally Invasive Surgery, Hanover Hospital, Roesebeckstrasse 15
Siloah, 30449 Hannover, Germany

ISBN 978-3-540-66929-6

Cataloging-in-Publication Data applied for

Die Deutsche Bibliothek – CIP-Einheitsaufnahme
Reymond, Marc A.: Port site and wound recurrences in cancer surgery : incidence -
pathogenesis - prevention / Marc A. Reymond ; H. J. Bonjer ; F. Köckerling. Foreword by
Alfred Cuschieri. Transl. from the German by A. Jack. - Berlin ; Heidelberg ; New York ;
Barcelona ; Hong Kong ; London ; Mailand ; Paris ; Singapur ; Tokio : Springer, 2000
ISBN 978-3-540-66929-6   ISBN 978-3-642-57028-5 (eBook)
DOI 10.1007/978-3-642-57028-5

The use of general descriptive names, registered names, trademarks, etc. in this publication does not imply, even in the absence of a specific statement, that such names are ex-
empt from the relevant protective laws and regulations and therefore free for general
use.
Product liability: The publishers cannot guarantee the accuracy of any information
about the application of operative techniques and medications contained in this book. In
every individual case the user must check such information by consulting the relevant
literature.

Cover design: design & production GmbH, D-69121 Heidelberg
Typesetting: FotoSatz Pfeifer GmbH, D-82166 Gräfelfing
SPIN: 10755673   24/3135 – 5 4 3 2 1 0

Foreword

During the past 9 years, reports of 'port-site' deposits following laparoscopic surgery for malignancy, especially laparoscopic resection of colonic cancer, have cast a shadow on the wisdom of the laparoscopic approach in the surgical management in patients with cancer. Those reports of port-site deposits, some 90 cases reported in the literature up to 1999, have opened a 'can of worms' and highlighted the scarcity of our knowledge on cancer cell migration from solid tumors and the factors that underlie their successful implantation in surgical wounds both in the presence and absence of a positive pressure pneumoperitoneum. The jury is out even in relation to the effect of the healing surgical access wound – do the biochemical and cellular repair processes and the associated growth factors enhance or prevent implantation of exfoliated viable tumor cells? Whatever the answer to this question, it is clear that tumor cells do implant in healing surgical wounds and the key question is whether this is facilitated by laparoscopic surgery with CO_2 pneumoperitoneum compared to the traditional surgical exposure. It is known that tumors shed malignant cells into the blood stream, the peritoneal cavity and in the case of hollow organs, intraluminally. Equally there is good evidence that surgical and instrumental manipulation of tumors induce exfoliation of viable tumor cells.

The entire subject has been be-devilled by imponderable questions such as 'What is the nature of port-site/wound deposits in strict pathological terms? What it the gold standard technique for detection and quantitation of exfoliated tumor cells? What are the appropriate tumor models and animals for experimental investigation of this important problem, and how does the inevitable non-specific immune depression caused by surgery impact on the optimal surgical approach for resection of operable cancer?' The controversy on port-site/wound deposits has also demonstrated, as never before, that it is easy to formulate a hypothesis on presumed mechanisms of cancer cell migration and implantation but much more difficult to prove what actually happens even with meticulous and planned animal experimentation. Furthermore, in taking a clinical problem such as port-site deposits to the laboratory, the appropriateness of the model used is crucial to the valid extrapolation of the experimental results to the clinical situation.

It is not surprising, therefore, that practicing surgeons have been confused by the vast reported literature, at times seemingly contradictory, on clinical and experimental work on port-site tumor deposits since the early reports of such occurrences. A detailed reappraisal of the subject of port-site and wound deposits in all their aspects based on the published clinical and experimental work was necessary and long overdue. This is precisely what the editors of this monograph 'Port-Site and Wound Recurrence in Cancer' have done with considerable success. The account is comprehensive, written by authors who have been involved in research in the field and covers both the experimental work and the „clinical aspects of port-site/wound deposits. The monograph evaluates critically what is known and equally what is conjectural at this stage of our knowledge on the subject. From a research standpoint, the limitations of the various tumor models used and the useful conclusions that can be drawn are clearly and objectively outlined in this book. There is much information and sound advice in this book for both researchers and clinical surgeons.

In the final analysis 'port-site and wound deposits' have to be considered as local recurrence and as with other instances of treatment failure, the surgeon factor is important if not paramount. Rather than being a specific complication of laparoscopic surgery, port-site deposits have in part to be regarded as the aftermath of poor surgical technique that is at least as much to blame as some poorly understood biological mechanism. This to me is an important message that is repeatedly stressed in this seminal monograph. Its success as a reference manual on the subject is assured as the editors and their contributors have addressed this important subject in an objective fashion based on evidence and not conjecture.

Prof. Sir Alfred Cuschieri

Preface

Application of laparoscopic surgery to cancer has been associated with an increased number of secondary tumors implanted into the abdominal wall, termed „port-site recurrences". This complication reported for hundreds of patients in the literature could discourage many surgeons to apply minimally invasive surgery to cancer. However, in the meantime, the pathogenesis of port-site recurrences has been systematically addressed in basic and clinical research, and a number of efficient preventive strategies have been developed. The large number of published studies makes it difficult for the laparoscopic surgeon, the general surgeon, the gastroenterologists, and the interested oncologist to get a synthetic and critical overview over this novel field.

In this book we have united chapters from most of the groups which are active worldwide in experimental and clinical research on port-site recurrences. The problem of wound recurrence in open cancer surgery is also discussed in detail. This should allow the reader to get an organized insight into the different pathogenic mechanisms of port-site recurrences, notably as to where the cells from which the secondary tumor arises come from, how they are dispersed, and how local effects in the port-site wound can favor implantation. Moreover, the book contains well illustrated guidelines to show preventive measures applicable by any surgeon. These can reduce substantially the incidence of port-site recurrence, allowing a safer application of minimally invasive surgery in cancer.

Contents

List of Contributors

Aprahamian, Marc, M.D., Department of Surgery, University Hospital
B.P. 426, 67091 Strasbourg Cedex, France

Balli, Jorge, M.D., Texas Endosurgery Institute
4242 East Southcross, Suite # 1, San Antonio, TX 78222, USA

Buchmann, Peter, M.D., Professor of Surgery and Head, Departement of Surgery
Waid City Hospital, 8037 Zurich, Switzerland

Christen, Daniel, M.D., Departement of Surgery, Waid City Hospital
Tièchestr. 99, 8037 Zurich, Switzerland

Diaz-E, José A., M.D., Texas Endosurgery Institute
4242 East Southcross, Suite # 1, San Antonio, TX 78222, USA

Downey, Robert J., M.D., Thoracic Surgery, Memorial Sloan Kettering Cancer
Center, 1275 York Avenue, New York, NY 100121, USA

Fleshman, James W., M.D., Associate Professor of Surgery, Washington University School of Medicine, 216 South Kingshighway, St. Louis, MO 63110, USA

Franklin, Morris E., M.D., Professor of Surgery, University of Texas, Director
Texas Endosurgery Institute, 4242 East Sothcross, Suite # 1
San Antonio, TX 78222, USA

Hewett, Peter J., M.B.B.S., M.D., F.R.A.C.S.
Department of Surgery, The Queen Elisabeth Hospital, The University of
Adelaide, The Queen Elisabeth Hospital
Woodville Road, Woodwille, South, 5011 Australia

Inan, Ihsan, M.D., Dept. of Surgery, University Hospital of Geneva
Av. Micheli-du-Crest 14, CH - 1211 Geneva 14, Switzerland

Jacobi, Christoph A., M.D., Associate Professor, Dept. of Surgery, Humboldt-University of Berlin, Schumannstrasse 20/21, 10098 Berlin, Germany

Lee, Sang W., M.D., Departement of Surgery, Beth Israel-Deaconess Hospital
Boston, MA, USA

Milsom, Jeffrey, M.D., Chief, Division of Colorectal Surgery, Mount Sinai Medical
Center, 1 Gustave L.Levy Place Box 1259, New York, NY 10029, USA

Mutter, Didier, M.D. Ph.D., Associate Professor of Surgery
University Hospital, B.P. 426, 67091 Strasbourg Cedex, France

Nelson, Heidi, M.D., F.A.C.S., Professor and Chair, Division of Colon and
Rectal Surgery, Mayo Clinic, 200 First Street SW, Rochester, MI 55905, USA

Neuhaus, Susan, M.B.B.S., University of Adelaide Department of Surgery
Royal Adelaide Hospital, Adelaide, South Australia, 5000, Australia

Pross, Matthias, M.D., Department of Surgery, University Hospital of Magdeburg
Leipziger Str. 44, 39120 Magdeburg, Germany

Ridwelski, Karsten, M.D., Department of Surgery, University Hospital of
Magdeburg, Leipziger Str. 44, 39120 Magdeburg, Germany

Schneider, Claus, M.D., Department of Surgery and Center for Minimally
Invasive Surgery, Hanover Hospital, Roesebeckstr. 15, Siloah,
30449 Hannover, Germany

Schug, Christine, M.D., Department of Surgery and Center for Minimally
Invasive Surgery, Hanover Hospital, Roesebeckstr. 15, Siloah,
30449 Hannover, Germany

Sonoda, Toyooki, M.D., Research Fellow, Division of Colorectal Surgery
Mount Sinai Medical Center, 1 Gustave L.Levy Place Box 1259
New York, NY 10029, USA

Stocchi, Luca, M.D., Division of Colon and Rectal Surgery
Mayo Clinic, 200 First Street SW, Rochester, MI 55905, USA

Tannapfel, Andrea, M.D., Institute of Pathology, University of Leipzig
Liebigstr. 26, 04103 Leipzig, Germany

Texler, Michael L., M.D., Department of Surgery, The Queen Elisabeth Hospital
The University of Adelaide, The Queen Elisabeth Hospital
Woodville Road, Woodwille, South, 5011, Australia

Watson, David I., M.B.B.S., M.D., F.R.A.C.S, Director, the Royal Centre for
Endoscopic Surgery, University of Adelaide Department of Surgery,
Royal Adelaide Hospital, Adelaide, South, 5000, Australia

Whelan, Richard L., M.D., Associate Professor of Surgery, Columbia University
Columbia-Presbyterian Medical Center
161 Fort Washington Avenue, New York, NY 10032, USA

Wittekind, Christian, M.D., Professor and Head, Institute of Pathology, University of Leipzig, Liebigstr. 26, 04103 Leipzig, Germany

Wittich, Philippe, M.D., Department of Surgery, University Hospital Rotterdam
Dijkzigt Hospital, P.O. Box 2040, 3000 CA Rotterdam, The Netherlands

CHAPTER 1

Definition of Port-Site and Wound Recurrences in Cancer Surgery

A. Tannapfel, C. Wittekind

Introduction

The specific benefits of laparoscopic surgery over laparotomy have been well enumerated, and a laparoscopic approach is now considered the most suitable way of care for many surgical diseases. In recent years, laparoscopic surgery has been increasingly performed in patients with malignant diseases. Not long after the increasing use of the new technique for malignant tumors, reports of tumor recurrences at the laparoscopic port-sites appeared in the literature (Wexner and Cohen 1995; Vukasin et al. 1996). A recent review of the printed matter revealed an incidence of 1–2% of recurrences in trocar wounds as well as laparoscopic and thoracoscopic incisions (Franklin et al. 1996; Lumley et al. 1996). Despite the numerous reports of this phenomenon, port-site recurrences have been poorly defined up to now (Reymond et al. 1998). To obtain data on the real incidence as well as to compare the information from prospective multicenter trials, a clear and distinct definition of port-site recurrences is absolutely necessary. A critical look at the cases of port-site recurrences reported in the literature revealed that a wide range of different situations are classified as "port-site recurrences" (Mathew et al. 1996; Lacy et al. 1997; Pearlstone et al. 1999). In some studies, the tumor recurrences were clinically detectable, but were only one of many other sites of recurrent or metastatic disease (Whelan et al. 1998). In many of the cases reported, widely disseminated or advanced disease was present at the time of primary laparoscopic surgery (Whelan et al. 1998). Several studies failed to give any information about the time interval between the time of first surgery and onset of port-site recurrences (Johnstone et al. 1996). In addition, the data presented so far concerning recurrence at port-sites reveals multiple other sites of metastatic disease, calling into question the clinical significance of the port-site recurrence itself in terms of the prognosis (Nduka et al. 1994). Besides this obvious lack of a clear definition of port-site recurrences, many studies have analyzed different malignant conditions, e.g., rectal cancer, gallbladder and ovarian cancer even within the same set of investigations without looking for stage and grade of the disease (Egan et al. 1997). Furthermore, the diagnostic criteria for port-site recurrences are different within the literature, ranging from "malignant ascitis" to "serosal invasion" and "positive peritoneal washings".

Therefore, we would like to define port-site recurrences in terms of morphological confirmation, anatomical site, time of onset and also location of the tumor cells. The definition given here is based on the data published in the literature as well as own experiences (Hermanek and Wittekind 1994; Köckerling et al. 1997a,b). The incidence and also the time-course of port-site recurrences after laparoscopic surgery are comparable with those reported for needle track metastases after fine needle biopsies, mediastinoscopy or drainage tracts after cancer operations (Collins 1962; Chapman 1989; Solin 1983; Sharma 1994; Voravud et al. 1992).

Biological Basis of Port-Site Recurrences

In wound recurrences after open surgery as well as in port-site recurrences after endoscopic surgery, the biological basis of the tumor growth seems to be identical. The wound healing as a complex, but ordered phenomenon includes regeneration of parenchymal cells, migration and proliferation of parenchymal and connective tissue, synthesis of proteins of the extracellular matrix and remodeling as well as collagenization of the wound tissue. Traumatized and also healing tissue are therefore preferred sites for (metastatic) tumor growth. The local granulation tissue is rich in growth factors, which promote cellular growth and differentiation. The migration and proliferation of fibroblasts, deposition of extracellular matrix, formation of blood vessels and maturation is dependent on various growth factors and receptors. Within the granulation tissue, growth factors like vascular endothelial growth factor (VEGF), epithelial growth factor (EGF) and several others are expressed at high levels (Majno and Joris 1996; Hofer et al. 1999). The mitogenic and also morphogenic effects of these factors promote not only the growth of fibroblasts but also the proliferation of possibly viable shed tumor cells within these areas. Therefore, viable tumor cells from any source (after inoculation, manipulation or cells from the peritoneal surface or even systemic circulating tumor cells) are capable of producing a tumor growth within the "fertile environment" of the wound. The granulation tissue of a healed wound is a permissive environment, a favorable "soil" as an illustration of the "seed versus soil" paradigm. If the port-site is the preferential site for tumor growth over the laparotomy incision, as some animal data seem to imply, differences in vascular supply and healing properties between a midline incision and a puncture wound may exist.

From the histopathological point of view, another important question is whether the tumor cells responsible for port-site recurrences, arise from systemically circulating cells or free intraperitoneal cells. The latter case can be avoided by a gentle tumor preparation. Viable tumor cells released in the circulation may not only depend on the surgical procedure (Majno and Joris 1996; Berends et al. 1994; Collard and Reymond 1996; Champault et al. 1997).

Location and Diagnosis of Port-Site Recurrences

Port-site recurrences are defined as local, circumscribed tumor growths at the site of one or more trocar sites or at an incision wound after laparoscopic or thoracoscopic surgery for cancer. Port-site recurrences are localized within the abdominal or thoracic wall within the scar tissue and involve initially the dermis and the subcutaneous fat, usually not the muscular layer (Fig. 1.1). Port-site recurrences are not cutaneous metastases, as in advanced cancers. Therefore the terminology of "port-site metastases" should be avoided.

The diagnosis of port-site recurrences should be proven by biopsy. Peritoneal washings or ascitis showing malignant cells could reflect peritoneal metastases rather than port-site recurrences. The histological confirmation is necessary to differentiate the port-site recurrence from hyperplastic gran-

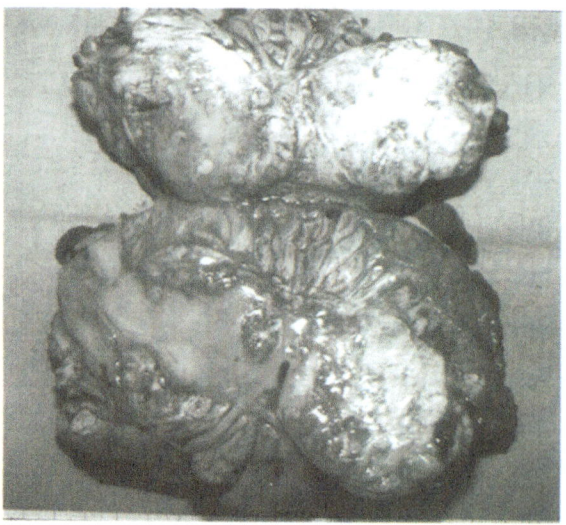

Fig. 1.1. Port-site recurrence after laparoscopic resection of a gallbladder carcinoma. Note that the subcutaneous tissue is primarily involved. Courtesy of M. Pross, M.D., University Hospital, Magdeburg, Germany

ulation tissue or cheloid scars. These two features are common situations particularly in the case of healing by second intention. Especially for multicenter trials we would therefore recommend to diagnose port-site recurrences only in the case of a localized histologically proven tumor growth within the fibrous tissue of the trocar scar.

The development of port-site recurrences is independent of stage and grade of the individual tumor but occurs usually more often in advanced stage of disease.

Histologically, the tumor cells grow localized within the fibrous tissue or the subcutaneous fat of the incision or trocar wound or scar (Figs. 1.2, 1.3 and 1.4). A peritumorous inflammatory infiltrate is

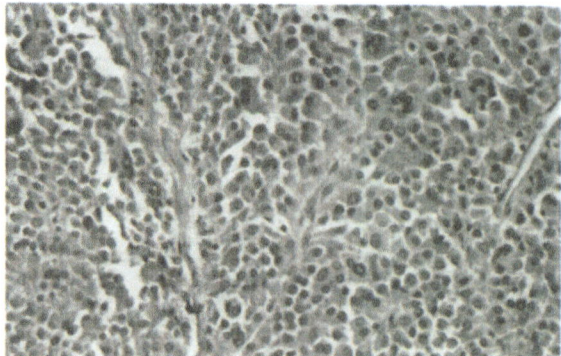

Fig. 1.2. Infiltrates of a pheochromocytoma within the subcutaneous tissue (hematoxylin & eosin, original magnification, ×40)

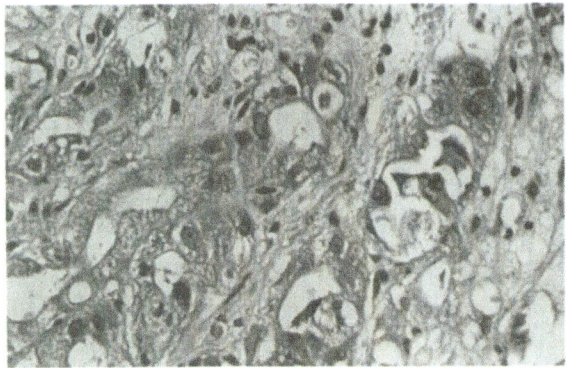

Fig. 1.3. Infiltrates of poorly differentiated adenocarcinoma within the subcutaneous tissue with PAS-positive intracytoplasmic mucin deposits (PAS, original magnification, × 40)

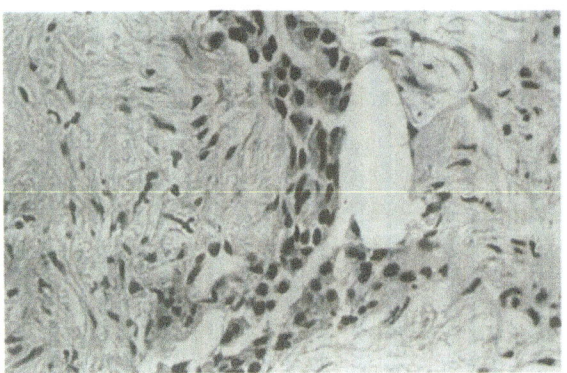

Fig. 1.4. Infiltrates of a poorly differentiated adenocarcinoma within the subcutaneous tissue (HE, original magnification,× 40)

usually also present and could be the morphological correlation of the clinical presentation of a nodular painful infiltration of the scar. The tumor cells are of the same tumor type as the primary tumor, the grade of cellular differentiation (grading) may be different. In some cases, port-site recurrences are less well differentiated than the primary tumor.

Time of Presentation of Port-Site Recurrences

Port-site recurrences are early recurrences, occurring within a few months after primary endoscopic surgery (Fig. 1.5). They are neither "residual tumor cells" nor "peritoneal", "cutaneous" or "skin" metastases. Very early recurrence, a case reported in the literature occurred 14 days after surgery, might reflect an advanced stage of disease with peritoneal metastases rather than port-site recurrences (Johnstone et al. 1996; Litynski and Paolucci 1998). In the case of peritoneal metastases present at the time of

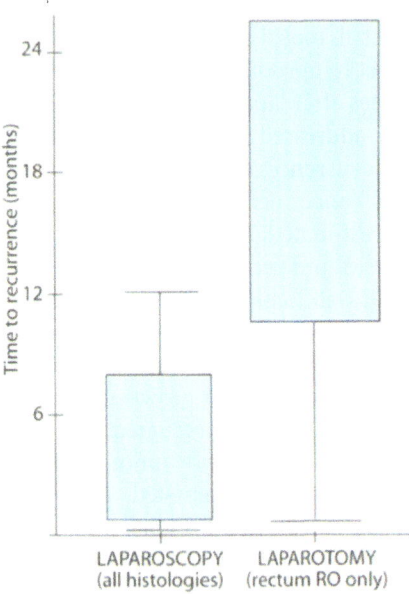

Fig. 1.5. Time elapsed between laparoscopy and clinical diagnosis of a port-site recurrence (*left box*) compared to the time of detection of distant metastasis after curative surgery for rectal cancer. Note that most port-site recurrences occur within the first 200 days, whereas distant metastasis are rare during the first postoperative year

primary surgery, the terminology of port-site recurrences should be avoided. Given the biological evidence of a tumor cell doubling time of 100 days for colorectal metastases, a single tumor cell requires 30 cell doublings to reach a palpable size of 1 g (10^9 cells) (Collins 1962). Massive initial inoculation of tumor cells at the time of surgery is therefore suggested, if port-site recurrences were clinically evident 200 days after surgery.

Port-site recurrences should be clearly differentiated from peritoneal metastases or serosal invasion.

The diagnosis of port-site recurrences should strictly follow these criteria to avoid bewilderment and confusion in future studies. Reviewing the literature, many of the reported port-site recurrence cases showed widely disseminated stages of disease. In some studies, next to the port-site recurrences, multiple other sites of metastatic disease were overt. This may raise the question if port-site recurrences have any impact on the outcome of the patients rather than the endoscopic surgical procedure (Wille et al. 1997; Hughes et al. 1983; Reilly et al. 1996).

Most ongoing clinical trails compare open vs. minimal surgery procedures. Therefore, a firm definition of tumor recurrences at laparotomy wounds or port-sites is absolutely mandatory. However, isolated incision recurrences after open laparotomy for malignant diseases appear to be very rare events (Schaeff et al. 1998; Lee et al. 1998; Reilly et al. 1996). In contrast to port-site recurrences, the question of recurrences after laparotomy at the laparotomy site has been addressed infrequently in the literature. Incision recurrences after conventional treatment of colorectal cancer are uncommon, although probably underestimated. This may be due to the clinical view that wound recurrences usually reflect widespread intra-abdominal, fatal disease. Furthermore, data about tumor recurrences in laparotomy wounds are difficult to interpretate because of the possibility that the tumor growth might precede or even succeed laparotomy recurrence. A recent study of a comparison of wound tumor recurrence after open and laparoscopic-assisted splenectomy in a murine model revealed a higher mortality rate in the laparoscopic group, without however gaining statistical significance (Reilly et al. 1996). The fact that many patients may have "silent" wound implants in laparotomy incisions was elucidated in those patients undergoing either staged second look or symptomatic second look surgery (Reilly et al. 1996). We would therefore recommend that the above stated criteria for recurrences be applied to laparotomy wounds as well as port-site recurrences.

The application of a strict definition of port-site recurrences seems in our opinion the basis of an analysis of the true incidence of port-site recurrences. A stage-by-stage comparison of recurrences and outcomes between patients who underwent endoscopic surgery and those who did not seems only feasible if port-site recurrences were diagnosed strictly relying on (morphological and clinical) criteria. Port-site recurrences should be clearly differentiated from serosal invasion, peritoneal metastases and positive peritoneal washings. Port-site recurrences are not "peritoneal" or "skin" metastases (Berends et al. 1994). These features are well known poor prognostic indicators. A multivariate analysis of risk factors of port-site recurrences is absolutely necessary for the interpretation of the findings in laparoscopic surgery. The distinct diagnosis of port-site recurrences should give answers to the most important question if laparoscopic minimal surgery is superior to laparotomy in terms of patients outcome. Rejection of laparoscopic surgery for malignant conditions is not justified without performing multivariate analysis with clearly defined variables. Strict adherence to the definition of port-site recurrences may help to assess the risk of this event and weigh it against any potential benefit of the laparoscopic procedure to the individual patient.

Summary

The occurrence of port-site recurrences is a well known, but ill defined surgical complication in the laparoscopic treatment of cancer. Therefore, port-site recurrences should only be diagnosed if:

- The diagnosis is histologically proven
- A localized, circumscribed subcutaneous tumor growth of the abdominal or thoracic wall occurs within the fibrous tissue of the scar as a consequence of a trocar or other incision sites after laparoscopy, thoracoscopy or mediastinoscopy for cancer
- Early tumor recurrence is observed within a time-span of a few months only (up to approx. 200 days)
- Port-site recurrences are not identical with peritoneal metastases, serosal invasion, skin metastases.

The diagnosis should be histologically proven at least in cases where this is the only site of tumor recurrence. Malignant cells in peritoneal washings or malignant ascitis fail to be secure indicators of port-site recurrences.

The adherence to the definition will enable multicenter trials with stage-to-stage comparison to assess the risk of port-site recurrences and weigh it against any potential benefit of the laparoscopic procedure.

References

Berends FJ, Kazemier G, Bonjer HJ, Lange JF (1994) Subcutaneous metastases after laparoscopic colectomy [letter]. Lancet 344: 58

Champault G, Taffinder N, Ziol M, Riskalla H, Catheline JMC (1997) Cells are present in the smoke created during laparoscopic surgery. Br J Surg 84: 993–995

Chapman WC (1989) Tumor seeding from percutaneous biliary catheter tract. Ann Surg 209: 1989

Collard JM, Reymond MA (1996) Video-assisted thoracic surgery (V.A.T.S.) for cancer: risk of parietal seeding and of early local recurrence. Int Surg 81: 343–346

Collins VP (1962) Time of occurrence of pulmonary metastasis from carcinoma of colon and rectum. Cancer 15: 387–395

Egan C, Knolmayer TJ, Bowyer MW, Asbun HJ (1997) Port-site recurrences: a current review of the literature (Abstract). Surg Endosc 11: 196

Franklin ME, Rosenthal D, Abrego-Medina D, Dorman JP, Glass JL, Norem R, Diaz A (1996) Prospective comparison of open vs. laparoscopic colon surgery for carcinoma. Dis Colon Rectum 39: S35–46

Hermanek P, Wittekind C (1994) To what extent are laparoscopic procedures defensible in oncologic surgery? Chirurg 65: 23–28

Hofer SOP, Molema G, Hermens RAEC, Wanebo HJ, Reichner JS, Hoekstra HJ (1999) The effect of surgical wounding on tumor development. Eur J Surg Oncol 25: 231–243

Hughes ESR, McDermott FT, Polgase A, Johnson WR (1983) Tumor recurrence in the abdominal wall scar after large-bowel cancer durgery. Dis Colon Rectum 26 : 571–572

Johnstone PAS, Rohde DC, Swartz SE, Fetter JE, Wexner SD (1996) Port-site recurrences after laparoscopic and thoracoscopic procedures in malignancy. J Clin Oncol 14: 1950–1956

Köckerling F, Reymond MA, Schneider C, Hohenberger W (1997a) Mistakes and hazards in oncological laparoscopic surgery. Chirurg 68: 215–224

Köckerling F, Schneider C, Scheidbach H, Reymond MA, Wittekind C, Hohenberger W, Laparoscopic Colorectal Surgery Group (1997b) Laparoscopic colorectal surgery: indications and design of a multicentre study. In: Farthmann EH, Meyer C, Richter HA (eds) Current aspects of laparoscopic colorectal surgery – Indications – Methods – Results. Springer, Berlin Heidelberg New York, pp 56–63

Lacy AM, Delgado S, Garcia-Valdecasas JC, Castella A, Grande L, Fuster J, Visa J (1997) Port-site recurrences and recurrence after laparoscopic colectomy in malignancy(Abstract). Randomized trial. Surg Endosc 11: 170

Lee SW, Whelan RL, Southall JC, Bessler M (1998) Abdominal tumor wound recurrence after open and laparoscopic-assisted splenectomy in a murine model. Dis Colon Rectum 41: 824–831

Litynski GS, Paolucci V (1998) Origin of laparoscopy: coincidence or surgical interdisciplinary thought ? World J Surg 22: 899–902

Lumley JW, Fielding GA, Rhodes M, Nathanson LK, Siu S, Stitz RW (1996) Laparoscopic-assisted colorectal surgery. Lessons learned from 240 consecutive patients. Dis Colon Rectum 39: 155–159

Majno G, Joris I (1996) Cells, tissues, and disease. Blackwell Science, New York

Mathew G, Watson DI, Rofe AM, Baigrie CF, Ellis T, Jamieson GG (1996) Wound metastases following laparoscopic and open surgery for abdominal cancer in a rat model. Br J Surg 83: 1087–1090

Nduka CC, Monson JR, Menzies-Gow N, Darzi A (1994) Abdominal wall metastases following laparoscopy. Br J Surg 81: 648–652

Pearlstone DB, Mansfield PF, Curley SA, Kumparatana M, Cook P, Feig BW (1999) Laparoscopy in 533 patients with abdominal malignancy. Surgery 125: 67–72

Reilly WT, Nelson H, Schroeder G, Wieand HS, Bolton J, O'Connell MJ (1996) Wound recurrence following conventional treatment of colorectal cancer. Dis Colon Rectum 39: 200–207

Reymond MA, Schneider C, Kastl S, Hohenberger W, Köckerling F (1998) The pathogenesis of port-site recurrences. J Gastrointest Surg 2: 406–414

Schaeff B, Paolucci V, Thomopoulos J (1998) Port-site recurrences after laparoscopic surgery. A review. Dig Surg 15: 124–134

Sharma P (1994) Metastatic implantation of an oral squamous-cell carcinoma at a percutaneous endoscopic gastrostomy site. Surg Endosc 8: 1232–1235

Solin L (1983) Subcutaneous seeding of pancreatic carcinoma along a transhepatic biliary catheter tract. Br J Radiol 56: 83–84

Voravud N, Shin DM, Dekmezian RH, Dimery I, Lee JS, Hong TW (1992) Implantation metastasis of carcinoma after percutaneous fine-needle aspiration biopsy. Chest 43: 1533–1540

Vukasin P, Ortega AE, Greene FL, Steele GD, Simons AJ, Anthone GJ, Weston LA, Beart RW (1996) Wound recurrence following laparoscopic colon cancer resection. Results of The American Society of Colon and Rectal Surgeons Laparoscopic Registry. Dis Colon Rectum 39: S20–23

Wexner SD, Cohen SM (1995) Port-site recurrences after laparoscopic colorectal surgery for cure of malignancy. Br J Surg 82: 295–298

Whelan RL, Allendorf JD, Gutt CN, Jacobi CA, Mutter D, Dorrance HR, Bessler M, Bonjer HJ (1998) General oncologic effects of the laparoscopic surgical approach. Surg Endosc 12: 1092–1095

Wille GA, Gregory R, Guernsey JM (1997) Tumor implantation at port-site of video-assisted thoracoscopic resection of pulmonary metastasis. West J Med 166: 65–66

CHAPTER 2

A Case Report

I. Inan, M.A. Reymond

The patient, a 67-year-old man, presented with nonspecific abdominal pain over the last 3 weeks. The personal history was uneventful with the exception of a known diverticulosis. Abdominal examination was normal. Barium enema revealed a large caecal tumor, that was suspected to be malignant (Fig. 2.1). Coloscopy showed the presence of an unique, bulky tumor, and histopathological analysis of the biopsy confirmed the malignant nature. A computerized tomography of the abdomen detected no distant metastases, locally the tumor was described to infiltrate the pericolic fatty tissue.

A laparoscopic right hemicolectomy was performed. The procedure was uncomplicated, being performed with standard port-sites, one at the umbilicus, one in the right upper quadrant, two in the right lower quadrant, and the specimen was extracted through a minilaparotomy in the right flank (Fig. 2.2). Resection and anastomosis were performed extracorporeally. No intraabdominal dissemination was noticed. The patient made an uneventful recovery.

Histopathology of the right colon showed a moderately differentiated adenocarcinoma, partly mucinous, infiltrating the subserosa. One lymph node was metastatic out of 17 harvested. The pathologist classified the tumor as pT3N1M0, Dukes C, Jass III. The patient received a postoperative adjuvant therapy.

Sixteen months later, he re-presented with a nodule at the minilaparotomy site (Fig. 2.3). This was excised and proved to be a subcutaneous metastasis of a mucinous adenocarcinoma (Fig. 2.4). During the operation, a liver metastasis in the segment VII was discovered. After uneventful recovery, the patient was scheduled for a new chemotherapy.

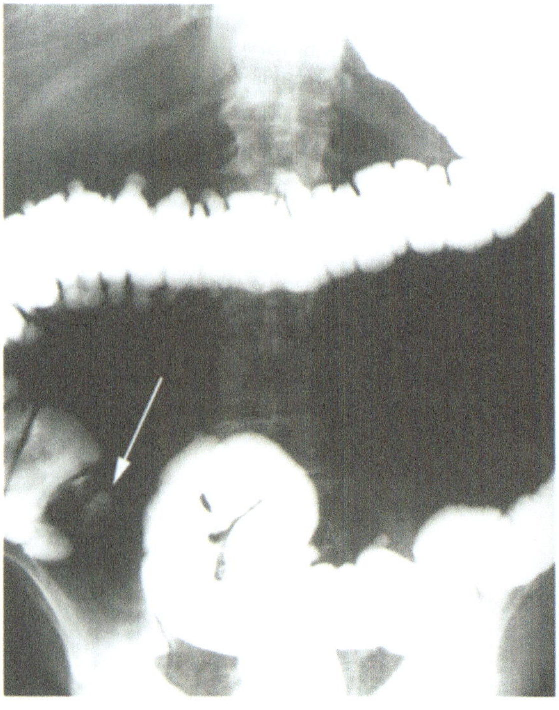

Fig. 2.1. Barium enema demonstrating a filling defect in the caecum. At coloscopy, the presence of a adenocarcinoma of the colon was histologically confirmed

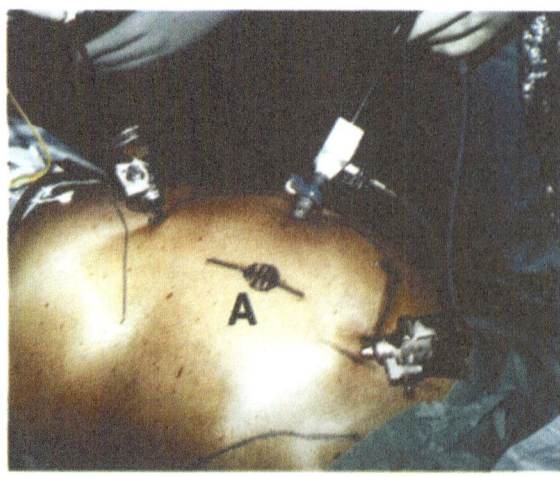

Fig. 2.2. Position of the trocars and of the minilaparotomy (A) at the initial procedure

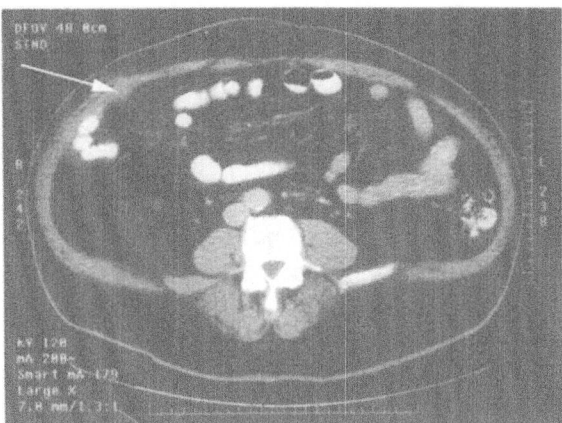

Fig. 2.3. Abdominal CT demonstrating a port-site recurrence at the site of extraction in the right lower quadrant (*arrow*), 16 months after the initial curative resection

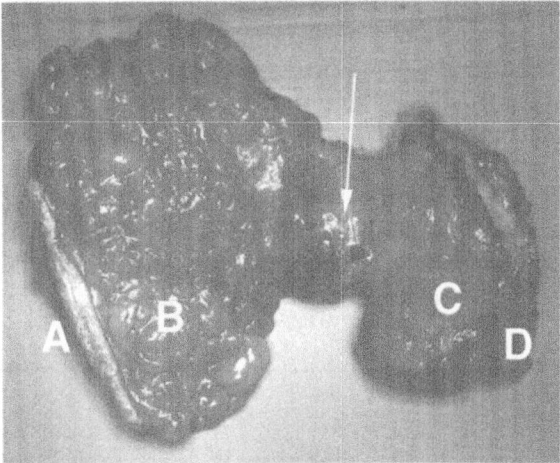

Fig. 2.4. Macroscopic appearance of the resected specimen, showing the subcutaneous location of tumor recurrence (*arrow*). *A*, skin; *B*, subcutaneous tissue; *C*, muscle layer; *D*, fascia and peritoneum

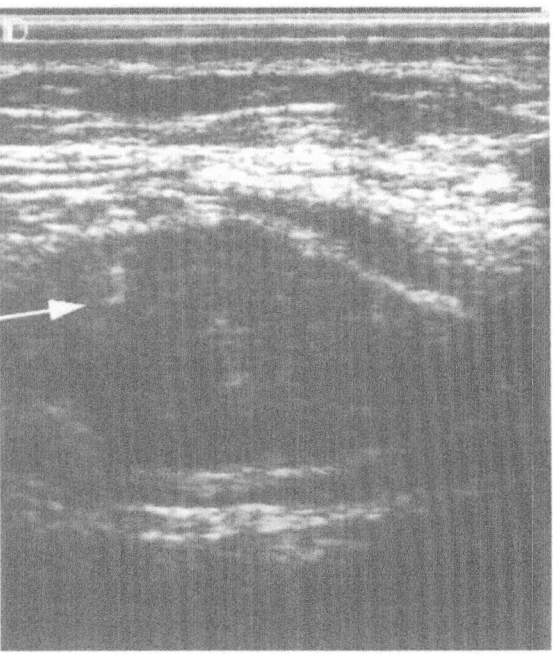

Fig. 2.5. Ultrasound demonstrating a second colon cancer recurrence at the port-site resection site (*arrow*), 14 months later

Fourteen months later, a second tumor recurrence was discovered at the same extraction site (Fig. 2.5). This was excised in toto, and histopathology showed again a metastasis of the primary adenocarcinoma, involving the muscle.

Eight months later, the patient is still alive, with evidence of disseminated disease.

CHAPTER 3

Abdominal Wall Recurrences in Open Surgery

L. Stocchi, H. Nelson

Introduction

An increasing interest in the topic of abdominal wall recurrences has followed the surge of minimally invasive surgery, principally due to concerns regarding early reports of an increased risk of port-site and incisional wound metastases associated with the pneumoperitoneal technique (Berends 1994). Whether this complication is an inevitable consequence of the laparoscopic approach per se or can be considered as an error in judgement or technique and/or part of the learning phase is still a matter of debate. Regardless, as a consequence the incidence of wound recurrence after open surgery has been investigated in the attempt to establish a standard with which laparoscopic surgery should be compared. The purpose of this overview is to examine the possible pathogenic mechanisms, review current reports on abdominal wall recurrences of colorectal cancer, in particular the correlations between cytology of peritoneal fluid and survival, and compare them with analogous experiences reported in the literature for other types of malignancies.

Abdominal Wall Recurrence in Colorectal Cancer

Tumor recurrence at the abdominal wall after colorectal resection is a rare event. Abdominal wound recurrences after open colonic resection range from 0.8% to 2.5% (Cass et al. 1976; Hughes et al. 1983; Reilly et al. 1996). A number of variables affect the incidence of wound recurrences, including the tumor stage and the methodology of analysis adopted. It has been shown that advanced stage tumors are associated with an increased incidence of wound recurrence, which is generally associated with peritoneal carcinomatosis. However, cases of abdominal wound recurrences following resection of stage II (Dukes' B) colon and rectal cancer have been reported. In the report by Hughes et al. the staging was

B in 8 and C in 3 out of the 11 cases where the pathology of the resected tumor was available (Hughes et al. 1983). This suggests that the pattern of recurrence is not exclusively related to the stage of the tumor. In addition, since the detection of abdominal wall recurrence frequently occurs as an incidental finding at surgery, i.e., these lesions are often asymptomatic, it is reasonable to presume that the true incidence of this phenomenon is underestimated. In fact, this is supported by autopsy studies where higher rates of abdominal wall recurrences are reported when compared with recurrences discovered at follow-up. The mechanism of detection of abdominal wall recurrence is variable. No doubt, the sensitivity of abdominal wall recurrence detection depends on the intensity and focus of the investigations.

Autopsy Studies

Autopsy studies are accurate in detecting the presence of abdominal wall recurrences, but are unable to provide data regarding the timing of recurrence and therefore cannot detail whether the abdominal wall has been the first recurrence site. Cass and colleagues reported 7 wound recurrences out of 78 local recurrences following resection of colorectal cancer in 280 patients, corresponding to 2.5% of the overall and 9% of the local recurrences (Cass et al. 1976). Although not specifically addressed in the study, it is reasonable to presume that most wound recurrences occurred in association with local recurrences described as "contiguous to the operative site". In another autopsy study, Welch and Donaldson encountered a total of 24 cases of abdominal wall recurrences following 145 cases of colorectal cancer resection (16.6%), all of them associated with other sites of recurrence (Welch and Donaldson 1979). Autopsy studies are useful to show that the abdominal wall metastases become increasingly likely to occur as the tumor advances. However, even when detected at autopsy, it is difficult to prove where the first site of recurrence was, or whether the recurrence extended secondarily, spreading from other areas. Sites of distant spread can often be more readily detected before the sites of locoregional failure are detected, even though the latter may be the initial site of recurrence.

Second-Look Laparotomy

At a time when CT was not available, the second-look surgery was promoted as an opportunity to detect recurrent colorectal cancer when excision with curative intent was still possible. The advantage of this approach is that initial sites of recurrence can be noted when they are still solitary and provide a more accurate estimation of the high-risk areas and patterns of spread; they are also more likely to be amenable to complete resection. As it might be expected, wound implants were more frequent in symptomatic patients (5.3%, 4/75) than in planned second-look operations (3/91, 3.3%) (Gunderson and Sosin 1974).

Data from Prospective Adjuvant Therapy Trials

The North Central Cancer Treatment Group performed a retrospective review of wound recurrence after open surgery for colon and rectal cancer using patients entered on prospective, randomized adjuvant trials. This report is instructive for a number of findings. Firstly, it provides a long-term follow-up on a wide number of patients with high-risk tumors who also received adjuvant chemotherapy and/or radiation treatments. Advanced stage tumors were not included in the analysis, since the clinical relevance of incisional wound recurrence in the context of widespread metastatic disease was considered circumspect. Out of 1,711 patients with primary adenocarcinoma of the colon or rectum treated for cure, 25 had an abdominal wound recurrence, and 11 had a documented incisional wound recurrence. While 8 patients were diagnosed by clinical examination and confirmed by local excision, 18 patients were operated for recurrent disease. Patients with stage II (Dukes' B) disease had in this study a wound recurrence rate comparable to stage III (Dukes' C) patients. Wound recurrences were generally associated with poor outcome, with 9 out of the 11 above-mentioned patients having multiple sites of recurrence along with their surgical wounds (Reilly et al. 1996).

In contrast with it, in a retrospective analysis on 372 laparoscopic colectomies, trocar site recurrences occurred in 4 cases and resection of the recurrence was successfully accomplished in 3 of them. In the fourth one, the tumor recurred at the midline wound following a converted resection of a T4N1 cancer which was adherent to the pancreas. Therefore, it seems reasonable to presume that the type of recurrence occurring at a trocar site could be biologically different from a similar occurrence in a major laparotomy wound and generally be associated with a better prognosis, at least in colorectal cancer (Fleshman et al. 1996). However, this is still speculative.

There are insufficient data and follow-up to warrant a definitive statement on whether laparotomy vs. laparoscopy wound tumors are really different in terms of outcome. This will be interesting to follow-up if clear-cut differences are substantiated, and it would implicate different mechanisms of tumor spread between the two surgical approaches.

Abdominal Wall Recurrence After Malignancies Other than Colorectal Cancer

Abdominal wound recurrence has been reported following surgery for a number of malignancies, including adrenocortical (Fig. 3.1), esophageal (Recht et al. 1989), endometrial (Curtis et al. 1994; Barter 1986), hepatocellular, gallbladder, ovarian carcinoma (La Fianza et al. 1997), and pancreatic carcinoma following percutaneous biliary drainage (Cutherell et al. 1986; Doctor et al. 1997; Charnley et al. 1995). Similar recurrences have also been observed following percutaneous drainage after gastric cancer surgery (Fig. 3.2). Recently, the interest in abdominal wall recurrences has sharply increased following isolated reports of port-site recurrences following laparoscopic procedures, similar to what has been reported for laparoscopic resection of colorectal cancer. In other cases abdominal wall recurrences have long been described as a phenomenon associated with percutaneous needle biopsies (Kruitwagen et al. 1996) or standard treatment of malignancies with open surgery.

In a multicenter study on pathologic and surgical variables on 4,765 primary liver cancers conducted by the Liver Cancer Study Group of Japan, "skin metastases" were encountered at autopsy in 24 out of 1832 cases of hepatocellular carcinoma (1.3%) and 8 out of 108 cholangiocarcinomas (7.4%). Of note, these skin metastases were found to frequently coexist with other multiple distant metastases, which sug-

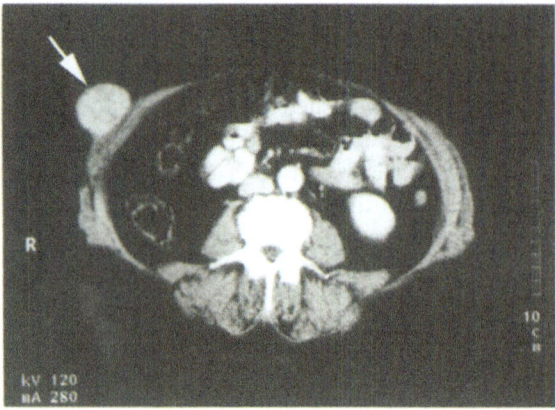

Fig. 3.1. Pre-operative computered tomography of an abdominal wall recurrence (*arrow*) after conventional resection of adrenocortical adenocarcinoma using a retroperitoneal approach in a 64-year-old patient. Courtesy of H.J. Bonjer, Rotterdam, The Netherlands

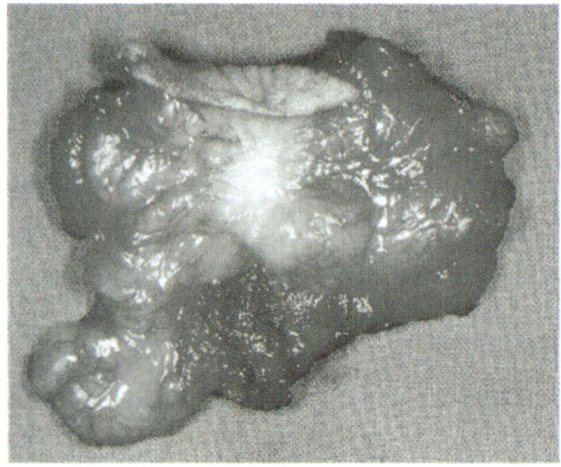

Fig. 3.2. Drainage tract tumor recurrence after gastric cancer surgery. Courtesy of P. Buchmann, Zurich, Switzerland

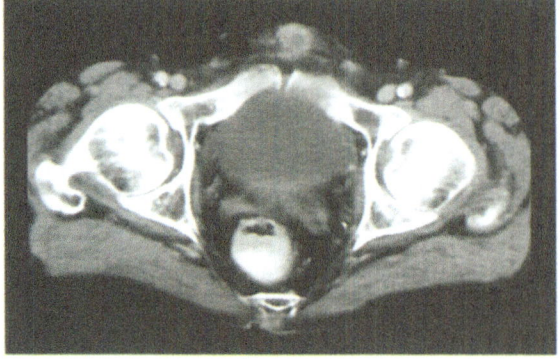

Fig. 3.3. Pre-operative computerized tomography of an abdominal wall recurrence 6 months after conventional resection of an pT3N1M0 adenocarcinoma of the right colon in a 61-year-old patient. This recurrence was not associated with peritoneal carcinomatosis.

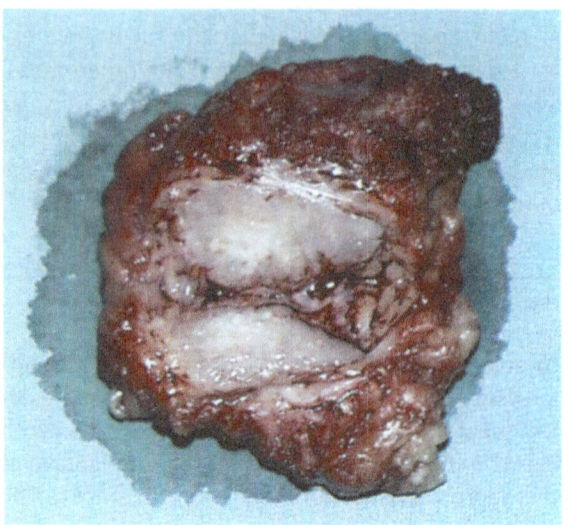

Fig. 3.4. Operative specimen of the abdominal wall recurrence shown in Fig. 3.3. The recurrence is located in the subcutaneous tissue, with no infiltraton of the muscle layer.

gest that abdominal wall recurrence occurs in the context of widespread metastatic disease (Liver Cancer Study Group of Japan, 1990). Conversely, in an anecdotal report on abdominal wall recurrences after hepatocellular carcinoma, excision of the local recurrence was followed by long-term survival in 2 out of 3 cases, suggesting that abdominal wall recurrences

were not always associated with either advanced or diffuse metastatic disease (Koffi et al. 1996). However, the prevalence of abdominal wall recurrence in the series was comparable with the Japanese audit mentioned above, at 1.2%. Although not specifically addressed in the study, it is presumed the manipulation of the tumor may cause implantation at the wound site. A similar hypothesis has been advocated for perineal wound recurrence, although this location cannot be strictly considered as an abdominal wall recurrence. This kind of complication has been reported even in specialized unit with large experience and low local recurrence rates after anterior resection of the rectum (Heald et al. 1997). In addition, recurrence at the site of Gelpi retractor after coloanal anastomosis has been reported (Zinzindohoue et al. 1997).

In a series on 93 patients with gallbladder carcinoma, the subgroup analysis comparing rates of abdominal wall recurrence of cancers discovered following laparoscopic, open cholecystectomy and cases requiring conversion to open surgery did not disclose any significant difference among the 3 groups (6 out of 21, 29%; 8 out of 26, 31%; 5 out of 16, 31%, respectively). This would suggest that intraperitoneal exfoliation of neoplastic cell would have occurred, irrespective of the technical approach adopted. As an alternative hypothesis, the authors consider the abdominal wall recurrence as a pure expression of aggressive disease. This would be further supported by the occurrence of one further case of umbilical metastasis, which was present even before surgery (Ricardo et al. 1997).

The comparison between abdominal wall recurrences following resection of colorectal cancer versus other malignancies offers various clinical scenarios and therapeutic options, suggesting that although occurring at the same site, aggressiveness and biologic behavior could still be different according to the histologic type of tumor.

Summary

There is scant data in the literature concerning abdominal wall recurrence after surgical treatment of intraabdominal malignancies, especially colorectal cancer. Studies which have been carried out with renewed emphasis following the development of laparoscopic port-site recurrences have clarified that the event is rare, but possibly and probably overlooked by most investigators. Its pathogenesis and natural history are still unclear.

References

Anonymous (1990) Primary liver cancer in Japan. Clinicopathological features and results of surgical treatment. Liver Cancer Study Group of Japan. Ann Surg 211: 277–287

Barter JF, Hatch KD, Orr JW, Jr., and Shingleton HM (1986) Isolated abdominal wound recurrence of an andometrial adenocarcinoma confined to a polyp. Gynecol Oncol 25: 372–375

Berends FJ, Kazemier G, Bonjer HJ, Lange JF (1994) Subcutaneous metastases after laparoscopic colectomy. Lancet 344: 58

Cass AW, Million RR, Pfaff WW (1976) Patterns of recurrence following surgery alone for adenocarcinoma of the colon and rectum. Cancer 37: 2861–2865

Charnley RM, Banerjee AK, Whitaker SC, Spiller RC, Doran J (1995) Peritoneal seeding of pancreatic cancer following transperitoneal biliary procedures. Br J Surg 82: 393

Curtis MG, Hopkins MP, Cross B, Tantri MD, Jenison EL, Rehmus E (1994) Wound seeding associated with endometrial cancer. Gynecol Oncol 52: 413–415

Cutherell L, Wanebo HJ, and Tegtmeyer CJ (1986) Catheter tract seeding after percutaneous biliary drainage for pancreatic cancer. Cancer 57: 2057–2060

Doctor N, Dafnios N, Dick R, Davidson BR (1997) Peritoneal seeding of pancreatic head carcinoma following percutaneous transhepatic drainage and stenting. Br J Surg 84: 197

Fleshman JW, Nelson H, Peters WR, et al, (1996) Early results of laparoscopic surgery for colorectal cancer. Retrospective analysis of 372 patients treated by Clinical Outcomes of Surgical Therapy (COST) Study Group. Dis Colon Rectum 39: 53–58

Gunderson LL, Sosin H (1974) Areas of failure found at reoperation (second or symptomatic look) following "curative surgery" for adenocarcinoma of the rectum. Clinicopathologic correlation and implications for adjuvant therapy. Cancer 34: 1278–1292

Heald RJ, Smedh RK, Kald A, Sexton R, Moran BJ (1997) Abdominoperineal excision of the rectum – an endangered operation. Norman Nigro Lectureship. Dis Colon Rectum 40: 747–751

Hughes ES, McDermott FT, Polglase AL, Johnson WR (1983) Tumor recurrence in the abdominal wall scar tissue after large-bowel cancer surgery. Dis Colon Rectum 26: 571–572

Koffi E, Moutardier V, Sauvanet A, Noun R, Flejou JF, Belghiti J (1996) Wound recurrence after resection of hepatocellular carcinoma. Liver Transpl Surg 2: 301–303

Kruitwagen RF, Swinkels BM, Keyser KG, Doesburg WH, Schijf CP (1996) Incidence and effect on survival of abdominal wall metastases at trocar or puncture sites following laparoscopy or paracentesis in women with ovarian cancer. Gynecol Oncol 60: 233–237

La Fianza A, Di Maggio EM, Preda L, Schifino MR, and Campani R (1997) Infiltrative subcutaneous metastases from ovarian carcinoma after paracentesis: CT findings. Abdom Imaging 22: 522–523

Recht MP, Coleman BG, Barbot DJ, Rosato EF, Aronchick JM, Epstein DM, Gefter WB, Millewr WT (1989) Recurrent esophageal carcinoma at thoracotomy incisions: diagnostic contributions of CT. J Comput Assist Tomogr 13: 58–60

Reilly WT, Nelson H, Schroeder G, Wieand HS, Bolton J, O'Connell MJ (1996) Wound recurrence following conventional treatment of colorectal cancer. A rare but perhaps underestimated problem. Dis Colon Rectum 39: 200–207

Ricardo AE, Feig BW, Ellis LM, Hunt KK, Curley SA, MacFadyen BV Jr, Mansfield PF (1997) Gallbladder cancer and trocar site recurrences. Am J Surg 174: 619–622

Welch JP, Donaldson GA (1979) The clinical correlation of an autopsy study of recurrent colorectal cancer. Ann Surg 189: 496–502

Zinzindohoue F, Penna C, Parc R (1997) Adenocarcinoma arising on the site of a Gelpi retractor after coloanal anastomosis for rectal cancer. Br J Surg 84: 362

CHAPTER 4

Port-Site Recurrences in Laparoscopic Surgery

Ph. Wittich, H.J. Bonjer

Introduction

Tumor growths at port-sites after laparoscopic surgery for abdominal cancer have caused major concern among doctors and patients in the early 1990s (Wexner and Cohen 1995). Laparoscopic surgery was considered less traumatic for the patient but appeared deceiving in malignancies in some patients. Many surgeons have abandoned the laparoscopic approach in patients with malignant tumors for fear of port-site recurrences. A wide variety of experimental studies have been instigated to unravel the pathogenesis of port-site recurrences in laparoscopic surgery. Are we facing a novel problem caused by a surgical technique that had been accepted to be superior to conventional open surgery too readily? Browsing through ancient medical literature revealed some interesting communications. In 1903, von Mikulicz published an article entitled "Small contributions to the surgery of the intestinal tract". The Mikulicz procedure involved exteriorization of a colonic cancer through a small incision to allow extracorporeal resection. The incentive of this procedure was to minimize fecal spill in the peritoneal cavity to prevent abdominal abscesses in an era devoid of antibiotics. More than half of the patients developed a cancerous recurrence in the abdominal wall within 4 years. Ninety years later, this phenomenon was encountered again at narrow extraction sites employed for laparoscopic removal of cancerous specimens (Drouard et al. 1991). In 1907 Charles Ryall stated in an article on "Cancer infection and cancer recurrence: a danger to avoid in cancer operations" that "…cancer cells must have been liberated during manipulation of the growth and carried to the abdominal incisions by the instruments, suture or surgeon's hands…". Almost one century later, the great vision of Ryall was confirmed in the laboratory by Hewett et al. (1996) who detected cancer cells on laparoscopic instruments after manipulation in rats with tumor cell infested abdominal cavities.

The present literature on cancer recurrence at port-sites involves a large volume of case reports, small series and attempts to review all these individual cases. Thorough analysis of these case histories can provide guidance in resolving the complex pathogenesis of port-site recurrences. In this chapter, port-site recurrences of gynecological malignancies, colon cancer, gallbladder cancer, urological malignancies and after diagnostic laparoscopy will be discussed subsequently.

Gynecological Malignancies

Port-site recurrences after gynecological laparoscopy have been reported for all cancers of the female reproductive organs. However, laparoscopy for ovarian cancer is most commonly associated with port-site recurrences. In a review of 19 cases of metastases at the trocar insertion after laparoscopy for gynecological malignancy, 14 occurred after surgery for ovarian cancer. Curiously, 3 of these 14 ovarian tumors were borderline tumors (Wang et al. 1997). Most of the procedures that were followed by port-site recurrences involved laparoscopic puncture or biopsy of ovarian tumors. The true incidence of port-site recurrences after laparoscopy for ovarian cancer is difficult to assess. Other authors noted only one metastasis at a trocar site in 70 women with ovarian cancer accounting for an incidence of 1.4% (Childers et al. 1994). Reports of port-site recurrences after laparoscopy for cervical cancer are rare (Naumann and Spencer 1997). Only two reports exist of metastases of cervical cancer in surgical scars after open surgery. One in the abdominal incision after radical hysterectomy for stage Ib squamous cell carcinoma, and another at the site of a retroperitoneal drain in a patient with a stage IIa squamous cell carcinoma of the cervix (Boulez and Herriot 1994). One case report has been published on port-site recurrences after laparoscopic surgery for endometrial cancer (Wang et al. 1997). In this case, laparoscopy-assisted vaginal hysterectomy had been done combined with laparoscopic pelvic and aortic lymphadenectomy for stage IIIc disease. Metastases occurred after an interval of 6 months at multiple port-sites and at the episiotomy that had been employed for extraction of the specimen. Relaparotomy for bowel obstruction revealed diffuse peritoneal carcinomatosis. Kadar showed in a retrospective review of 24 patients who had laparoscopic surgery for metastatic gynecological disease, port-site recurrences in 16% of all patients (Kadar 1997). Advanced stages of disease clearly predispose to port-site recurrences.

Colorectal Cancer

The first laparoscopic resections for colorectal cancer were performed in 1991 (Jacobs et al. 1991). The striking reduction of morbidity after laparoscopic removal of the gallbladder ignited great enthusiasm for laparoscopic colorectal surgery. However, in 1993 several alarming case reports on port-site recurrences after laparoscopic resection of colorectal cancer (Fig. 4.1) startled general surgeons and evoked great criticism among conventional surgeons about the application of laparoscopic techniques in the treatment of colorectal cancer (Alexander et al. 1993; Berends et al. 1994; Guillou et al. 1993). Particularly, reports of port-site recurrences after laparoscopic resection of Dukes A carcinomas caused major turbulence (Fingerhut 1995; Lauroy et al.1994; Prasad et al. 1994). In one of these cases, a polypectomy was performed after colotomy (Lauroy et al. 1994). At microscopy, this polyp contained a Duke's A carcinoma. Possibly, either inadvertent grasping of an occult tumor, that was not visible on the serosal side of the bowel, or tumor cell seeding through the lumen caused port-site recurrences in these Dukes A cases. Although port-site recurrences had been reported by the end of 1994 in less than 30 patients worldwide, laparoscopic treatment of colorectal malignancy became and remains very controversial. Many suggested that abdominal wall recurrence after colorectal cancer resection occurred exclusively after laparoscopy while tumor recurrence at the abdominal wall after conventional resection of colorectal cancers has been suggested to occur rarely. Reilly reported in a study of 1171 patients who had open curative resections for colorectal cancers that the incidence of abdominal wall recurrence varied from 0.6% to 0.9% for either Dukes B or C stages

(Reilly et al. 1996). These figures are in agreement with the 0.8% incidence rate of abdominal wall recurrence that had been documented by Hughes et al. in 1983. However, the method of detection appears to play an important role in determining the true incidence of abdominal wall recurrences. Welch and Donaldson (1979) discovered 16.6% wound recurrence in 145 autopsies performed in patients with recurrent colorectal cancer. Others encountered cancer recurrence in the abdominal wall of more than 3% of patients who underwent a second look operation after a curative resection of colorectal cancer (Gunderson et al. 1974). Two-thirds of these abdominal wall recurrences were at the level of the fascia and had not been found at physical examination.

Extensive review of the literature until 1999 revealed 82 port-site recurrences after laparoscopic colorectal surgery (Table 4.1). Port-site recurrences occurred after all types of colorectal resections. In this overview, a predominance of laparoscopic right hemicolectomy appeared to be present. The tumor stages were known in 72 cases in our review and of these 5 were classified as Dukes A, 11 as Dukes B, 42 as Dukes C and 14 as Dukes D. Disseminated disease at the time of diagnosis of the port-site recurrences was reported in 15 patients. All these patients had colorectal cancers staged as either Dukes C or Dukes D at the primary colorectal operation. Port-site recurrences were found at ports either used for instrumentation or the laparoscope and at extraction sites. The median interval until discovery of port-site recurrences was 6 months. The earliest documentation of a port-site recurrence was 1 month after sur-

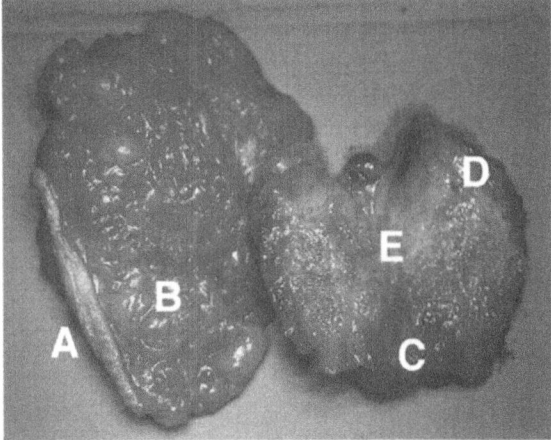

Fig. 4.1. Port-site recurrence at the extraction port 15 months after laparoscopic hemicolectomy for cancer *A*, skin; *B*, subcutaneous tissue; *C*, muscle; *D*, fascia and peritoneum; *E*, tumor. Courtesy from I. Inan and P. Petropoulos, Fribourg, Switzerland

Table 4.1. Port-site metastases after laparoscopic resection of colorectal malignancy

Reference	Patients	Stage	No. and location p.s.m. (+ available details)	Interval
Alexander et al. (1993)	1	Duke's C	1: unspec. port	3 months
Barrat et al. (1998)	1	Duke's D	1: unspec. port (dissem. disease)	n.m.
Berends et al. (1994)	3	Duke's BII Duke's CII Duke's D	1 p.s.m. each patient: 2 umbilical ports, 1 unspec. port	n.m.
Bokey et al. (1997)	1	Duke's B	1: RLQ port (excised)	12 months
Boulez and Herriot (1994)	3	n.m.	n.m.	n.m.
Christen et al. (1995)	1	T4NxMx	1: unspec. port	n.m.
Cirocco et al. (1994)	1	T3N2M0	5: 4 ports + excorp. wound (dissem. disease)	9 months
Cook and Dehn (1996)	2	Duke's C + liver metas. Duke's C	1: umbilical port 1: unspec. port	9 months 15 months
Fielding et al. (1997)	2	Duke's C Duke's D	1: unspec. port (dissem. disease) 1: unspec. port (dissem. disease)	n.m.
Fingerhut (1995)	3	1x Duke's A 2x Duke's B	n.m.	n.m.
Fleshman et al. (1996)	4	T4N1M0 T3N1M0 T3N0M0 T2N0M0	1: conversion laparotomy 1: unspec. port (excised) 1: unspec. port (excised) 1: unspec. port (excised)	n.m.
Fodera et al. (1996)	1	n.m.	1: right paraumbilical port	7 months
Fusco et Paluzzi (1993)	1	T3N1M0	1: RLQ port (excised)	10 months
Gellman et al. (1996)	1	Carcinosis	1: unspec. port (dissem. disease)	4 months
Gionnone cited in Wexner and Cohen (1995)	1	Duke's C	1: unspec. port	2 months
Gould cited in Wexner and Cohen (1995)	1	n.m.	n.m.	4 months
Guillou et al. (1993)	1	Duke's C	n.m.	n.m.
Jaquet et al. (1995a)	2	Duke's C T3N0M0	1: left port 1: excorp. wound	1 month 10 months
Jaquet et al. (1995b)	1	T3N0M0	2: right + left port	9 months
Kwok et al. (1996)	2	Duke's D n.m.	1: excorp. wound (dissem. disease) 1: unspec. port (dissem. disease)	n.m.
Lauroy et al. (1994)	1	Duke's A	1: right paraumbilical port	9 months
Leung et al. (1999)	1	n.m.	1: unspec. port (dissem. disease)	n.m.
Lumley et al. (1996)	1	Duke's D	1: unspec. port (dissem. disease)	n.m.
Montorsi et al. (1995)	1	T3N0M0	1: excorp. wound (excised)	2 months
Newman cited in Wexner and Cohen (1995)	1	Duke's C	1: unspec. port	6 months
Nduka et al. (1994)	1	Duke's C	3: right paraumbilical + umbilical port + perineal wound	3 months
Ng et al. (1996)	1	n.m.	2: scope port + right port	n.m.

Table 4.1. (Fortsetzung)

Reference	Patients	Stage	No. and location p.s.m. (+ available details)	Interval
Ngoi cited in Wexner and Cohen (1995)	1	Duke's B	1: unspec. port	n.m.
Prasad et al. (1994)	2	Duke's B Duke's A	1: RLQ port (excised) 1: excorp. wound	6 months 26 months
Ramos et al. (1994)	3	Duke's C Duke's C Duke's C	2: unspec. port + excorp. wound (dissem. disease) 2: unspec. port + excorp. wound (dissem. disease) 1: excorp. wound	6 months 8 months 21 months
Rosato et al. (1998)	10	2x Stage I 2x Stage II 5x Stage III 1x Stage IV	1 p.s.m. each patient: 8x unspec. port (1x dissem. disease) 2x excorp. wound (1x dissem. disease)	Stage I: 18 and 44 months
Schaeff et al. (1998)	12	8x Stage III 4x Stage IV	1 p.s.m. each patient: 8x unspec. port, 3x excorp. wound, 1x perineal wound (7 p.s.m. excised)	n.m.
Stitz cited in Wexner and Cohen (1995)	1	Duke's D	n.m.	n.m.
Ugarte (1995)	1	Duke's C	1: unspec. port	9 months
Vukasin et al. (1996)	5	Stage III Stage III Stage III Stage III Stage III	1: excorp. wound 1: unspec. port 1: unspec. port (2x dissem. disease) 1: unspec. port 1: excorp. wound	2 months 3 months 7 months 15 months 21 months
Walsh et al. (1993)	1	n.m.	1: RLQ port	6 months
Wexner and Cohen (1995)	5	2x Duke's B 3x Duke's C	1 p.s.m. each patient: unspec. ports	3-6 months 6-12 months
Wilson (1994)	1	n.m.	1: unspec. port	n.m.

p.s.m. = port-site metastasis, unspec. = unspecified, n.m. = not mentioned, RLQ = right lower quadrant
(dissem. disease) = disseminated disease at discovery of port-site metastasis
(excised) = port-site metastasis was excised

Table 4.2. All studies with more than 50 patients included 3547 patients in total. In these studies, 30 patients with port-site metastases were found (0.85%).

Reference	Study	Patients	Follow-up	P.S.M
Ballantyne (1995)	Registry	498	n.s.	3 (0.6%)
Bokey et al. (1997)	Retrospective	66	Median 26 months	1 (1.5%)
Fielding et al. (1997)	Retrospective	149	n.s.	2 (1.3%)
Fleshman et al. (1996)	Registry	372	n.s.	4 (1.1%)
Franklin et al. (1996)	Prospective	191	>30 months	0
Gellman et al. (1996)	Retrospective	58	n.s.	1 (1.7%)
Hoffman et al. (1996)	Retrospective	39	at least 24 months	0
Huscher et al. (1996)	Retrospective	146	Mean 15 months	0
Khalili et al. (1998)	Retrospective	80	Mean 21 months	0
Kwok et al. (1996)	Retrospective	83	n.s.	2 (2.5%)
Leung et al. (1999)	Retrospective	179	Mean 19.8 months	1 (0.65%)
Lord et al. (1996)	Retrospective	71	Mean16.7	0
Lumley et al. (1996)	Retrospective	103	n.s.	1 (1.0%)
Milsom et al. (1998)	Prosp. rand.	42	Median 18 months	0
Rosato et al. (1998)	Registry	1071	n.s.	10 (0.93%)
Vukasin et al. (1996)	Registry	480	>12 months	5 (1.1%)

gery while the longest interval was 44 months. In 33 patients, the interval between surgery and the discovery of the port-site recurrence was recorded. Of interest is that only 5 (15%) of these 33 patients developed port-site recurrences more than 1 year after the colorectal resection. The treatment and outcome of port-site recurrences after laparoscopic colorectal surgery has been reported in very few cases.

Surgical inexperience appears an important etiologic factor for port-site recurrences considering the high incidences reported in early small series and the far lower rates in later reports on groups with more patients (Berends et al. 1994; Franklin et al. 1996). Therefore, it appears appropriate to only consider studies with more than 50 cases for assessment of the incidence of port-site recurrences after laparoscopic colorectal surgery. In 3547 patients, culled from series with more than 50 cases, port-site recurrences were recorded in 30 patients accounting for an incidence of 0.85% (Table 4.2).

Gallbladder Cancer

Laparoscopic cholecystectomy is the most common endoscopic procedure in general surgical practice. The incidence of gallbladder cancer in cholecystectomy specimens varies from 0.18% to 0.81% of all cholecystectomies (Pezet et al. 1992). Although thickening of the gallbladder wall and solitary polypoid lesions greater than 1 cm in diameter can indicate malignancy of the gallbladder, approximately half of all gallbladder cancers is not suspected before surgery (Fig. 4.2).

During laparoscopy, small tumors that do not invade the muscular layer, T1 tumors, can easily be missed, particularly because tactile senses are less during laparoscopic surgery. In one study of 24 patients with proven gallbladder cancer, 14 out of 24 were not suspected during the operation. Of these 14 cases 9 were classified as either T2 or T3 tumors (Yamaguchi et al. 1996). When laparoscopic cholecystectomy is performed in those cases with undetected malignancy, tumor cells can be disseminated in the peritoneal cavity due to inadvertent grasping of the tumor or perforation of the gallbladder. The incidence of gallbladder perforation during laparoscopic dissection and removal of the gallbladder has been reported to vary from 24% to 33%. In a series of 2616 laparoscopic cholecystectomies, 24 gallbladder cancers were identified, accounting for an incidence of 0.9% (Yamaguchi et al. 1996). Three abdominal wall recurrences were observed (13%), all in patients with either T2 or T3 tumors. In another series of

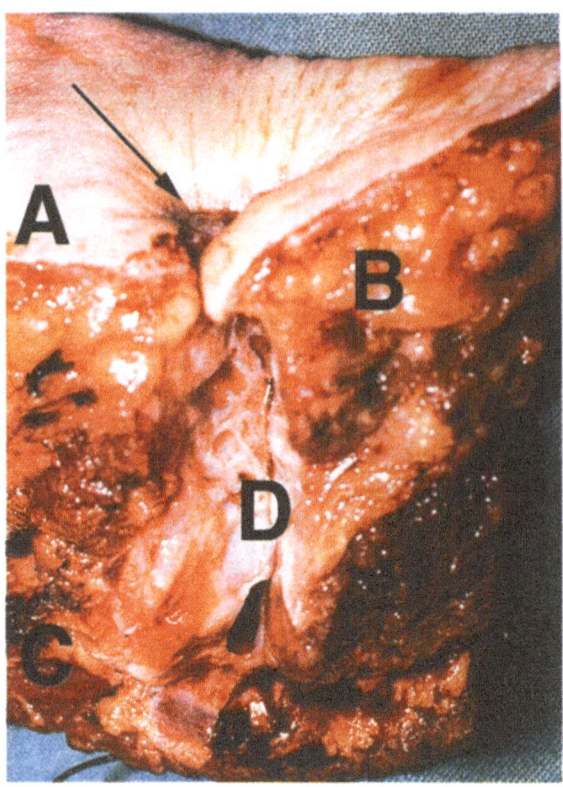

Fig. 4.2. Port-site recurrence at the umbilical port (*arrow*) 8 weeks after laparoscopic cholecystectomy. The recurrence is located in the subcutaneous tissue *A,* skin; *B,* subcutaneous tissue; *C,* muscle; *D,* tumor. Courtesy from H. Lippert, Magdeburg, Germany

10925 laparoscopic cholecystectomies, 37 patients had adenocarcinoma of the gallbladder (0.34%) (Z'graggen et al. 1998). Besides one patient, who had a polyp on preoperative ultrasonography of the gallbladder, malignancy was not suspected preoperatively in any of these cases. In 46% of all gallbladder cancers, malignancy was recognized during operation. Port-site recurrences occurred in 14% of the patients with gallbladder cancer after an interval of 6–16 months. These metastases were encountered at equal rates in all tumor stages, but accidental gallbladder perforations significantly increased the chance of port-site recurrences. Suzuki et al. (1998) reviewed 3566 patients who had undergone laparoscopic cholecystectomy and 30 patients with unexpected gallbladder carcinoma were identified. Malignancy was noted in only one patient during laparoscopic surgery. Bile spillage occurred in half the patients with gallbladder cancer. Port-site recurrences were documented in three cases (10%), staged as T2 and T3 cancers. The 3-year survival rate for T1 disease was 100%, and for T2 disease 70%.

These rates appear comparable to those of hidden gallbladder cancer in open surgery (Suzuki et al. 1998). Ricardo et al. (1997) reported their experience with 91 patients who were diagnosed with gallbladder cancer and of these patients 90% had advanced disease (T2 or T3 cancers). They analyzed the incidence of port-site recurrences in patients who had laparoscopic cholecystectomy, open cholecystectomy or converted procedures. In advanced gallbladder cancer, the operative technique appeared not to affect the rate of abdominal wall recurrence. One patient in this study presented with an umbilical metastasis prior to surgery. Such rare umbilical metastases from intra-abdominal tumors are known as "Sister Mary Joseph's nodules" and can be the first sign of malignant disease in a patient (Khan and Cook 1997). Though its pathogenesis may be different from the pathogenesis of port-site metastases, the Sister Mary Joseph's nodule in this patient illustrated the avidity of gallbladder cancer cells for the abdominal wall.

In this laparoscopic era, thorough ultrasonographic evaluation of the gallbladder is mandatory to prevent any dismal consequences of laparoscopic cholecystectomy. In suspect cases, laparoscopy can be performed to assess the macroscopic appearance of the gallbladder. When the serosal aspect of the gallbladder appears normal, laparoscopic ultrasonography should be performed subsequently to identify abnormal thickening of the gallbladder wall, polyps or enlarged lymph nodes in the hepatoduodenal ligament. In case of any remaining suspicion, laparoscopy should be converted to open surgery.

Urological Malignancy

Laparoscopy plays an important role in the diagnosis and treatment of urological malignancy. In several centers with laparoscopic and oncological expertise, laparoscopic nephrectomy has become the procedure of choice in patients with renal cell cancer staged as T 1 or T 2. In a registry of 157 patients who had undergone laparoscopic radical nephrectomy, abdominal wall recurrence was not observed at a mean follow-up period of more than 2.5 years (Cadeddu et al. 1998). Obviously, a longer follow-up is mandatory to draw final conclusions about the incidence of abdominal wall recurrence since renal cell cancer is known for its late metastases. Of interest is the technique for specimen removal in laparoscopic radical nephrectomy. Unlike general surgeons, urologists do not refrain from morcellating cancerous specimens in a plastic bag. In spite of this technique,

port-site recurrences have not been reported after laparoscopic radical nephrectomy. In the registry of 157 patients, only 1 patient had a local recurrence located in the ureteral stump. Retrograde embolization of tumor cells or implantation of exfoliated renal cancer cells were considered possible mechanisms of the ureteral recurrence. Similar ureteral recurrence after radical nephrectomy has been reported after open procedures (Remis and Halverstadt 1992). Therefore, laparoscopy does not appear instrumental in ureteral recurrence. Laparoscopic pelvic lymphadenectomy is commonly employed to assess the lymphatic spread of prostatic cancer. In this procedure lymph nodes are frequently removed without use of a protecting bag. Surprisingly, only few reports exist on port-site recurrences after laparoscopic pelvic lymphadenectomy (Bangma et al. 1995; Stolla et al. 1994). Direct laparoscopic biopsy of bladder cancer was followed by a port-site recurrence (Andersen and Steven 1995).

Janetschek et al. (1999) reported that they did not observe any port-site recurrences in 24 patients who had had laparoscopic lymphadenectomy for non-seminomatous testicular cancer at a mean follow-up of 2 years. Non-seminomatous testicular cancer requires chemotherapy prior to abdominal lymphadenectomy. Thus, possibly, chemotherapy reduced the risk of port-site recurrences.

Diagnostic Laparoscopy

Diagnostic laparoscopy, frequently in combination with laparoscopic ultrasonography and biopsy, is a valuable tool to identify the cause of ascites or assess the resectability of abdominal cancers. It may prevent unnecessary laparotomies in up to 32% of patients with gastrointestinal malignancies, or modify the treatment in up to 34% (Barrat et al. 1998; McCulloch et al. 1998; Nieveen van Dijkum et al. 1999). However, the occurrence of port-site recurrences after diagnostic laparoscopy raises the question if this procedure in known or suspected malignancy, exposes patients with resectable malignant disease to the risk of cancer dissemination.

Reports on port-site recurrences after diagnostic laparoscopy are scarce and the population of patients is seldom mentioned. Furthermore, there is considerable heterogeneity of underlying diseases in the studied patients. Nieveen van Dijkum et al. described in 1996 a series of 250 patients who had undergone a laparoscopy for staging of gastrointestinal malignancy including 121 periampullary tumors, 66 esophageal tumors, 26 proximal bile duct cancers, 21 liver tumors and 13 other intra-abdominal malignancies and 4 patients (1.6%) developed a port-site recurrence. In two of these patients, intraoperative biopsy showed metastatic disease, but in the other two, no metastases were seen. These latter patients underwent exploratory laparotomy which revealed locally advanced non-resectable tumors. Interestingly, metastases developed at the port-sites but not in the laparotomy wound. In another study, 3 out of 40 patients undergoing laparoscopy for staging (40 esophageal and 10 gastric cancers) developed port-site recurrences (7.5%) (Cook and Dehn 1996). Two patients had gastric carcinoma (20% of all gastric cancers) and one patient had esophageal cancer (3.3% of all esophageal cancers).

In a French study of 109 patients with gastrointestinal malignancy, no port-site recurrences after diagnostic laparoscopy with intra-abdominal ultrasonography were reported (Barrat et al. 1998). A British series reported 49 patients who underwent diagnostic laparoscopy for gastric cancer (McCulloch 1998). Port-site recurrence occurred in one patient with intraoperatively assessed disseminated disease (2%). In a large Dutch study of 286 patients that had had laparoscopy and laparoscopic ultrasonography for periampullary and pancreatic cancers, 7 patients with port-site recurrences were identified (2.4%) (Nieveen van Dijkum et al. 1999) All patients had disseminated disease at the time of laparoscopy and the port-site tumors developed after a mean period of 8 months. Although all port-site recurrences after a diagnostic procedure were seen in patients with non-resectable tumors or disseminated disease, some of them required excision for patient comfort. Muensterer et al. (1997) recommended midline placement of trocars, which should facilitate port-site excision at the time of cytoreductive surgery.

References

Alexander RJT, Jacques BC, Mitchell KG (1993) Laparoscopically assisted colectomy and wound recurrence. Lancet 341: 249

Andersen JR, Steven K (1995) Implantation metastasis after laparoscopic biopsy of bladder cancer. J Urol 153: 1047–1048

Ballantyne GH (1995) Laparoscopic-assisted colorectal surgery: review of results in 752 patients. Gastroenterologist 3: 75–89

Bangma CH, Kirkels WJ, Chada S, Schroder FH (1995) Cutaneous metastasis following laparoscopic pelvic lymphadenectomy for prostatic carcinoma. J Urol 153: 719–723

Barrat C, Champault G, Catheline JM (1998) Is laparoscopic evaluation of digestive cancer legitimate? A prospective study of 109 cases. Ann Chir 52: 602–606

Berends FJ, Kazemier G, Bonjer HJ, Lange JF (1994) Subcutaneous metastases after laparoscopic colectomy. Lancet 344: 58

Bokey EL, Moore WE, Keating JP, Zelas P, Chapuis PH, Newland RC (1997) Laparoscopic resection of the colon and rectum for cancer. Br J Surg 84: 822–825

Boulez J, Herriot E (1994) Multicentric analysis of laparoscopic colorectal surgery in FDCL group: 274 cases. Br J Surg 81: 527

Cadeddu JA, Ono Y, Clayman RV, Barrett PH, Janetschek G, Fentie DD, McDougall EM, Moore RG, Kinukawa T, Elbahnasy AM, Nelson JB, Kavoussi LR (1998) Laparoscopic nephrectomy for renal cell cancer: evaluation of efficacy and safety: a multicenter experience. Urology 52: 773–777

Childers JM, Aqua KA, Surwit EA, Hallum AW, Hatch KD (1994) Abdominal-wall tumor implantation after laparoscopy for malignant contitions. Obstet Gynecol 84 (5): 765–769

Christen D, Buchmann P, Klingler K (1995) Wie sicher ist die laparoskopische Kolonchirurgie? Schweiz Med Wochenschr 125: 1597–1601

Cirocco WC, Schwartzman A, Golub RW (1994) Abdominal wall recurrence after laparoscopic colectomy for colon cancer. Surgery 116: 842–846

Cook TA, Dehn TC (1996) Port-site recurrences in patients undergoing laparoscopy for gastrointestinal malignancy. Br J Surg 83 :1419–1420

Drouard F, Delamarre J, Capron JP (1991) Cutaneous seeding of gallbladder cancer after laparoscopic cholecystectomy. N Engl J Med 325: 1316

Fielding GA, Lumley J, Nathanson L, Hewitt P, Rhodes M, Stitz R (1997) Laparoscopic colectomy. Surg Endosc 11: 745–749

Fingerhut A (1995) Laparoscopic colectomy. The French experience. In: Jager R, Wexner SD (eds) Laparoscopic colorectal surgery. Churchill Livingstone, New York

Fleshman JW, Nelson H, Peters WR, Kim HC, Larach S, Boorse RR, Ambroze W, Leggett Ph, Bleday R, Stryker S, Christenson B, Wexner S, Rattner D, Sutton J, Fine AP (1996) Early results of laparoscopic surgery for colorectal cancer. Retrospective analysis of 372 patients treated by clinical outcomes of surgical therapy (Cost) study group. Dis Colon Rectum 39: 53–58

Fodera M, Pello M, Atabe k U, Spence RK, Alexander JB, Camishion RB (1995) Trocar site tumor recurrence after laparoscopic-assisted colectomy. J Laparoendosc Surg 5: 259–262

Franklin ME, Rosenthal D, Abrego-Medina D, Dorman JP, Glass JL, Norem R, Diaz A (1996) Prospective comparison of open vs. laparoscopic colon surgery for carcinoma. Five-year results. Dis Colon Rectum 39: 35–46

Fusco MA, Paluzzi MW (1993) Abdominal wall recurrence after laparoscopic-assisted colectomy for adenocarcinoma of the colon. Dis Colon Rectum 36: 858–861

Gellman L, Salky B, Edye M (1996) Laparoscopic assisted colectomy. Surg Endosc 10: 1041–1044

Guillou PJ, Darzi A, Monson JRT (1993) Experience with laparoscopic colorectal surgery for malignant disease. Surg Oncol 36: 858–861

Gunderson LL, Sosin H, Sevitt S (1974) Areas of failure found at reoperation (second or symptomatic look) following "curative surgery" for adenocarcinoma of the rectum: clinicopathologic correlation and implications for adjuvant therapy. Cancer 34: 1278–1292

Hewett PJ, Thomas WM, King G, Eaton M (1996) Intraperitoneal cell movement during abdominal carbon dioxide insufflation and laparoscopy. An in vivo model. Dis Colon Rectum 39: S62–66

Hoffman GC, Baker JW, Doxey JB, Hubbard GW, Ruffin WK, Wishner JA (1996) Minimally invasive surgery for colorectal cancer. Initial follow-up. Ann Surg 223: 790–798

Hughes ES, McDermott FT, Polglase AL, Johnson WR (1993) Tumor recurrence in the abdominal wall scar tissue after large-bowel cancer surgery. Dis Colon Rectum 26: 571–572

Huscher C, Silecchia G, Croce E, Farello GA, Lezoche E, Morino M, Azzola M, Feliciotti F, Rosato P, Tarantini M, Basso N (1996) Laparoscopic colorectal resection. A multicenter Italian study. Surg Endosc 10: 875–879

Jacobs M, Verdeja JC, Goldstein HS (1991) Minimally invasive colon resection (laparoscopic colectomy). Surg Laparosc Endosc 1: 144–150

Jacquet P, Averbach AM, Jacquet N (1995a) Abdominal wall metastasis and peritoneal carcinomatosis after laparoscopic-assisted colectomy for cancer. Eur J Oncol 21: 568–570

Jacquet P, Averbach AM, Stephens AD, Sugarbaker PH (1995b) Cancer recurrence following laparoscopic colectomy. Report of two patients treated with heated intraperitoneal chemotherapy. Dis Colon Rectum 38: 1110–1114

Janetschek G, Hobisch A, Hittmair A, Holtl L, Peschel R, Bartsch G (1999) Laparoscopic retroperitoneal lymphadenectomy after chemotherapy for stage IIB nonseminatous testicular carcinoma. J Urol 161: 477–481

Kadar N (1997) Port-site recurrences following laparoscopic operations for gynecological malignancies. Br J Obstet Gynecol 104: 1308–1313

Khahili ThM, Fleshner PhR, Hiatt JR, Sokol ThP, Manookian C, Tsushima G, Philips EH (1998) Colorectal cancer: comparison of laparoscopic with open approaches. Dis Colon Rectum 41: 832–838

Khan AJ, Cook B (1997) Metastatic carcinoma of umbilicus: "Sister Mary Joseph's nodule". Cutis 60: 297–298

Kwok SPY, Lau WY, Carey PD, Kelly SB, Leung KL, Li AKC (1996) Prospective evaluation of laparoscopic-assisted large-bowel excision for cancer. Ann Surg 223: 170–176

Lauroy J, Champault G, Risk N, Boutelier P (1994) Metastatic recurrence at the trocar site: should digestive carcinomas still be managed by laparoscopy? Br J Surg 81: 31

Leung KL, Yiu RYC, Lai PBS, Lee JFY, Thung KH, Lau WY (1999) Laparoscopic-assisted resection of colorectal carcinoma. Five-year audit. Dis Colon Rectum 42: 327–333

Lord SA, Larach SW, Ferrara A, Williamson PR, Lago CP, Lube MW (1996) Laparoscopic resections for colorectal carcinoma. A three year experience. Dis Colon Rectum 39: 148–153

Lumley JW, Fielding GA, Rhodes M, Nathanson LK, Siu S, Stitz RW (1996). Laparoscopic-assisted colorectal surgery. Lessons learned from 240 consecutive patients. Dis Colon Rectum 39: 155–159

McCulloch P, Johnson M, Jairam R, Fischer W (1998) Laparoscopic staging of gastric cancer is safe and affects treatment strategy. Ann R Coll Surg Engl 80: 400–402

Mikulicz Von J (1903) Small contributions to the surgery of the intestinal tract. Boston M & S J 148: 608–611

Milsom JW, Bohm B, Hammerhofer KA, Fazio V, Steiger E, Elson P (1998) A prospective, randomized trial comparing laparoscopic versus conventional techniques in colorectal cancer surgery: a preliminary report. J Am Coll Surg 187: 46–57

Montorsi M, Fumagalli U, Rosati R, Bona S, Chella B, Huscher

C (1995) Early parietal recurrence of adenocarcinoma of the colon after laparoscopic colectomy. Br J Surg 82: 1036–1037

Muensterer OJ, Averbach AM, Jacquet P, Otero SE, Sugarbaker PH (1997) Malignant peritoneal mesothelioma. Case-report demonstrating pitfalls of diagnostic laparoscopy. Int Surg 82: 240–243

Naumann RW, Spencer S (1997) An umbilical metastasis after laparoscopy for squamous cell carcinoma of the cervix. Gynecol Oncol 64: 507–509

Nduka CC, Monson JRT, Menzies-Gow N, Darzi A (1994) Abdominal wall metastases following laparoscopy. Br J Surg 81: 648–652

Ng WT, Yeung HC, Koh GH, Ng WF (1996) Mechanism for port-site recurrence after laparoscopic cancer surgery. Br J Surg 83: 1478

Nieveen van Dijkum EJM, De Wit LTh, Obertop H, Gouma DJ (1996) Port-site recurrences after laparoscopic surgery for gastrointestinal malignancies. Br J Surg 83: 1793–1794

Nieveen van Dijkum EJM, De Wit LTh, Van Delden OM, Rauws EAJ, Van Lanschot JJB, Obertop H, Gouma DJ (1997) The efficacy of laparoscopic staging in patients with upper gastrointestinal tumors. Cancer 79: 1315–1319

Nieveen van Dijkum EJM, Romijn MG, Van Eijck CJHJ, Gouma DJ (1999) Rapport van ontwikkelingsgeneeskunde project van de ziekenfondsraad (unpublished)

Pezet D, Fondrinier E, Rotman N, Guy L, Lemesle P, Lointier P, Chipponi J (1992) Parietal seeding of carcinoma of the gallbladder after laparoscopic cholecystectomy. Br J Surg 79: 230

Prasad A, Avery C, Foley RJE (1994) Abdominal wall metastases following laparoscopy. Br J Surg 81: 1697

Ramos JM, Gupta S, Anthone GJ, Ortega AE, Simons AJ, Beart RW (1994) Laparoscopy and colon cancer. Is the port-site at risk? A preliminary report. Arch Surg 129: 897–900

Reilly WT, Nelson H, Schroeder G, Wieand HS, Bolton J, O'Connell MJ (1996) Wound recurrence following conventional treatment of colorectal cancer. Dis Colon Rectum 39: 200–207

Remis RE, Halverstadt DB (1992) Metastatic renal cell carcinoma to the bladder: case report and review of the literature. J Urol 147: 1358–1360.

Ricardo AE, Feig BW, Ellis LM, Hunt KK, Curley SA, MacFadyen BV, Mansfield PF (1997) Gallbladder cancer and trocar site recurrences. Am J Surg 174: 619–623

Rosato P, Silecchia G, De Leo A, Carlini M, Azzola M, Giraudo G, Franzato GB, Tamborrino E (1998) Port-site and wound metastases following laparoscopic resection of colorectal carcinoma. The experience of the Italian registry. Data presented at the 33rd Congress of the European Society for Surgical Research (ESSR)

Ryall C (1907) Cancer infection and cancer recurrence: a danger to avoid in cancer operations. Lancet: 1311–1316

Schaeff B, Poalucci V, Thomopoulos J (1998) Port-site recurrence after laparoscopic surgery. Dig Surg 15: 124–134

Stolla V, Rossi D, Bladou F, Rattier C, Ayuso D, Serment G (1994) Subcutaneous metastases after coelioscopic lymphadendectomy for vesical urothelial carcinoma. Eur Urol 26: 342–343

Suzuki K, Kimura T, Ogawa H (1998) Is laparoscopic cholecystectomy hazardous for gallbladder cancer? Surgery 123: 311–314

Ugarte F (1995) Laparoscopic cholecystectomy port seeding from a colon carcinoma. Am Surg 61: 820–821

Vukasin P, Ortega AE, Greene FL, Steele GD, Simons AJ, Antho- ne GJ, Weston LA, Beart RW (1996) Wound recurrence fol- lowing laparoscopic colon cancer resection. Results of the American society of colon and rectal surgeons laparoscopic registry. Dis Colon Rectum 39: 20–23

Walsh DC, Wattchow DA, Wilson TG (1993) Subcutaneous me- tastases after laparoscopic resection of malignancy. Austr N Z J Surg 63: 563–564

Wang PH, Yen MS, Yuan CC, Chao KC, Ng HT, Lee WL, Chao HT (1997) Port-site recurrence after laparoscopic-assisted vaginal hysterectomy for endometrial cancer: possible mechanisms and prevention. Gynecol Oncol 66: 151–155

Welch JP, Donaldson GA (1979) The clinical correlation of an autopsy study of recurrent colorectal cancer. Ann Surg 189: 496–502

Wexner SD, Cohen SM (1995) Port-site recurrences after lapa- roscopic colorectal surgery for cure of malignancy. Br J Surg 82: 295–298

Wilson JP (1994) Discussion. Ann Surg 219: 742

Yamaguchi K, Chijiiwa K, Ichimiya H, Sada M, Kawakami K, Nishikata F, Konomi K, Tanaka M (1996) Gallbladder carci- noma in the era of laparoscopic cholecystectomy. Arch Surg 131: 981–985.

Z'graggen K, Birrer S, Maurer CA, Wehrli H, Klaiber C, Baer HU (1998) Incidence of port-site recurrence after laparo- scopic cholecystectomy for preoperatively unsuspected gall- bladder carcinoma. Surgery 124: 831–838

CHAPTER 5

Port-Site Recurrences in Thoracoscopic Surgery

R. Downey, M.A. Reymond

Video-assisted thoracic surgery (VATS) procedures have been rapidly adopted by thoracic surgeons for the management of thoracic surgical problems. In relation to cancer, and for example, radical esophagectomies (Collard et al. 1993) and pulmonary lobectomies (Roviaro et al. 1992; Kirby et al. 1993; Walker et al. 1993) have been performed with success. However, only incomplete information is available as to effectiveness, and possible complications of VATS utilized for the management of cancer. Both parietal seeding and early local recurrence have been anecdotally reported in the surgical literature after such operations. This chapter will review the most serious concern about thoracoscopy when used for the potentially curative resection of a thoracic malignancy, which is that it may be associated with an increased risk of tumor implantation within the operative field.

A surgeon competent at performing a thoracotomy for the resection of a lung malignancy may feel at considerable disadvantage when first performing VATS procedures because of the markedly diminished ability to palpate the lung. With VATS procedures, the target lesion often can only be visualized on a video monitor if it distorts the pleural surface, as palpation is limited to the structures that can be reached with as much of a finger as can be inserted through the chest wall. This limited ability to define the margins of the disease to be resected has raised concerns that either unrecognized inadequate tissue margins may lead to an increased rate of local recurrence, or with disruption of the malignancy lead to implantation into either the pleural cavity or the tissues of the chest wall.

Dissemination After Fine Needle Puncture

Mesothelioma has been noted to commonly grow along any incision or puncture site (Table 5.1) and malignant effusions have been noted to implant into

Table 5.1. Reports of port-site recurrences after thoracoscopy

Author	Year	Histology	Delay
Boutin and Rey	1993		
Buhr et al.	1995	Lung cancer 1 Metastasis 1	?
Dixit et al.	1997	Esophageal cancer	
Downey et al.	1996	Lung cancer 9 Mesothelioma 5 Metastases 5 Small cell lung 1 Esophagus cancer 1	2 weeks-29 months
Fondrinier et al.	1998	Metastasis	5 months
Fry et al.	1995	Lung cancer	5 months
Johnstone et al.	1996	Review : 23 cases	
Sartorelli et al.	1996	Metastasis (sarcoma)	
Thurer	1993	Lung cancer	
Walsh and Nesbitt	1995	Metastasis (sarcoma)	3 months
Wille et al.	1995	Metastasis	?
Yim	1995	Lung adenocarcinoma	

chest tube insertion sites (Sugi et al. 1997), but otherwise mechanical dissemination of disease has been held to be a rare event. Needle biopsy tracks are associated with a low risk of implantation: Sinner and Zajicek (1979) reported that out of 1264 biopsies, only one led to an implant. Procedures associated with even gross disruption of malignant tissues, such as mediastinoscopy, have been associated with similarly low rates being noted in 8 out of 6490 procedures (Auschbaugh 1970).

Chest Wall Recurrence After Thoracotomy

Chest wall implants have until now been considered rare events in thoracic surgery for cancer. Three case reports of incisional implants following resection of esophageal malignancies can be found in the literature (Haverback and Smith 1959; Recht 1989; Collard and Reymond 1996). Two reports of implants into a thoracotomy incision after a lung resection for a primary lung malignancy have been published (Table 5.2). We are aware of another such patient referred to Memorial Sloan-Kettering Cancer Center after a pneumonectomy performed elsewhere for bronchioalveolar cancer, where the first site of recurrent disease was a string of subcutaneous nodules along the length of the surgical incision. The operative note suggested that the bronchus was sharply divided, re-resected to the level of the carina, and then oversewn. It is tempting to think that the implant was due to contamination of the wound with tumor-laden airway secretions, as are often present with bronchioalveolar carcinoma.

Table 5.2. Reports of wound recurrences after thoracotomy

Author	Year	Histology	Delay
Lewis et al.	1997	Lung cancer	
Yokoi et al.	1996	Lung cancer	9 months

Port-Site Recurrences After VATS

Reports of malignant implants occurring in incisions utilized for minimally invasive procedures have become relatively common. Such reports include extrathoracic procedures involving such malignancies as gallbladder carcinoma (Drouard et al. 1991; Pezet et al. 1992), hepatocellular carcinoma (Keate and Schaffer 1992), gastric adenocarcinoma (Cava et al. 1990), trophoblastic tissue (Tatcher et al. 1989) and colon carcinoma (Wexner 1995). In 1993, a

Author	Year	Histology	Delay
Hix	1990	Lung cancer	
McDonald and Baird	1994	Lung cancer	
Migueres et al.	1975	Malignant mesothelioma 4, other pleural neoplasm 1	
Moloo et al.	1985	Bronchogenic carcinoma	13 months
Muller et al.	1986	Bronchogenic carcinoma	
Paik et al.	1994	Squamous lung carcinoma	
Sacchini et al.	1989	Lung cancer	
Sing et al.	1996	Lung cancer	4 months
Sinner and Zajicek	1976	Lung cancer	
Voravud et al.	1992	Lung adenocarcinoma	

report of a lung cancer chest wall implant after an apparently uneventful VATS resection was also published (Thurer 1993). Since that report, additional case reports of port-site recurrences following VATS for cancer have been published (Table 5.3).

Concerns raised by these reports led us (Downey et al. 1996) to send a survey to the members of the Video-Assisted Thoracic Surgery Study Group (VATSSG), which began with the question: 'Have you participated in the care of any patient who underwent a VATS procedure for the biopsy or resection of a thoracic malignancy and whose subsequent course suggests either subcutaneous implantation, pleural seeding or staple line recurrence of the malignancy?'. Out of 55 surgeons 48 responded, of whom 16 reported 21 cases in which the surgeon felt that it was likely that the manner of appearance of recurrent disease was most consistent with dissemination at the time of the VATS procedure.

The histologies involved were non-small cell lung cancer in nine patients, small cell carcinoma in 1, mesothelioma in 5, esophageal cancer in 1, and pulmonary metastases of varied histology in 5. The site of apparent implantation was the incision in 14, the pleural surface in 2, the pulmonary parenchymal suture line in 2, and multiple sites in 3, so that only 14 cases fulfill the criteria of port-site recurrences defined earlier in this book. The median time from performance of the VATS procedure to recognition of implantation was 4 months (range 2 weeks to 29 months). A variety of salvage measures were undertaken, such as chest wall resection, radiation, chemotherapy, and combinations thereof; the material provided by the responsible physicians did not allow assessment of the possible effectiveness of such steps.

We emphasized in our report (Downey et al. 1996) that the denominator of total number of VATS procedures performed was not known, as the surgeons reporting the cases may have cared for the patient after a procedure performed by another surgeon, and therefore, these cases should be considered as a series of anecdotes. Thus, it was difficult to define with this data the incidence of port-site recurrences after VATS. Since that time there have been three publications examining the incidence of dissemination. Jancovici et al. (1996) reported 2 port-site recurrences in 148 procedures (incidence 1.4%). One year later, Swanson et al. (1997) reported 475 consecutive thoracoscopies performed for malignant disease without any port-site recurrences.

In small animal models, CO_2 pneumoperitoneum has been shown to increase the incidence of port-site recurrences as compared to anesthesia alone (Jones et al. 1995; Jacobi et al. 1996a,b; Bouvy et al. 1996; Dorrance et al. 1996; Hubens et al. 1996; Mathew et al. 1996). Port-site recurrences reported after VATS cannot be related to the use of CO_2 since no gas is applied to inflate the pleural cavity (Fig. 5.1 and 5.2). Interestingly, the time elapsed between the surgical procedure and the clinical diagnosis of the port-site recurrence is not significantly different between laparoscopy and thoracoscopy, suggesting that the adjuvant role of CO_2 pneumoperitoneum on tumor growth might be modest in clinical practice (Fig. 5.3).

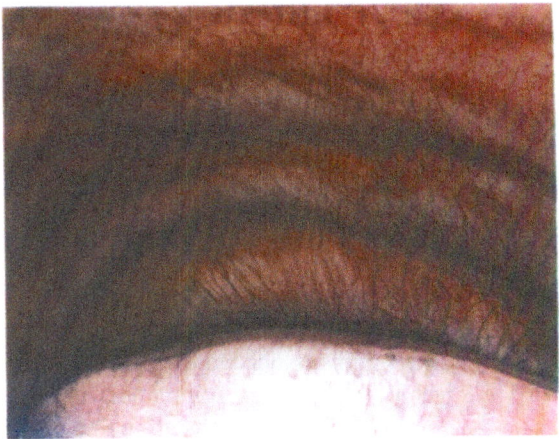

Fig. 5.2. In thoracoscopy – as opposed to laparoscopy – no CO_2 pneumoperitoneum is applied. There is enough working space after exsufflation of the lung (*image bottom*)

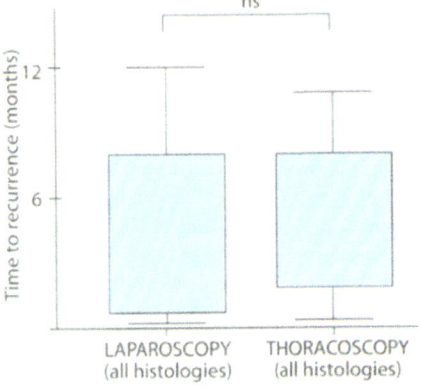

Fig. 5.3. Time elapsed between the surgical procedure and diagnosis of the port-site recurrence is not significantly different between laparoscopy (with CO_2 pneumoperitoneum) and thoracoscopy (without insufflation)

Preventive Measures

It appears that the problem of chest wall implantation after VATS procedures performed with the manipulation of malignant tissue can be dealt with by proper surgical technique. Appropriate protective measures have been proposed elsewhere (Collard et al. 1996):

- Extraction of the neoplastic tissue using a protective device (e.g.,thoracoport, glove, bag, sheet)
- Enlargement of the incision through which the tumor is extracted
- Copious irrigation of the chest cavity and aspiration of the washing fluid at the end of the procedure

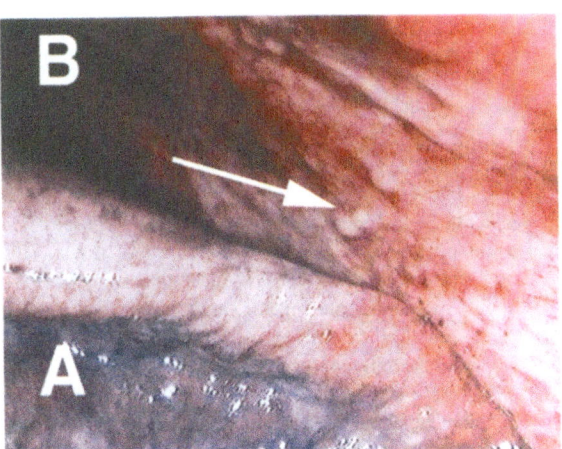

Fig. 5.1. By definition, a port-site recurrence is not associated with pleural carcinomatosis (*arrow*, tumor implants of the serosa; *A*, lung; *B*, chest wall)

- Retraction of the intrathoracic structures with smooth instruments instead of using grasping forceps (no-touch dissection)
- Not trying to remove poorly-delineated lesions
- Not hesitating to convert into thoracotomy

Many issues still remain open, such as the concern of the margins obtained in the lung parenchyma, and the possibility of an increased rate of staple line recurrences, or of disruption and implantation onto the surfaces of the pleural cavity. A full evaluation of the risks and benefits associated with the utilization of VATS techniques for the manipulation of malignant disease will require demonstration that, stage-for-stage, disease-free, and overall survival are identical or better than those achieved with more traditional 'open' techniques. Until that time, the possible benefits of diminished pain, shortened hospitalization, and preserved postoperative pulmonary function should be considered secondary issues.

References

Auschbaugh DG (1970) Mediastinoscopy. Arch Surg 100: 568–573

Boutin C, Rey F (1993) Thoracoscopy in pleural malignant mesothelioma: a prospective study of 188 consecutive patients. Part 1: Diagnosis. Cancer 72: 389–393

Bouvy ND, Marquet RL, Lambert SWJ, Jeekel J, Bonjer HJ (1996) Laparoscopic bowel resection in the rat: earlier restoration of IGF-1 and less tumor growth (abstract). Surg Endosc 10: 567

Buhr J, Hurtgen M, Kelm C, Schwemmle K (1995) Tumor dissemination after thoracoscopic resection for lung cancer. J Thorac Cardiovasc Surg 110: 855–856

Cava A, Roma J, Gonzales Quintela A (1990) Subcutaneous metastasis following laparoscopy in gastric adenocarcinoma. Eur J Surg Oncol 16: 63–67

Collard JM, Reymond MA (1996) Video-assisted thoracic surgery (V.A.T.S.) for cancer: risk of parietal seeding and of early local recurrence. Int Surg 81: 343–346

Collard JM, Lengele B, Otte JB, Kestens PJ (1993) En bloc and standard esophagectomies by thoracoscopy. Ann Thorac Surg 56: 675–679

Dixit AS, Martin CJ, Flynn P (1997) Port-site recurrence after thoracoscopic resection of osophageal cancer. Aust N Z J Surg 67:148–149

Dorrance HR, Oein K, O'Dwyer PJ (1996) Laparoscopy promotes tumor growth in an animal model. Surg Endosc 10: 559

Downey RJ, McCormack P, LoCicero III J, and the Video-Assisted Thoracic Surgery Study Group (1996) Dissemination of malignancies following video-assisted thoracic surgery. J Cardiovasc Thorac Surg 111: 954–960

Drouard F, Delamarre J, Capron JP (1991) Cutaneous seeding of gallbladder cancer after laparoscopic cholecystectomy [letter]. N Engl J Med 325: 1316

Fondrinier E, Lorimier G, Cellier P, Gamlin E (1998) Parietal tumor seeding after thoracoscopic surgery: apropos of a case. Chirurgie 123: 612–615

Fry WA, Siddiqui A, Pensler JM, Mostafavi H (1995) Thoracoscopic implantation of cancer with a fatal outcome (see comments). Ann Thorac Surg 59: 42–45

Haverback CZ, Smith RR (1959) Transplantation of tumor by suture and its prevention. Cancer 12:1029–1042

Hix WR (1990) Chest wall recurrence of lung cancer after transthoracic fine needle aspiration biopsy. Ann Thorac Surg 50: 1020–1021

Hubens G, Pauwels M, Hubens A, Vermeulen P, Van Marck E, Eyskens E (1996) The influence of pneumoperitoneum on the peritoneal implantation of free intraperitoneal colon cancer cells. Surg Endosc 10: 181

Jacobi CA, Sabat R, Ordemann J, Müller JM (1996a) Influence of different gases on the tumor cell growth in laparoscopic surgery. Preliminary results of an experimental study in a rat model. Langenbecks. Arch Chir Suppl 1: 381

Jacobi CA, Sabat R, Böhm B, Zieren HU, Volk HD, Müller JM (1996b) Pneumoperitoneum with CO_2 stimulates malignant tumor growth. Surg Endosc 10: 551

Jancovici R, Lang-Lazdunski L, Pons F (1996) Complications of video-assisted thoracic surgery: a five year experience. Ann Thorac Surg 61: 533–537

Johnstone PAS, Rohde DC, Swartz SE, Fetter JE, Wexner SD (1996) Port-site recurrences after laparoscopic and thoracoscopic procedures in malignancy. J Clin Oncol 14: 1950–1956

Jones DB, Guo LW, Reinhard MK, Soper NJ, Philpott GW, Connet J, Fleshman JW (1995) Impact of pneumoperitoneum on trocar site implantation of colon cancer in hamster model. Dis Colon Rectum 38:1182–1188

Keate RF, Shaffer R (1992) Seeding of hepatocellular carcinoma to peritoneoscopy insertion site [letter]. Gastrointest Endosc 38: 203–204

Kirby TJ, Mack MJ, Landreneau R, Rice TW (1993) Initial experience with video-assisted thoracoscopic lobectomy. Ann Thorac Surg 56:1248–1253

Lewis RJ, Caccavale RJ, Sisler GE, Bocage JP (1997). Does VATS favor seeding of carcinoma of the lung more than a conventional operation? Int Surg 82: 127–130

Mathew G, Watson DI, Rofe AM, Baigrie CF, Ellis T, Jamieson GG (1996) Wound metastases following laparoscopic and open surgery for abdominal cancer in a rat model. Br J Surg 83: 1087–1090

McDonald CF, Baird L (1994). Risk of needle tract metastasis after fine needle lung aspiration in lung cancer – a case report. Respir Med 88: 631–632

Migueres J, Jover A, Krempf M (1975) Note sur les incidents et accidents de la biopsie pleurale à l'aiguille: l'ensemencement néoplastique de la paroi. Poumon Coeur 31: 347–349

Moloo Z, Finley RJ, Lefcoe MS, Turner-Smith L, Craig ID (1985) Possible spread of bronchogenic carcinoma to the chest wall after a transthoracic fine needle aspiration. A case report. Acta Cytol 29: 167–169

Muller NJ, Bergin CJ, Miller RR, Ostow DN (1986) Seeding of malignant cells into the needle track after lung and pleural biopsy. Can Assoc Radiol J 37: 192–194

Paik HC, Lee DY, Lee HK, Kim SJ, Lee KB (1994) Chest wall implantation after fine needle aspiration biopsy. Yonsei Med J 35: 349–354

Pezet D, Fondrinier E, Rotman N, Guy L, Lemesle P, Lointier P, Chipponi J (1992) Parietal seeding of carcinoma of the gallbladder after laparoscopic cholecystectomy (see comments). Br J Surg 79: 230

Recht MP (1989) Recurrent esophageal carcinoma at thoracotomy incisions: diagnostic contributions of CT. J Comput Assist Tomogr 13: 58–60

Roviaro G, Rebuffat C, Varoli F, Vergani C, Mariani C, Mariocco M (1992) Video-endoscopic pulmonary lobectomy for cancer. Surg Laparosc Endosc 2: 244–247

Sacchini V, Galimberti V, Marchini S, Luini A (1989) Percutaneous transthoracic needle biopsy: a case report of implantation metastasis. Eur J Surg Oncol 15: 179–183

Sartorelli KH, Partrick D, Meagher DP Jr (1996) Port-site recurrence after thoracoscopic resection of pulmonary metastasis owing to osteogenic sarcoma. J Pediatr Surg 31: 1443–1444

Sing RF, Kefalides PT, Mette SA, Fallahnejad M (1996) Chest wall metastasis after percutaneous fine-needle aspiration biopsy. J Am Osteopath Assoc 96: 546–547

Sinner WN, Zajicek J (1979) Pulmonary neoplasms diagnosed with transthoracic needle biopsy. Cancer 43: 1533–1540

Sugi K, Nawata K, Ueda K, Kaneda Y, Nawata S, Oga A, Kesato K (1997) Chest wall implantation of lung cancer at the drainage tube site: report of a case. Surg Today 27: 666–668

Swanson SJ, DeCamp MM Jr, Mentzer SJ (1997) Thoracoscopic resection of lung malignany without port-site recurrence. Chest 112: 9

Tatcher SS, Grainger DA, True LD (1989) Pelvic trophoblastic implants after laparoscopic removal of a tubal pregnancy. Obstet Gynecol 74: 514–515

Thurer RL (1993) Video-assisted thoracic surgery (letter). Ann Thorac Surg 56: 199–200

Voravud N, Shin DM, Dekmezian RH, Dimery I, Lee JS, Hong WK (1992) Implantation metastasis of carcinoma after percutaneous fine-needle aspiration biopsy. Chest 102: 303–315

Walker WS, Carnochan FM, Tin M (1993) Thoracoscopy assisted pulmonary lobectomy. Thorax 48(9): 921–924

Walsh GL, Nesbitt JC (1995) Tumor implants after thoracoscopic resection of a metastatic sarcoma (see comments). Ann Thorac Surg 59: 215–216

Wexner SD (1995) Laparoscopic resection of colorectal cancer. Contemp Surg 46: 93–111

Wille GA, Gregory R, Guernsey JM (1997) Tumor implantation at port-site of video-assisted thoracoscopic resection of pulmonary metastasis. West J Med 166: 65–66

Yim AP (1995) Port-site recurrence following video-assisted thoracoscopic surgery. Surg Endosc 9: 1133–1135

Yokoi K, Miyazawa N, Imura G (1996) Isolated incisional recurrence after curative resection for primary lung cancer. Ann Thorac Surg 61: 1236–1237

CHAPTER 6

Port-Site Recurrences in Colon and Rectal Cancers: Randomized Studies

T. Sonoda, J.W. Milsom

Port-site recurrence (PSR), or the metastasis of cancer cells to incisional sites of the abdominal wall, has been reported after curative laparoscopic operations for many gastrointestinal malignancies. This has probably been the single most important factor which has discouraged the widespread use of laparoscopy in the treatmen t of colorectal cancers so far. Malignant cell implantation in incisional sites has long been known to occur after conventional surgery, but whether laparoscopy actually increases the risk of wound implantation remains unclear.

Prospective Data

The phenomenon of port-site recurrence was first described in 1993 in a 67-year-old woman who, 3 months after a curative laparoscopic-assisted right hemicolectomy for a Dukes C carcinoma, developed a wound recurrence (Alexander et al. 1993). In the meantime, many cases of PSR have been reported in the literature (see chap. 4). The incidence of PSR has ranged from 0% to 21% depending on the study (Wexner and Cohen 1995; Tomita et al. 1999) but the true incidence still remains unknown, since most reports to date have been sporadic cases and no single series has a large enough denominator to accurately make this assessment (Vukasin et al. 1996).

Tumor recurrence in the abdominal wall after curative resection of colorectal malignancies has been known to occur even in conventional open surgery. There have been two large series to date examining this incidence. Hughes et al. in 1983, reported 11 cases of incisional recurrence in 1603 cases of colorectal cancers, for an overall incidence of 0.68%. Similarly, Reilly et al. in 1996, reported an incisional site recurrence rate of 0.64% in 1711 patients.

As expected, the incidence of wound implantation varies according to the intensity of the follow-up regimen. Gunderson and co-workers found incisional recurrences in 3.3%–5.3% of patients who had reo-perations either as a second look or symptomatic look (Gunderson and Sosin 1974; Gunderson et al. 1985). Studies of autopsies on patients with recurrent colorectal cancers have reported rates of wound recurrence as high as 16.6% (Welch and Donaldson 1979). Furthermore, in the study of Reilly et al., only 4 out of the 11 wound recurrences were detected clinically, while the other 7 were found at relaparotomy.

A review of recent, non-randomized larger series of laparoscopic colorectal cancer surgery (Vukasin et al. 1996; Kwock et al. 1996; Huscher et al. 1996; Franklin et al. 1996; Fleshman et al. 1996; Lord et al. 1996) has revealed the incidence of port-site metastasis to be in the range of 0–1.1%, closer to the incidence found in open surgery. The range of follow-up in these studies has been short, however, ranging from 12 months (Vukasin et al. 1996) to 30–36 months (Franklin et al. 1996).

Randomized Studies

There have been 3 randomized prospective studies published to date comparing open with laparoscopic treatment of colorectal malignancies (Table 6.1):

Table 6.1. Prospective randomized data on the incidence of port-site recurrences

Author	Year	No. lap opera-tions	No. recur-rences (%)	Median follow-up (range)
Lacy et al.	1995	25	0 (0%)	6.5 months (1–12)
Stage et al.	1997	15	0 (0%)	14 months (7–19)
[a]Milsom et al.	1998	55	0 (0%)	17 months (1.5–46)

[a] Two local abdominal recurrences were seen in the open group, both in the setting of disseminated disease

Judging from these randomized prospective studies, at least in the short term, there is no increased risk of port-site recurrence after laparoscopic resection of colorectal cancers. Since about 80% of cancer recurrence occurs within the first year (Vukasin et al. 1996) we can estimate that most port-site metastasis will present during this time period. In Hughes et al. study of open colorectal cancer recurrences, however, 2 of the 11 incisional recurrences were diagnosed after a period of 24 months (Hughes et al. 1983). Therefore, the true rate of port-site recurrence will not be known until the maturation of 5- and 10-year follow-up data from these randomized prospective trials.

Influence of the Surgeon on the Incidence of Port-Site Recurrences

While incisional recurrence after colorectal cancer operations can be the result of systemic malignant disease (Hughes et al. 1983) or even hematogenous seeding (Jewell and Romsdahl 1965) the fact that malignant wound implants have occurred after stage I colorectal cancers suggests that it is likely to be a result of direct inoculation of exfoliated tumor cells from traumatic mobilization, resection, and removal of the cancer (Nudka et al. 1994; Tomita etal. 1999; Whelan et al. 1998). Indeed, several studies have confirmed the presence of free malignant cells in peritoneal cavity washings sampled during colorectal cancer surgery (Wong et al. 1996; Leather et al. 1994; Ambrose et al. 1989). However, in the only randomized, prospective study to date comparing tumor cell exfoliation in open vs. laparoscopic colectomies for cancer, no malignant cells were detected in the peritoneal washings of either group before and after specimen resection (despite a 30% incidence of positive cytology in the pilot study) (Kim et al. 1998). This study implied that tumor cell spillage in both laparoscopy and conventional surgery should be minimal when colorectal cancer operations are performed according to strict oncologic principles.

There is increasing evidence that surgical technique may influence the outcome in colorectal cancers, even in open surgery. For example, in the recent German Study Group Colo-Rectal Carcinoma (SGCRC) analysis of 1121 cases of rectal cancer, the treating department and the individual surgeon were found to be independent variables in both locoregional recurrence and 5-year survival (Kessler and Hermanek 1998). If poor surgical technique affects outcome in open colorectal cancer surgery, it is

safe to assume that it will affect outcome in laparoscopic colorectal cancer resections as well. We are convinced that poor surgical technique is the most important factor contributing to PSR.

If the pathogenesis of PSR is indeed a technically related issue, what are the possible measures of prevention? On a more practical level, laparoscopic surgery adhering to sound oncologic principles is probably the only precautionary measure one needs to take. We strive for 1) early ligation of the major blood vessels, 2) early isolation of the tumor by dividing the bowel proximal and distally to the tumor, therefore minimizing the lateral spread of malignant cells, 3) minimal manipulation of the tumor bearing segment, and 4) extraction of the mobilized specimen in an impermeable bag.

Irrigation of wounds with a tumorcidal agent such as iodine or ethanol is also easy and safe, and may be beneficial.

Conclusion

Examined critically, there seems to be little in terms of sound scientific data to justify the reputation of laparoscopy that it leads to high rates of PSR when used to treat colorectal carcinomas. PSR in the setting of curative operations is most likely related to poor surgical technique. When performed by experienced surgeons using good oncologic technique, laparoscopy should have rates of PSR comparable with rates of abdominal wall recurrences in open surgery.

References

Alexander RJT, Jacques BC, Mitchell KG (1993) Laparoscopically assisted colectomy with wound recurrence (letter). Lancet 342: 368

Ambrose NS, MacDonald F, Young J, Thompson H, Keighley MR (1989) Monoclonal antibody and cytological detection of free malignant cells in the peritoneal cavity during resection of colorectal cancer – can monoclonal antibodies do better? Eur J Surg Oncol 15: 99–102

Fleshman JW, Nelson H, Peters WR, Kim HC, Larach S, Boorse RR, Ambrose W, Legett P, Bleday R, Stryker S, Christenson B, Wexner S, Senagore A, Rattner D, Sutton J, Fine AP (1996) Early result of laparoscopic surgery for colorectal cancer: a retrospective analysis of 372 patients treated by Clinical Outcomes of Surgery Therapy (COST) study group. Dis Colon Rectum 39: 53-58

Franklin ME, Rosenthal D, Abrego-Medina D, Dorman JP, Glass JL, Norem R, Diaz A (1996) Prospective comparison of open vs. laparoscopic colon surgery for carcinoma. Five year results. Dis Colon Rectum 10: 35-46

Gunderson LL, Sosin H (1974) Areas of failure found at reoperation (second or symptomatic look) following "curative surgery" for adenocarcinoma of the rectum: clinicopathologic correlation and implications for adjuvant therapy. Cancer 34: 1278–1292

Gunderson LL, Sosin, H, Sevitt S (1985) Extrapelvic colon-areas of failure in a reoperation series: implications for adjuvant therapy. Int J Radiat Oncol Biol Phys 11: 731–741

Hubens G, Pauwels M, Hubens A, Vermeulen P, VanMarck E, Eyskens E (1996) The influence of a pneumoperitoneum on the peritoneal implantation of free intraperitoneal colon cancer cells. Surg Endosc 10: 809–812

Hughes ESR, McDermott FT, Polgase AL, Johnson WR (1983) Tumor recurrence in the abdominal wall scar tissue after large-bowel cancer surgery. Dis Colon Rectum 26: 571–572

Huscher C, Silecchia G, Croce E, Farello GA, Lezoche E, Morino M, Azzola M, Feliciotti F, Rosato P, Tarantini M, Basso N (1996) Laparoscopic colorectal resection: a multicenter Italian study. Surg Endosc 10: 875–879

Jewell WR, Romsdahl MM (1965) Recurrent malignant disease in operative wounds not due to surgical manipulation from the resected tumor. Surgery 58: 806–809

Kessler H, Hermanek P (1998) Outcomes in rectal cancer surgery are directly related to technical factors. Semin Colon Rectal Surg 9: 247–253

Kim SH, Casillas S, Milsom JW, Dietz DW, Vladesavlejevic A (1997) Data presented at the First Workshop on Experimental Laparoscopic Surgery, Frankfurt

Kim SH, Milsom JW, Gramlich TL, Toddy SM, Shore GI, Okuda J, Fazio VW (1998) Does laparoscopic vs. conventional surgery increase exfoliated cancer cells in the peritoneal cavity during resection of colorectal cancer? Dis Colon Rectum 41: 971–978

Kwok SP, Lau WY, Carey PD, Kelly SB, Leung KL, Li KA (1996) Prospective evaluation of laparoscopic-assisted large bowel excision for cancer. Ann Surg 223: 170–176

Lacy AM, Garcia-Valdecasas JC, Pique JM, Delgado S, Campo JM, Bordas JM, Taura P, Grande L, Fuster J, Pacheco JL, Visa J (1995) Short-term outcome analysis of a randomized study comparing laparoscopic vs. open colectomy for colon cancer. Surg Endosc 9: 1101–1105

Leather AJ, Kocjan G, Savage F, Hu W, Yui CY, Boulos PB, Northover JMA, Phillips RKS (1994) Detection of free malignant cells in the peritoneal cavity before and after resection of colorectal cancer. Dis Colon Rectum 37: 814–819

Lord SA, Larach SW, Ferrara A, Williamson PR, Lago CP, Lube MW (1996) Laparoscopic resections for colorectal carcinoma: a three year experience. Dis Colon Rectum 39: 148–154

Mathew G, Watson DI, Ellis T, DeYoung N, Rofe AM, Jamieson GG (1997) The effect of laparoscopy on the movement of tumor cells and metastasis to surgical wounds. Surg Endosc 11: 1163–1166

Mathew G, Watson DI, Ellis TS, Jamieson GG, Rofe AM (1999) The role of peritoneal immunity and the tumour-bearing state on the development of wound and peritoneal metastases after laparoscopy. Aust NZ J Surg 69: 14–18

Milsom JW, Bohm B, Hammerhofer K, Fazio V, Steiger E, Elson P (1998) A prospective, randomized trial comparing laparoscopic versus conventional techniques in colorectal cancer surgery: a preliminary report. J Am Coll Surg 187: 46–57

Nduka CC, Monson JRt, Menzies-Gow N, Darzi A (1994) Abdominal wall metastasis following laparoscopy. Br J Surg 81: 648–652

Reilly WT, Nelson H, Schroeder G, Wieand S, Bolton J, O'Connell MJ (1996) Wound recurrence following conventional treatment of colorectal cancer: a rare but perhaps underestimated problem. Dis Colon Rectum 39: 200–207

Stage JG, Schulze S, Moller P, Overgaard H, Andersen M, Rebsdorf-Pedersen VB, Nielsen HJ (1997) Prospective randomized study of laparoscopic versus open colonic resection for adenocarcinoma. Br J Surg 84: 391–396

Tomita H, Marcello PW, Milsom JW (1999) Laparoscopic surgery of the colon and rectum. World J Surg 23: 397–405

Vukasin P, Ortega A, Greene F, Steele G, Simons AJ, Anthone GJ, Weston LA, Beart RW (1996) Wound recurrence following laparoscopic colon cancer resection. Results of the American Society of Colon and Rectal Surgeons Laparoscopic Registry. Dis Colon Rectum 39: 20–23

Welch JP, Donaldson GA (1979) The clinical correlation of an autopsy study of recurrent colorectal cancer. Ann Surg 189: 496–502

Wexner SD, Cohen SM (1995) Port site metastases after laparoscopic colorectal surgery for cure of malignancy. Br J Surg 82: 295–298

Whelan RL, Sellers GJ, Allendorf BA, Laird D, Bessler MD, Nowygrod R, Treat MR (1996) Trocar site recurrence is unlikely to result from aerosolization of tumor cells. Dis Colon Rectum 39: 7–13

Whelan RL, Allendorf JD, Gutt CN, Jacobi CA, Mutter D, Dorrance HR, Bessler M, Bonjer HJ (1998) General oncologic effects of the laparoscopic surgical approach. 1997 Frankfurt international meeting of animal laparoscopic researchers. Surg Endosc 12: 1092–1095

Wong LS, Morris AG, Fraser IA (1996) The exfoliation of free malignant cells in the peritoneal cavity during resection of colorectal cancer. Surg Oncol 5: 115–121

CHAPTER 7

Pathogenesis: Tumor Cell Lines and Application in Experimental Animal Studies

J.W. Fleshman

Introduction

Numerous models have been used in the search for a clue to the cause of trocar site implants after laparoscopic colectomy for cancer. On the surface, each of these models can give us some insight into the issue. However, as the editors of this book are suggesting, different models have different inherent features that may influence the outcome of studies focusing on the impact of conditions found during laparoscopic colectomy. Only if we can evaluate the models critically can we evaluate the conclusions drawn from the experiments present in the literature. Only if we can determine the part that each model plays, by knowing the behavior of the tumor cell lines, can we reliably identify those features of laparoscopy which have fostered implantation of cancer in small wounds.

It is difficult to relate all of the published experimental animal protocols to the clinical setting. Knowledge of the specific details of experimental conditions allows one to determine whether the findings can be used as representative of the human clinical setting. The factor that is most difficult to interpret and understand its influence on outcomes, is the "tumor model." Each tumor model is derived from a separate source of malignant cells having an unique metastatic potential, invasive tendency, immunogenicity, requirements for growth, speed of growth and response to external conditions such as pressure, heat, CO_2, etc. Therefore, before concluding that we have identified the cause of laparoscopically-induced small wound implantation, a discussion of these features of individual tumor models will be useful. The reader will also note that not all of the parameters mentioned above are known for each tumor model. That discussion, within the limits of a surgical text, follows.

Tumor Xenografts/Tissue Type

Cells and pieces from tumor derived from numerous species and tissues have been used to study trocar implants after laparoscopy. Mouse tumor models are the most commonly used. These include melanoma (B16), colon cancer (C 26), neurofibroma (TBJ-NB), and mammary cancer (MMC). Rat models include colon cancer (C-531 and DHD/K12/TRb), mammary cancer (Dark Agouti mammary adenocarcinoma – DAMA), and osteosarcoma (ROS-1). Human tissue models include colon cancer (Lim 1215, GW39), lung mesothelioma (H.Messo.1a), and cervical cancer (HeLa). Each of these has its own growth characteristics and requirements that influence outcomes of the study. Immediately one can see a problem in trying to draw conclusions about the clinical development of wound implants after a resection of colon cancer or response of the host to laparoscopy when a breast cancer model is used in an immune incompetent host.

Tumor Cell Lines (Table 7.1)

Mouse

Mouse Melanoma (B16)

Mouse melanoma B16 is an aggressive tumor cell line. It is a mouse melanoma which arose spontaneously in a C57BL/6 mouse in 1954 (Bystryn et al. 1974). Only 10 cells are needed in culture to establish in vitro growth (Whelan et al. 1996). The tumor line is carried in culture using Dulbecco's modified Eagles Media (DMEM) with 10% bovine serum and added penicillin and streptomycin. Viability after separation from the culture plates with a trypsinization process is 95%. After a latent period, tumors will grow at a standard rate regardless of the inoculum size (Bystryn et al. 1974) (Fig. 7.1) When 10^6 cells are injected intradermally into a syngeneic mouse

Table 7.1. Mouse tumor lines

Name	Source	Immuno-genicity	Metastatic potential	Viabi-lity	Affected by CO_2	Affected by pressure	Growth character	Carcino-matous IP	Suspended in media
B16	Melanoma	Moderate	+	95%	–	–	10^6 cells 95% tumor	?	DMEM + 10% BS
C26	Colon cancer	Slightly	+ liver	95%	?	?	10^5 cells 95% tumor	–	RPMI 1640 + 10% FCS
MMC	Mammary ca	Highly	?	95%	?	?	10^6 cells 95% tumor	?	RPMI 1640 + 10% FCS
TBJ-NB	Neurofibroma	Minimally	+	95%	?	?	5×10^5 cells 95% tumor	–	RPMI 1640 + 10% FCS

strain C57/BL/6, tumors will develop in 95% of animals (Southall et al. 1998). The cancer cell line has been classified as moderately immunogenic by Prehn and Main (1957), indicating a potential for modulating T-cell response in the recipient host. B16 readily metastasizes to the lung depending on the number of cells injected (Fidler 1973).

The B 16 melanoma line has exhibited variability in malignant potential from generation to generation (Bystryn 1974). However, palpable tumor development more frequently varies based on variable tumor viability from tumor preparation to tumor preparation (Southall et al. 1998). Therefore, it is imperative to insure a viability which is consistently 95%+ for all experiments. The tumor doubling time is unknown. The tumor does not appear to be adversely affected by CO_2 or pressure to 15 mmHg (Whelan et al. 1996).

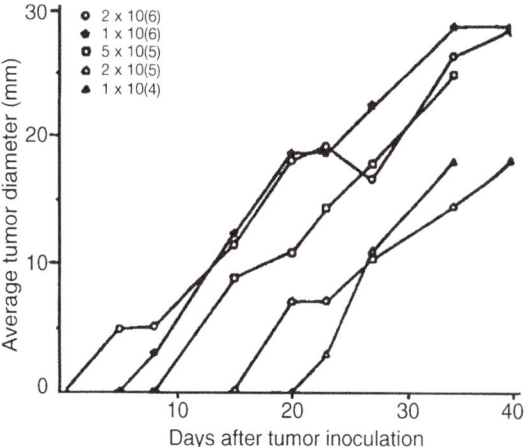

Fig. 7.1. Average growth of B-16 melanoma in groups of 10 C57BL/6 mice inoculated with varying numbers of viable B-16 melanoma cells obtained from tissue culture (reproduced from Bystryn et al. 1974)

Mouse Colon Cancer C-26

C-26 mouse colon cancer is maintained by serial transfer in Balb/C syngeneic mice dorsal skin and suspended in RPMI (Roswell Park Media Institute) 1640 with 10% fetal calf serum and penicillin/streptomycin for transfer or experimental injection. More is known about C-26 growth patterns and 10^5 cells injected into a mouse spleen tip result in tumors measuring 0.5–2.7 cm after 8 days (Lee et al. 1998a). If 10^5 cells are used, 92% of animals develop tumors as compared to only 20% tumor growth when 10^4 are injected (Lee et al. 1998b). Viability can be maintained at 95% levels or better during experiments according to vital trypan blue testing. C-26 has also been transferred as solid chunks weighing 150 mg (Whelan et al. 1996). Unfortunately, all of the cells in a solid tumor cannot be assumed to be viable, unless converted to a suspension and sampled. C-26 has been classified as slightly immunogenic (Southall et al. 1998).

Liver metastases will develop in two-thirds of mice after splenic injection of 10^5 cells. Tumors usually occur only at wound sites and do not cause carcinomatosis when spilled into the intraperitoneal cavity. The response to CO_2 and pressure are unknown.

Mouse Mammary Cancer

Mouse mammary cancer (MMC) derived from a cancer line MC2 established in 1983 (Bugelski et al. 1983) has been used in studies with C3H/H mice (Allendorf et al. 1998). The tumor and mice are syngeneic and thus require no immunosuppression. MMC is a highly immunogenic cell line and as a result develops a plateau of maximal growth in 12–14 days (Vaage and Pepin 1985). Rejection occurs in 20% of mice after tumor is established to a 10 mm size. The tumors develop a capsule of surrounding mononuclear cells, eosinophils, and collagen. This interesting feature can have a positive or negative affect on a study's outcome and must be carefully considered when planning a protocol. The cells are suspended in RPMI 1640 + 10% fetal calf serum and penicillin and streptomycin. Injection of 10^4 cells into the dorsal skin of a mouse results in tumor growth in more than 10% of animals, whereas injection of 10^6 cells produces tumor growth in 95% of animals (Allendorf et al. 1998). Data regarding response to CO_2, pressure, and intraperitoneal growth characteristics are not available.

Mouse Neurofibroma TBJ-NB

The mouse neurofibroma C1300 NB was established in 1940 as a spinal cord tumor in strain A mice. The TBJ-NB line as a clone of C1300-NB is minimally immunogenic and aggressively metastasizing. The cell line is carried either in vitro in RPMI 1640 with 10% fetal calf serum and penicillin/streptomycin/amphotericin B or by in vivo passage. An inoculum of 5×10^5 cells in the flank of A/J mice produces a 12–15 mm diameter tumor in 14 days. Intraperitoneal tumor (10^4 cells) only produces tumors at wound sites and carcinomatosis does not occur (Iwanaka et al. 1998). However, TBJ-NB has been reported to cause metastatic spread to lung, liver, kidney and spleen in A/J mice (Choi et al. 1989). Intravenous injection of tumor (10^4 cells) does not cause wound site implantation (Iwanaka et al. 1998). Response to pressure and CO_2 are not known. Strain A mice do not produce antitumor response to TBJ-NB. The tumor does not produce class I major histocompatibility antigens (MHCI) and is resistant to natural killer-mediated (NK) tumor killing. It is considered minimally immunogenic.

Rat (Table 7.2)

Colon Cancer (CC531)

CC531 is a 1,2 dimethylhydrazine-induced, moderately differentiated adenocarcinoma of the rat colon (Martin et al. 1973). The tumor is syngeneic to WAG rats and transplantable when injected in RPMI 1640 with 5% fetal calf serum and penicillin/streptomycin medium. The tumor is weakly immunogenic. Viability in the cell suspension is 95% by trypan blue exclusion. Intraperitoneal injection results in carcinomatosis and implantation anywhere within the peritoneal cavity (Bouvy et al. 1997). The tumor is felt to be sensitive to immunomodulation (Marquet et al. 1987). Tumor developed at intraperitoneal sites other than wounds and liver or lung with an intraperitoneal inoculum of 5×10^5 cells in RPMI. Metastasis did not develop otherwise. Metastasis requires intravenous injection (Paik et al. 1998). The affect of CO_2 on tumor growth is felt to be facilitative (Bouvy et al. 1996). The effect of pressure is unknown. Injection of 10^8 cells in the flank of WAG rats results in a 2.5 cm^3 tumor after 6 weeks. CC531 is a CD44 producing colon cancer.

Colon Cancer (DHD/K12/TRb)

DHD/K12/TRb rat colon cancer was originally chemo-induced in the BD IX rat in 1973 in Dijon, France (Martin et al. 1973). The tumor line is cultured in Dulbecco's MEM and Ham's F10 medium with 10% fetal bovine serum containing glutamine and penicillin/streptomycin. Only 10^4 cells are needed to establish growth of the tumor in culture medium or after subcutaneous or intraperitoneal injection (Lagadec et al. 1987; Reisser et al. 1991). The tumor line seems to be stimulated by air and carbon dioxide

Table 7.2. Rat tumor lines

Name	Source	Immuno-genicity	Metastatic potential	Viabi-lity	Affected by CO_2	Affected by pressure	Growth character	Carcino-matous IP	Suspended in media
CC531	Colon cancer	Weakly	-	95%	+	?	10^8 2.5 cm^3/6 weeks	+	RPMI + 5% FCS
DHD/KIZ/TRb	Colon cancer	?	+ liver	100%	+	+	?	+	DMEM + HANS F10 +Gluthamin + 10% FBS
DAMA	Mammary	?	?	100%	+	?	2×10^8 2.5 mm/ 7 days	+	PBS
ROS-1	Osteosarcoma	?	?	95%	-	+	2×10^6 2.5 cm^3/ 3 weeks	?	RPMI + 5% FCS +levoglu-temide

under pressure (Jacobi et al. 1997a). Intraperitoneal injection results in implants in sites other than wounds. Jacobi et al. found that increasing the pressure of CO_2 decreased tumor growth in vitro but only at highest (15 mm Hg) levels in vivo (Jacobi et al. 1998). This tumor line grows preferentially in the subcutaneous tissue as compared to intraperitoneal sites when exposed to CO_2 independently of the intraperitoneal pressure (Jacobi et al. 1998). DHD/K12/TRb induces carcinomatosis with solid tumors which gives rise to hemorrhagic ascites (Lagadec et al. 1987). The rate of growth for this tumor line is unknown. Viability was assumed to be 100% by acridine orange and fluorescence microscopy counting prior to injection. Liver metastases occur in 10% of rats in the setting of carcinomatosis.

Mammary Cancer (DAMA)

Mammary cancer occurs spontaneously in Dark Agouti rats and has been maintained in carrier rats since 1972 (Coyle et al. 1990). The Dark Agouti mammary adenocarcinoma (DAMA) can be cultured in RPMI 1640 + 10% fetal calf serum + Hepes buffer, penicillin/gentamycin. Intraperitoneal injection of 2×10^7 cells causes carcinomatosis whereas a 10-fold reduction (2×10^6) yields only sparse growth. Tumor cell suspensions from the fresh tumor have been transferred in sterile phosphate buffer solution (PBS) after determining the number of viable cells with trypan blue and adjusting the concentration accordingly. The number of cells injected are assumed to be 100% viable (Mathew et al. 1996, 1997a; Neuhaus et al. 1998). DAMA has been shown to be growth inhibited by helium and stimulated by nitrous oxide, air and CO_2. The immunogenicity and response to pressure is unknown. Doubling time is 10 days during which a 1 g tumor will grow to 10 g. The model does not produce metastases.

Osteosarcoma (ROS-1)

A spontaneous osteosarcoma originating in the tibia of a WAG-Rij rat has been maintained in cell culture in RPMI 1640 with 5% fetal calf serum, 1% levoglutamide, and penicillin/ streptomycin since 1974 (Barendsen and Janse 1978). ROS-1 is thus syngeneic with the WAG-Rij strain rats. An inoculum of 2×10^6 cells in the flank of the rat yields a 2.5 cm^3 tumor after 3 weeks of growth. If a 1 mm^3 piece of tumor (8 mg) is placed under the renal capsule in a WAG rat, the tumor will grow to 20–30 mg over 7 days (Bouvy et al. 1998). Viability of the cells in suspension exceeds 95% with trypan blue exclusion. Doubling time has been shown to be 3.5 + 1 days at a volume of 0.5–1.0 cm^3 (Barendsen and Janse 1978). No distant metastases developed in the renal capsule model (Bouvy et al. 1998). Tumor growth has been shown to be increased in response to increased pressure but unaffected by exposure to air or CO_2 (Bouvy et al. 1998). The immunogenicity and metastatic potential for this tumor line is unknown. Data is not available regarding the effects of intraperitoneal injection.

Human (Table 7.3)

Colon Cancer (Lim 1215)

Colon cancer Lim 1215 was first cultured in 1984 from an omental metastasis in a patient with hereditary nonpolyposis colorectal cancer in Melbourne, Australia (Coyle et al. 1990). The tumor was poorly differentiated and caused carcinomatosis in the patient and subsequently in the BALB/c mice immunodeprived by thymectomy irradiation. The tumor cells are maintained in RPMI 1640 plus 10% fetal calf serum, hydrocortisone, thioglycerol and streptomycin/penicillin. Doubling time is 32 h. The tumor has been shown to produce CEA and differentiate to goblet cells. LIM 1215 has been shown to be respon-

Table 7.3. Human tumor lines

Name	Source	Immuno-genicity	Metastatic potential	Viabi-lity	Affected by CO_2	Affected by pressure	Growth character	Carcino-matous IP	Suspended in media
Lim 1215	Colon cancer	CEA +	+		?	?	10^5 1 cm @ 4 weeks 32 h double	+	RPMI-1640 = 10% FCS
GW39	Colon cancer	CEA reactive	–	90%	–	–	2×10^6 1 cm^3/ 2 weeks	–	McCoy's 5 A
H.Messola	Mesothelioma	?	?	?	+	–	?	+	Ringer's solution
HeLa	Cervical ca	?							MEM + glutamose + 4% FCS

sive to fluorouracil. The sensitivity of the cell line to CO_2 and pressure is unknown. The cell line is C-erb-2+ and considered highly metastatic and aggressive in vitro since low inocula produce growth.

Colon Cancer (GW 39)

A human signet ring cell cancer was established as a tumor cell line by injecting fresh tumor cells in the cheek pouch of the Golden Syrian Hamster by Goldenberg et al. in 1966. The cells secrete mucin and express carcino-embryonic antigen. The tumor has been carried since then in the thigh musculature of the hamster or frozen in liquid nitrogen as a single cell suspension in McCoy's 5 A medium containing 10–20% dimethyl sulfoxide. The frozen cells can be thawed, washed and resuspended in McCoy's 5 A as a volume-to-volume cell suspension for intraperitoneal injection (Wu et al. 1998a). Injection of the cells intraperitoneally in the hamster does not produce carcinomatosis, nor does the cell line metastasize hematogenously. Palpable tumors are established only at sites of direct intramuscular, serosal or mesothelial injection and wound sites exposed to cells. Viability of cells in suspension is >90% with trypan blue exclusion. GW39 yields 6.7×10^7 cells/g in solid tumor form. Injection of 2×10^6 cells in thigh of a Golden Syrian hamster yields a 1 g tumor in 2–3 weeks. The tumor line has shown no consistent growth response to exposure of CO_2 or pressure based on tumor mass (Wu et al. 1998a). The immunogenicity of tumor is unknown.

Lung Mesothelioma (H. Messo 1a)

A human lung mesothelioma has been established at the German Cancer Research Institute in Heidelberg from hemorrhagic ascites from a human subject. Injection intraperitoneally produces a solid tumor in nude mice, without ascites (Volz et al. 1996a). H. messo tumor cells in a 2 ml volume of Ringer's solution injected in the abdomen of nude mice will produce an intraperitoneal seeding rate >90% (Volz et al. 1996b) Based on animal survival data, there is no affect on tumor growth when exposed to helium, air or heated carbon dioxide. However, room temperature CO_2 promotes tumor growth and decreases animal survival (Volz et al. 1998). The immunogenicity and metastatic potential is unknown. There is no affect of pressure on growth of tumor. Viability data is not available.

Cervical Cancer (HeLa)

Cervical cancer cells from a human source have been maintained in culture in Minimal Essential Media plus Glutamine +4% fetal calf serum for years. The tumor line is an aggressive line and will grow under almost any condition to which it is subjected. The cell line has been used as a marker for cell distribution since it accepts Chromium[51] labeling and maintains the label even after fixation with Karnovski's fixative. Chromium labeling kills the cells (Reymond et al. 1999). Killed cells have no metastatic or implantation potential. The immunogenicity is unknown.

Summary

As one can see the tumor models used so far vary greatly in their invasiveness, immunogenicity, growth characteristics, and sources. Ideally, a solid tumor, displaying the same characteristics of a human colon cancer (even though these vary greatly), should be used to study the effect of laparoscopy on colon cancer in human patients. This is virtually impossible, and for this reason it is worth the effort to evaluate the data that is currently available from many laboratories around the world using different models, techniques and hypotheses.

Experimental Protocols

It is somewhat difficult to evaluate or even organize the results of the large amount of research that has been done to identify the cause of port-site implantation of tumors after laparoscopy. Reviewing only those papers dealing specifically with port-site recurrence in an animal model, one can grossly categorize the studies.

Broad categories can be established as follows:

1. Documentation that port-site recurrence is related to laparoscopy and the role techniques play on the occurrence
2. Investigation of the mechanism of cell movement to and establishment of tumor at port-sites
3. Evaluation of the effects of laparoscopic conditions on tumor growth
4. Identification of preventative maneuvers that will reduce port-site implants

This chapter will consider each of these areas with a specific view to relate the outcomes to the tumor model, the method of tumor utilization (intraperitoneal injection, retroperitoneal injection, dorsal injection), and tumor preparation (solid, cell suspension, operative intervention).

Documentation of Port-Site Recurrence Relationship to Laparoscopy

The initial report that suggested pneumoperitoneum may play a role in the development of trocar site recurrences appeared in 1995 (Jones et al.). A study undertaken at Washington University in St. Louis using hamsters and the human colon cancer GW 39 showed an increase in the incidence of trocar wound implantation of tumors from 26% in animals not receiving pneumoperitoneum to 75% in animals receiving pneumoperitoneum of 10 mm Hg for 10 min. A cell suspension containing $\sim 1.6 \times 10^6$ cells was injected into the abdominal cavity after placement of 5 mm trocars in all 4 quadrants. A CO_2 pneumoperitoneum was maintained for 10 min (Fig. 7.2) Trocar sites were harvested 6 weeks later and the incidence of trocar site implantation was calculated for the pneumoperitoneum group and controls (no pneumoperitoneum group) based on the presence of microscopic and macroscopic tumor implants. Since the GW 39 tumor line does not produce carcinomatosis or distant metastasis and only develops at wounds exposed to tumor cells, the incremental increase in trocar site implants was felt to be due to the presence of the pneumoperitoneum or the CO_2 environment. The mechanism of cell distribution was not clear since ordered removal of trocars from each quadrant did not cause preferential tumor occurrence.

This study had many flaws including non-randomization, an excessively high tumor inoculum, a high-pressure pneumoperitoneum and the possibility of high tumor variability due to multiple tumor cell preparations during the study. As a result, the data were highly questioned. Even so, a second study using 8×10^5 cells intraperitoneally, with lower pressure, performed in a randomized manner with 50 animals in each group (eliminating tumor variability as a source of error) and with sophisticated immunohistochemical evaluation of all available trocar sites, revealed a significant increase in tumor occurrence in the presence of a pneumoperitoneum (Wu et al. 1997). This alerted the laparoscopic surgery community to a potential problem with the technique and stimulated a flurry of research to seek the cause of these findings.

The tumor cell inoculum in the above study was still well above the amount of cell spillage presumed to occur in the clinical setting even in the worst of circumstances. A third study was completed using even smaller tumor inocula (3.2×10^5 and 1.6×10^5) (Wu et al. 1998a). The conclusion made from this last group of experiments showed that the effect of the pneumoperitoneum decreased proportional to the tumor cell inoculum decrease (Fig. 7.3). The obvious conclusion followed that maintenance of a very low level of tumor cells in the abdominal cavity can reduce trocar site recurrence to a minimal level in the clinical setting. The challenge would be to eliminate it altogether. Unfortunately, we do not know the response of GW 39 to CO_2 without pressure because it is not maintained in tissue culture. A facilitatory affect of CO_2 on GW 39 growth could be partially responsible for these findings.

Other groups of investigators around the world addressed the issue of pneumoperitoneum and trocar site recurrences using their available small animal models.

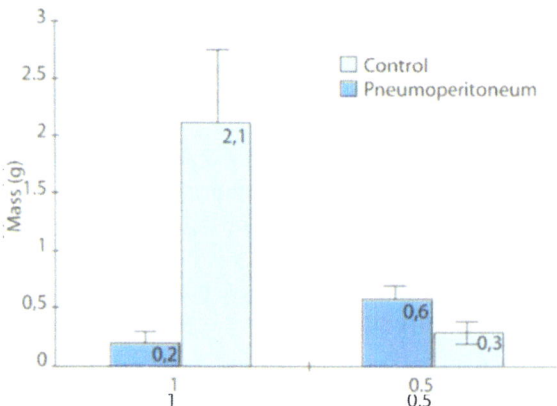

Fig. 7.2. Mass of palpable tumor implants at trocar sites. SEM = standard error of mean (reproduced from Wu et al. 1998)

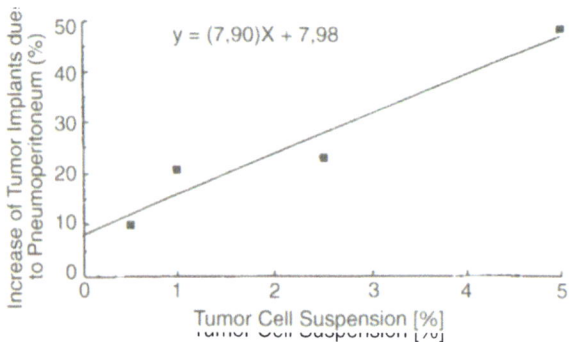

Fig. 7.3. Increasing effect of pneumoperitoneum on trocar site tumor implantation with increasing tumor cell suspensions. Linear regression analysis: correlation coefficient = 0.97; slope = 7.9; $p < 0.05$ (reproduced from Wu et al. 1998)

The group from Columbia-Presbyterian developed a solid tumor model in the tip of the spleen by injecting C-26 mouse colon cancer cells in the subcapsular layer (Lee et al. 1998b). After 10 days of growth, a splenectomy was performed with or without pneumoperitoneum and either with good technique or by damaging the tumor. Port-site implants were noted as were liver metastases. The four groups of animals (good technique/no pneumoperitoneum, crushed tumor/no pneumoperitoneum, good technique/+ pneumoperitoneum, crushed tumor/+ pneumoperitoneum) contained 8 animals each with 3 trocar sites (Fig. 7.4). The use of good technique reduced implants with or without pneumoperitoneum. Even though crush and pneumoperitoneum produced a higher incidence of trocar implants, it was not significantly higher than crushed with no pneumoperitoneum. This may be due to the small sample size since only 8 animals were used in each group (Fig. 7.5) The conclusion that technique influences implantation of tumor was justified based on the significant difference between crush and good technique groups. However, the conclusion that pneumoperitoneum had no influence was probably unjustified since there was a difference. This represents a type II statistical error. It should be noted that C-26 as a tumor model was well suited for this experiment. It rarely causes carcinomatosis, implants only at wound sites and implants to produce a tumor even at low inoculum levels (10^4 cells). Since this experiment involved crushing a solid tumor, the number of cells released into the peritoneal cavity could not be quantified.

The Rotterdam group compared a gasless laparoscopy approach to open laparotomy and laparoscopy with CO_2 pneumoperitoneum when a 350 mg solid lump of CC-531 rat colon cancer was placed in-

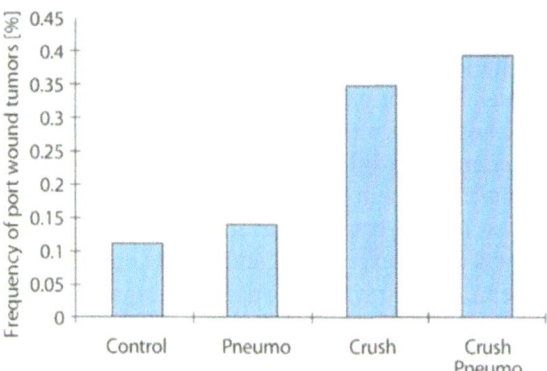

Fig. 7.5. Comparison of trocar site tumor incidence by intervention. $^*p < 0.001$, control versus crush. $^{**}p < 0.001$, pneumo versus crush pneumo (reproduced from Lee et al. 1998)

traperitoneally and removed and when a 5×10^5 cell suspension of CC-531 was injected intraperitoneally in WAG rats (Bouvy et al. 1996). This tumor model readily produces carcinomatosis and makes assessment of trocar site implantation difficult if the time frame for the experiment is inappropriate. The experiment assessed not only the growth of tumor in the peritoneal cavity but also the incidence of trocar site and wound implantation. In 6 small ($8 + 12$ animals in each group) groups of animals, there was a confusing difference in the response of tumor growth under these conditions. A minimally invasive approach resulted in less intraperitoneal tumor growth based on diameter and weight of tumor. CO_2 pneumoperitoneum seemed to increase tumor growth in the peritoneal cavity and the development of abdominal wall metastases compared to gasless laparoscopy. Even so, both types of laparoscopy (gasless and CO_2 pneumoperitoneum) resulted in less tumor growth than in the open laparotomy animals. The results make it difficult to draw a concrete conclusion because the results are dependent on differences in tumor weight/size. It is also possible that CO_2 itself increases tumor growth in the CC-531 model (Bouvy et al. 1996). The weight of evidence seemed to point to the gasless laparoscopy approach as the one with least tumor promotion effect.

Another comparison of gasless laparoscopy and CO_2 pneumoperitoneum laparoscopy was undertaken at the Royal Adelaide Hospital (Watson et al. 1997). The study used DAMA mammary cancer in Dark Agouti rats. Only 12 animals were used in each group to compare tumor implantation in trocar sites after laceration of a solid tumor in the retroperitoneum to release an unknown number of cells into the abdomen. There was a slight (but not statistical-

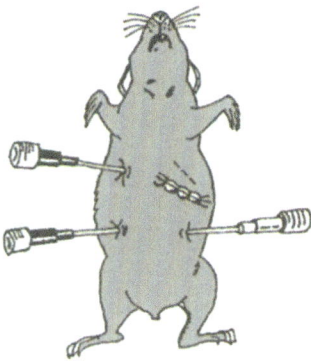

Fig. 7.4. Port and incision locations. Flank incision used for splenic injection of tumor shown as broken line (posteriorly) (reproduced from Lee et al. 1998)

ly significant) increase in tumor mass within the abdomen and a significant increase in trocar site implantation in the laparoscopy group. The tumor model does not produce metastases but does cause carcinomatosis and seems to be stimulated to grow by air, nitrous oxide and CO_2. The fact that CO_2 itself stimulates growth of DAMA mammary adenocarcinoma could be responsible for the increase in tumor growth in this experiment and not the pneumoperitoneum. Certainly, the use of gasless laparoscopy or minimally invasive approaches may reduce the risk of wound implantation of tumor. This protocol was the first one to use a solid tumor model to evaluate the circumstances causing port-site recurrences after laparoscopic colectomy for colorectal cancer. The drawbacks of a cell suspension model include the inoculation of tumor cells in a culture medium that can maintain viable cells ready to implant for long periods of time after the operation. A solid tumor model can simulate the clinical setting best, however, if the tumor is removed after the spillage of cells occurs. Unfortunately, a solid tumor model prohibits knowledge of the number of cells involved when manipulation of the tumor occurs.

A study from University of Southern California used a cell suspension model to once again compare laparoscopy and open procedures in their affect on wound implantation (Paik et al. 1998). The rat colon cancer DHD/K12/TRb was injected into BD IX rats followed by open incision or laparoscopy with a 15 mm Hg CO_2 pneumoperitoneum and trocar insertion on a randomized basis. A large number of animals were used to insure statistical significance of any difference. The results indicated a decrease in wound implantation in the laparoscopy group which only had trocar sites and no midline incision. The DHD/K12/TRb cell line is known to produce carcinomatosis when injected intraperitoneally, even though the authors reported no such occurrence in this study. The authors tried to identify only those tumors in the subcutaneous tissue as true wound implants to compensate for this. DHD/K12 has also been subsequently shown to be growth impeded by CO_2 pneumoperitoneum at 15 mm Hg (Paik et al. 1998). Even so, data suggested a clear protection against tumor implantation in the laparoscopic group.

Summary

It is difficult to draw a strong conclusion from any of these studies since they all had flaws and were not true reflections of the clinical setting. There seems to be some affect on the spread or implantation of cells by CO_2 pneumoperitoneum which enhances trocar site recurrence. There also seems to be a protective affect overall to a minimally invasive approach which reduces tumor growth. A balance of technical and immunological factors will need to be delineated before a final statement can be made regarding the etiology of trocar site implants.

Investigation of the Mechanism of Cell Movement to and Establishment of Tumor at Port-Sites

The movement of cells to an incision is influenced by many factors including the surgeon, abdominal cavity conditions, size of the wound and tumor factors. After the original reports of clinical trocar implants, speculation arose that the CO_2 pneumoperitoneum caused aerosolization of cells and movement of the cells to trocar sites. A number of studies have focused on this problem.

The Columbia-Presbyterian group provided the first evidence regarding aerosolization of cells (Whelan et al. 1996). An apparatus was developed using a pressure chamber, balloon and filters to determine whether B-16 melanoma and C-26 mouse colon cancer become aerosolized from a culture media, saline suspension or solid tumor piece under constant flow or static pressure of CO_2. (Fig. 7.6) This in vitro study showed that even 2×10^7 cells in a culture dish did not result in aerosolization of tumor cells. An animal model using Sprague-Dawley Rats and 10^5 cells of B-16 melanoma in a cell suspension was also able to show that desufflation from

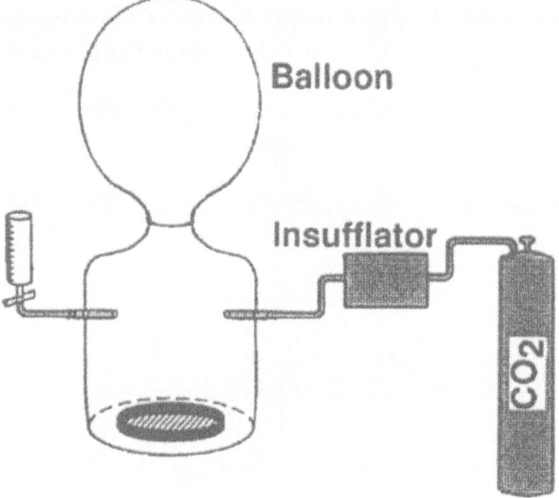

Fig. 7.6. Experimental apparatus used in the studies of Whelan (reproduced from Whelan et al. 1996)

15 mmHg CO_2 pneumoperitoneum and constant flow of CO_2 at a pressure of 5 mmHg and 10 mmHg did not produce aerosolization of cells. However, an interesting observation was made from an in vitro model using the balloon in the apparatus (Fig. 7.6) as a diaphragm through which trocars were placed and the cell suspension was made to coat the entire inner surface of the balloon. Cultures of the samples aspirated through the trocars grew B-16 in 5 of the 6 samples. Moderate agitation of tissue culture had produced no aerosolized cells before that experiment. B-16 requires only 10 cells to establish tumor growth in culture and is therefore a very sensitive model for this issue. A large number of samples and repeated e xperiments were done in this study to insure a correct result. The authors concluded that aerosolization of cells in a CO_2 pneumoperitoneum is probably not the mechanism by which cells reach the trocar sites. However, desufflation may expose the trocar sites to a cell-laden liquid. Rapid desufflation may cause transportation of cells throughout the abdomen in a liquid suspension, assuming that viable tumor cells are present in the peritoneal cavity in patients with colon cancer.

A second set of experiments using the apparatus shown in the figure above (Fig. 7.6) was undertaken with the same number of B-16 cells in culture exposed to higher CO_2 pressures of 15 and 30 mmHg (Sellers et al. 1998). Once again, no aerosolization of cells could be documented. The combination of these two experiments make aerosolization of cells an unlikely source of tumor spread.

A different approach was utilized by the group at the Royal Adelaide Hospital to evaluate aerosolization of cells as the mechanism of distributing cells in the abdominal cavity (Mathew et al. 1997b). Radiolabelled cells and viable cells from the DAMA mammary cancer were injected into the peritoneal cavity of Dark Agouti rats and a plastic tubing used to connect the tumor-bearing rats to a second animal with only a trocar in the abdominal cavity (Fig. 7.7). Cell suspensions containing $1-2 \times 10^8$ cells were added to the donor rats carefully to avoid aerosolization while the abdomen was insufflated to a pressure of 6 mmHg with CO_2 at a flow rate of 0.2 l/min. Recipient hamsters were also maintained at 6 mmHg pneumoperitoneum until the tumor cells were injected into the donor abdominal cavity and then the gas was vented through the insufflating trocar. The tips of all the trocars were kept clear of the liquid within the abdomen. The recipient rats were evaluated for tumor growth 3 weeks later. A second set of experiments utilized Cr^{51} labeled DAMA cells which

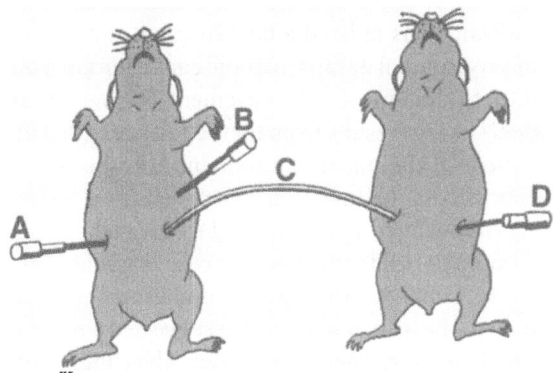

Fig. 7.7. Port placement for the experiment of Southall. *A*, primary insufflation port and minilaparoscope port; *B*, 20-gauge trocar for the introduction of tumor suspension; *C*, 14-gauge plastic tubing; *D*, 18-gauge venting trocar (adapted from Southall et al. 1998)

were collected from the connecting trocar from the first experiment to document the presence of label in vented gas. A gasless laparoscopy approach was also added to the experiment to determine whether the pneumoperitoneum was affecting distribution of cells. Tumor was found at the connecting tubing and venting trocar sites in the recipient rats in the first experiments when CO_2 was used. Approximately 3% of cells (by Cr^{51} label calculation) were recovered through the connecting tube in the second experiments. The gasless laparoscopy groups showed no transfer of tumor to recipient rats or recovery of labeled cells through the connecting tubing.

These experiments suggest that a high flow (0.2 l/min or 10–15 l/min in the clinical setting) and large tumor inoculum (2×10^8 cells) result in a pneumoperitoneum-dependent transfer of cells. Aerosolization may or may not be involved. The authors tried to control for liquid transfer by avoiding trocar contact with the liquid containing cells. However, they are unable to state conclusively what generated the cell transfer. The extremely high CO_2 leak rate and very high cell count are very artificial and do not mimic the clinical setting at all. They do suggest that technique is important since slippage of trocars causes high leakage rates of CO_2 and direct tumor injury is the only possible means of spilling 2×10^8 cells in the abdominal cavity. Removal of the CO_2 flow with a gasless approach eliminated the transfer of cells even in a high inoculum, suggesting the increase in importance of the pneumoperitoneum at high cell counts as suggested by Wu et al. (1998a).

The study group at the Queen Elizabeth Hospital in Adelaide has utilized a human colon cancer line LIM 1215 to simulate laparoscopic conditions in a pig model to document cell movement (Hewett et al. 1996). The first results from their efforts revealed little affect of the pneumoperitoneum on the movements of cells. An injection of 10% cells in 10 ml intraperitoneally in a porcine model only yielded laparoscopic port filter positive for cells in 30 determinations. However, they found numerous cells attached to the instruments which suggested a mechanism of direct transfer to port-sites. The clinical correlation was made with the inadvertent contact of the instruments with the tumor mass during colectomy as the major cause of trocar site implantation.

A more recent experiment, using the LIM 1215 cell line in the porcine model to video scintigraphically evaluate the movement of the cells through the abdomen with and without pneumoperitoneum, has shown that cells move slightly different under the two conditions (Hewett PJ, personal communication). A bolus of radiolabeled cells in the pelvis eventually migrate to the left subphrenic space and contaminate any instruments present and in contact with the abdominal fluid. The addition of a pneumoperitoneum more rapidly distributes the cells along the usual paths but also to other areas of the abdomen and once again results in instrument, and hence port-site, contamination. There is no evidence of aerosolization or alternate methods of cell movement other than traveling along the "gutters" of the abdomen. Instrument contamination remains the most important source of port-site contamination, according to their results.

Additional evidence that contamination of laparoscopic instruments is a major source of distributing tumor cells to port-sites was provided by the group in Christchurch, New Zealand. A porcine laparoscopic colectomy model, using Cr^{51} labeled, fixed HeLa cells injected intraperitoneally prior to the operation, revealed increased radiolabel in sections of the abdominal wall at the port-sites used by the operating surgeon regardless of the presence or absence (gasless laparoscopy) of pneumoperitoneum (Allardyce et al. 1996). The authors also found a direct relationship between the number of cells (10^7 or 5×10^6) and cell recovery from intra-abdominal tissues and port-sites.

A second set of experiments using the same model evaluated the use of peritoneal lavage, port venting – "chimney effect", instrument passage, aerosolization and gasless laparoscopy on the distribution of tumor cells (Allardyce et al. 1997). Vigorous port movement and port venting resulted in large numbers of cells recovered in the port-site but not in the filters applied to the port. Peritoneal lavage reduced, but did not eliminate, port-site contamination. Circumferential leakage of gas around a trocar ("chimney effect") seems to encourage the seepage of tumor-containing peritoneal fluid into the port-site. The "chimney effect" is related to activity (instrument passage, trocar movement, trocar replacement) at the port-site.

Finally, the location of the tumor cells and the surgical approach were evaluated as factors influencing tumor distribution in the HeLa cell-porcine model (Allardyce et al. 1998). Intraluminally and intramurally placed cells were less likely to result in port-site contamination than intraperitoneally placed HeLa cells regardless of the surgical approach (open vs. laparoscopic) to the sigmoid colectomy. This report suggested that laparotomy wound contamination may actually be higher for the open procedure than the laparoscopic procedure. This is somewhat surprising and may reflect the small number of animals in the experiment ($n = 4$) but brings another question into the controversy of port-site contamination. This set of experiments looked directly at the mechanical distribution of a non-viable tumor cell line and as such eliminates most of the biologic variability seen with a viable tumor cell line. It does not rely on tumor implantation or growth to a particular mass. The use of HeLa cells fixed in Karnovski's fixative may not allow direct clinical application of the findings since contamination does not necessarily translate to implantation and growth in the patient or even in the viable tumor experimental model. The "chimney effect" is certainly a frightening concept. No aerosolization is needed to induce movement of fluid containing tumor into the port around a trocar that is being actively used. Thus, special care should be taken to limit instrument exchange, unnecessary motion or trocar dislodgment.

Summary

The data so far suggest that aerosolization of cells during laparoscopy is not the source of tumor movement to wounds. However, pneumoperitoneum is a factor as it speeds movement of cells throughout the abdominal cavity and is responsible for the "chimney effect" seen around trocars. Instrument contamination and secondary seeding of the port-site is probably the most significant means of active delivery of cells to port-sites. Once again, the degree of port-site contamination correlates with the number of cells present in the abdominal cavity.

Factors Influencing Tumor Growth and Trocar Site Implantation

The immune effects of open and laparoscopic surgery will be dealt with in another section in this book. However, a number of studies have been performed which touch on the immune sparing properties of laparoscopic colectomy and the influence of such on trocar implantation. Other studies have assessed the influence of the conditions of laparoscopy (CO_2 pneumoperitoneum, early feeding, etc.) on tumor growth.

The group of Whelan has shown a decrease in remote tumor growth in laparoscopic colectomy cases as compared to open colectomy (Southall et al. 1998; Allendorf et al. 1998) A mouse model using immunocompetent mice and mouse mammary carcinoma (mmc) injected in the dorsal skin showed that an open cecectomy allowed more frequent growth of larger tumors than laparoscopic cecectomy (Allendorf et al. 1998). A large number of animals were used and the differences in frequency of tumor growth and mass of tumor were highly significant ($p < 0.01$). The mmc line was $> 95\%$ viable and 10^4 or 10^6 cells were injected in the dorsal skin to evaluate tumor establishment or tumor mass after 12 days respectively.

A second study, using colon-26 mouse adenocarcinoma and B16 melanoma in the Balbyc mouse model comparing laparotomy and laparoscopy without cecectomy, used tumor mass as the end point (Southall et al. 1998). C-26 adenocarcinoma produced larger tumors after laparotomy than after laparoscopy, and this difference was statistically significant ($p < 0.05$). However, B16 melanoma did not produce as clear a difference. Only after a second set of experiments could the differences be found to be significant between the laparotomy and laparoscopy groups. This may reflect an induced immune response or a variability of tumor viability between the experiments. For this reason, it is probably not as appropriate to use tumor mass as an end point. These findings in the mouse with colon cancer and melanoma confirmed previous findings from this laboratory using mammary cancer in a similar set of experiments (Allendorf et al. 1995).

These experiments thus far have been performed without tumor present in the abdominal cavity. The tumor has been injected in the dorsal skin and fat –

a rather artificial setting, but one designed to test the affects of laparotomy or laparoscopy on the immune system permission of tumor growth. However, a more realistic approach would seem to be one with tumor exposed to the conditions in the area of manipulation.

In order to address these issues, Whelan et al. (1996) produced a splenic tumor model in mice using C-26 colon cancer and then evaluated the influence of laparotomy/splenectomy or laparoscopy/splenectomy on the incidence of port-site tumors (Lee et al. 1998a). There was a higher incidence of port-site and left flank incision (used to establish the splenic tumor) tumor after laparoscopic than open splenectomy. The authors documented a decrease in port-site implants after laparoscopic splenectomy between the first study group of animals and a second study group. This may represent a learning curve. In the final analysis, there was a significantly higher incidence of port-site implants after laparoscopic splenectomy, but this was not significant when the number of animals with at least one port-site implant was compared between the open and laparoscopic splenectomy groups. The conclusion that operative technique may influence port-site implants is very appropriate. The issue of a learning curve may be particularly relevant to the early anecdotal reports of port-site recurrences in patients and the reason some laparoscopic surgeons have seen no port-site recurrences in their large series.

The influence of laparoscopy using air compared to CO_2 was evaluated in Berlin (Jacobi et al. 1997a). Initially, an in vitro study of tumor (DHD/KIZ/TRb Rat Colon Ca) growth was performed. Air and CO_2, bubbled through culture media, both increased growth compared to controls in this model. When the tumor cells were exposed to pneumoperitoneum of 8 mm Hg with air or CO_2, tumor growth in culture flasks was subsequently greater than a control group. The end point of the experiment was tumor mass in a relatively small group ($n = 5$) of animals. Finally, tumor growth in vivo in both the peritoneal cavity or subcutaneous sites of rats was increased by an 8 mm Hg pneumoperitoneum of air or CO_2 as compared to control without pneumoperitoneum. The influence of gas on tumor growth needs further investigation. The most interesting finding, however, is the affect of pressure on tumor growth. This study should be repeated using incidence of wound implants to eliminate growth variability as a potential source of error.

The influence of pressure during CO_2 laparoscopy on tumor growth was the next project from the group in Berlin (Jacobi et al. 1998). An in vitro culture of DHD/KIZ/TRb rat colon cancer cells was exposed to CO_2 for 3 h at pressures of 0, 5, 10 and 15 mm Hg. Growth suppression was found above 10 mm Hg as evidenced by counting of viable cells in culture 23 h later. A second experiment exposed DHD/KIZ/Trb tumor cells (10^4) in the abdomen of rats to pneumoperitoneum of 5, 10 and 15 mm Hg CO_2. The rats also had tumor cells injected into the dorsal skin. Pressures below 15 mm Hg led to increased intraperitoneal growth, but pressures 15 mm Hg or greater resulted in decreased growth. In contrast, CO_2 at all pressures resulted in increased subcutaneous growth of tumor compared to control (no laparotomy or laparoscopy). An increase in the number of port-site implants was also seen in rats receiving pneumoperitoneum of all levels ($p < 0.05$). The experiment used incidence as an end point and had a large number of animals in each group. Therefore, the results are less likely to be erroneous.

The group of Bonjer in Rotterdam evaluated the effect of laparoscopy on weight gain and tumor implantation in a rat model using another chemoinduced rat colon cancer (CC-531) (Bouvy et al. 1996). A small number of rats in each group in two experiments ($n = 11$) revealed a significant larger drop and slower recovery in weight, and a higher tumor implantation rate, after open small bowel resection than after laparoscopic small bowel resection. The authors concluded that CO_2 pneumoperitoneum stimulated CC-531 tumor growth intraperitoneally since laparoscopic procedures caused a greater tumor growth than the control groups with no CO_2 or resection. The evaluation of tumor implantation used a scoring system based on tumor diameter. This is less accurate than absolute incidence but does consider some of the biologic features of tumor growth. The scoring method has been compared to a radioactive method and found to correlate well (Ottow et al. 1987). Since the tumor is weakly immunogenic, a growth period of 4 weeks may be influencing the outcome of the tumor growth by immunomodulation. No data are provided regarding the number of sites of tumor growth. The authors repeated the experiment using CC-531 cells injected intraperitoneally or injected in the renal capsule. Tumor deposits were established initially and then the rats were subjected to either open small bowel resection, laparoscopic small bowel resection or anesthesia only. Once again, CO_2 pneumoperitoneum and laparoscopic resection (6 mm Hg) produced less tumor implantation than an open procedure, but more than anesthesia only. The authors conclud-

ed that laparoscopic bowel resection produces less stimulation of tumor growth. They were unable to determine the affect of preserved or suppressed immune response on the tumor growth.

Bouvy et al. (1998) repeated the solid tumor renal capsule model in rats with ROS-1 (a rat osteosarcoma). The tumor was established 3 days prior to CO_2 or air laparoscopic small bowel resection or gasless laparoscopic resection. A shorter tumor growth (7 days) was allowed and weights of tumor were used as the end point. Gasless laparoscopy produced significantly smaller tumor growth than air or CO_2 laparoscopy. The authors concluded that gasless laparoscopy may be indicated if patients with cancer are to be treated with laparoscopic techniques. Unfortunately, we do not know the effects of pressure on the growth of ROS-1, or the affect on the immune system of the rat.

A study from Dublin, Ireland, suggests that natural killer (NK) cell function is suppressed more after open laparotomy than laparoscopy, and this suppression is mediated in part by the generation of splenic suppressor cells (splenic macrophages) (Da Costa et al. 1998). B-16 melanoma cells were used to induce flank tumors in C57BL/6 mice. When excised, lung metastases developed. The spread to lungs could be enhanced by open laparotomy coincident with tumor excision. Laparoscopy resulted in a much smaller increase in lung metastases. An analysis of NK cell function in the spleen after laparotomy revealed marked suppression of reaction to B-16 cells. After laparoscopy, the NK cell function slowly returned to normal but was significantly better than after laparotomy and significantly worse than the control non-operated group. Splenic macrophages were found to actively suppress the NK cell function to varying degrees: laparotomy > laparoscopy > control. This study provides sound evidence that laparoscopy is less immune suppressive than laparotomy. The large number of animals and duplicated experiments yielded clear, believable results which have added another piece to the puzzle.

The use of various gases to establish pneumoperitoneum may affect tumor growth in different ways. A study from Mannheim, Germany, evaluated helium, CO_2 and heated CO_2 as pneumoperitoneum in a nude mouse model carrying human lung mesothelioma cells (Volz et al. 1998). Survival was the end point of the experiment for the groups of 15 animals. Helium pneumoperitoneum produced a better survival than CO_2 or heated CO_2.

The development of trocar site implants after intraperitoneal rat mammary tumor (DAMA) was evaluated in rats according to the use of CO_2, N_2O, helium, and air as pneumoperitoneum by Neuhaus et al. in 1998. The flank tumor could be incised via laparoscopic instrumentation to release tumor into the abdomen, simulating a solid tumor model. The study end point was incidence of implants at trocar sites as well as tumor mass. Helium produced fewer trocar site implants than CO_2, N_2O or air as pneumoperitoneum. These two studies suggest that there is a protective effect of helium against tumor growth after laparoscopy. It is hoped that these results are not tumor specific (mesothelioma, mammary).

Summary

There are many factors which influence the establishment of tumor cells at trocar sites and abdominal wounds. Thus far, only a few have been evaluated – pneumoperitoneum gas, immune response of the host, pressure, and operative technique. Further study is needed to evaluate the influence of local factors such as cytokine release, vascularization, adherence molecules, and growth factors.

Prevention of Tumor Implantation

Efforts to define the mechanism of tumor implantation after laparoscopic colectomy for cancer have ultimately turned to the prevention of implants. Some of these methods have identified specific "avoidances" while others have recommended "interventions" to counter the deposition and growth of tumor cells at the port-sites.

The first initiative was to define the nature of tumor injury which predisposed to implantation of cells. The group of Watson at the Royal Adelaide Hospital discovered that intentional laceration of an intraabdominal mammary tumor (DAMA) yielded markedly increased tumor implants in a rat model (Mathew et al. 1996). The combination of laparoscopy and tumor laceration was more frequently associated with implants than any combination of blunt injury and laparotomy or laparoscopy. Lack of tumor manipulation actually resulted in no tumor implantation after laparotomy or laparoscopy. This is profound evidence that tumor implantation is a mechanical problem. The rat mammary tumor is an aggressive adenocarcinoma but the technique used for these experiments assessed tumor implants at wounds within 7 days of intervention to prevent metastasis or carcinomatosis from being a factor. Therefore, good surgical technique is a critical factor in preventing trocar implants.

Local treatment of the port-sites would be an appropriate next step in preventing wound implants. We initially tried excision of trocar sites after laparoscopy in the presence of 8×10^5 cells of GW39 placed intraperitoneally in the Golden Hamster model (Wu et al. 1998b). This resulted in a 30% decrease in trocar site implants compared to no excision of the wounds after trocar removal (49% vs. 74%). The presence of trocar implants in 49% of trocar sites even after excision indicated that the continued presence of tumor cells after the procedure placed the wound at risk for tumor implantation. A simple addition of a local treatment such as povidone iodine swabbed in the trocar site or silver sulfadiazine coating the trocar and wound edges was found to reduce the incidence of trocar implants even further (75% to 29%) (Wu et al. 1998b). Therefore, a "local" treatment of small wounds may prevent a "local" phenomenon of tumor implantation at trocar sites. As previously mentioned, GW 39 does not spread hematogenously or metastasize. However, the presence of intraabdominal tumor cells even after local treatment must continue to expose the small port-site wounds to adequate tumor cell inocula to produce implants. The possibility of intraabdominal chemotherapy is therefore attractive.

The group in Berlin have tried several combinations of instilled agents to reduce cell implantation. Taurolidine (an aseptic) and heparin were found to reduce implants when instilled intraperitoneally and in vitro (Jacobi et al. 1997b). Taurolidine had a more profound affect than heparin. Taurolidine has antiadherence properties as well as an inhibitory function in the production of IL-1 in peripheral WBC. The chemoinduced DHD/K12/TRb rat colon cancer was found to be inhibited by taurolidine ± heparin, in vitro and when introduced intraperitoneally in the presence of pneumoperitoneum. The inhibition of tumor adherence may be an effective means of preventing trocar implants or tumor local recurrence due to tumor spillage.

Cytotoxic agents are obvious agents to consider for prevention of port-site recurrences. Watson et al. (1997) have used intraperitoneal povidone-iodine, isotonic saline, chlorhexidine and methotrexate to reduce port-site implants in the rat using intraperitoneal DAMA mammary cancer (produced by lacerating a left flank solid tumor transperitoneally). Only povidone iodine prevented implants completely but methotrexate was also very effective. The issue of post-treatment ileus and toxicity will need to be addressed before proceeding to clinical trials.

A second study was performed to evaluate cyclophosphamide as a protective agent (Iwanaka et al. 1998). Intraperitoneal or intravenous cyclophosphamide were shown to prevent the development of trocar site implants of neuroblastoma in A/J mice.

Summary

Good surgical technique, local treatment to prevent or destroy implanted cells and intraperitoneal chemotherapy are all means of preventing trocar implants. None of these techniques have been studied in a human model in a randomized way. Common sense dictates good technique. Local treatment with readily available, non-toxic agents may be the next step but should be evaluated in a randomized prospective trial.

Conclusions

Animal models and tumor cell lines have given us insight into the mechanism of port-site recurrence. These data need to be interpreted with the knowledge that each model and cell line carry a specific set of special parameters which may influence the outcome of a study unless controlled by the experimental design. Adequate numbers of animals are needed in each experimental group and should be determined prospectively with a power calculation for a randomized study. Tumor variability from day to day and experiment to experiment greatly influences outcome of a study if the end point is tumor weight or incremental growth. A more reliable measure is incidence of tumor occurrence, implantation or disappearance based on microscopic evaluation. The potential for continued increase in knowledge using these existing and other new cell line models is enormous. Not only will the mechanism and prevention of port-site recurrences be elucidated, but continued investigation should help us understand more fully the parameters of wound healing, tumor establishment, growth and mobility, physiologic parameters of surgical media/pneumoperitoneum, gases, incision length, etc., and help us define treatment methods for cancer in the future.

References

Allardyce R, Morreau P, Bagshaw P (1996) Tumor cell distribution following laparoscopic colectomy in a porcine model. Dis Colon Rectum 39: 47–52

Allardyce RA, Morreau P, Bagshaw PF (1997) Operative factors affecting tumor cell distribution following laparoscopic colectomy in a porcine model. Dis Colon Rectum 40: 939–945

Allardyce RA, Morreau PN, Frizelle FA, Bagshaw PF (1998) Tumor cell wound distribution after colectomy in a porcine model. Aust N Z J Surg 68: 363–366

Allendorf JD, Bessler M, Kayton ML, Osterling SD, Treat MR, Nowygrod R, Whelan RL (1995) Increased tumor establishment and growth after laparotomy versus laparoscopy in a murine model. Arch Surg 130: 649–653

Allendorf JDF, Bessler M, Horvath KD, Marvin MR, Laird DA, Whelan RL (1998) Increased tumor establishment and growth after open vs. laparoscopic bowel resection in mice. Surg Endosc 12: 1035–1038

Barendsen GW, Janse HC (1978) Differences in effectiveness of combined treatments with ionizing radiation and vinblastine, evaluated for experimental sarcomas and squamous cell carcinomas in rats. Int J Radiat Oncol Biol Phys 4: 95–102

Bouvy ND, Marquet RL, Hamming JF, Jeekel J, Bonjer HJ (1996) Laparoscopic surgery in the rat. Surg Endosc 10: 490–494

Bouvy ND, Marquet RL, Jeekel J, Bonjer HJ (1997) Laparoscopic surgery is associated with less tumor growth stimulation than conventional surgery: an experimental study. Br J Surg 84: 358–361

Bouvy ND, Giuffrida MC, Tseng LNL, Steyerberg EW, Marquet RL, Jeekel H, Bonjer HJ (1998) Effects of carbon dioxide pneumoperitoneum, air pneumoperitoneum, and gasless laparoscopy on body weight and tumor growth. Arch Surg 133: 652–656

Bugelski PJ, Kirsch RL, Poste G (1983) New histochemical method for measuring intratumoral macrophages and macrophage recruitment into experimental metastases. Cancer Res 43: 5493–5501

Bystryn J-C, Bart RS, Livingston P, Kopf AW (1974) Growth and immunogenicity of murine B-16 melanoma J Invest Dermatol 63: 369–373

Choi SH, Reynolds JL, Ziegler MM (1989) Systematic analysis of the immunoregulation of murine neuroblastoma. J Pediatr Surg 24: 15–19

Coyle P, Rofe AM, Bourgeois CS, Conyers AJ (1990) Biochemical manifestations of a rat mammary adenocarcinoma-producing cachexia: in vivo and in vitro studies. Immunol Cell Biol 68: 147–153

Da Costa ML, Redmond HP, Bouchier-Hayes DJ (1998) The effect of laparotomy and laparoscopy on the establishment of spontaneous tumor metastases. Surgery 124: 516–525

Fidler IJ (1973) The relationship of embolic homogeneity, number, size and viability to the incidence of experimental metastasis. Eur J Cancer 9: 223–227

Goldenberg DM, Witte S, Elster K (1966) GW 39: a new human tumor serially transplantable in the golden hamster. Transplantation 4: 760–763

Hewett PJ, Thomas WM, King G, Eaton M (1996) Intraperitoneal cell movement during abdominal carbon dioxide insufflation and laparoscopy: an in vivo model. Dis Colon Rectum 39: 62–66

Iwanaka T, Arya G, Ziegler MM (1998) Mechanism and prevention of port-site tumor recurrence after laparoscopy in a murine model. J Pediatr Surg 33: 457–461

Jacobi CA, Ordemann J, Bohm B, Zieren HU, Liebenthal C, Volk HD, Muller JM (1997a) The influence of laparotomy and laparoscopy on tumor growth in a rat model. Surg Endosc 11: 618–621

Jacobi CA, Ordemann J, Bohm B, Zieren HU, Sabat R, Muller JM (1997b) Inhibition of peritoneal tumor cell growth and implantation in laparoscopic surgery in a rat model. Am J Surg 174: 359–363

Jacobi CA, Wenger FA, Ordemann J, Gutt C, Sabat R, Muller JM (1998) Experimental study of the effect of intra-abdominal pressure during laparoscopy on tumor growth and port-site recurrence. Br J Surg 85: 1419–1422

Jones DB, Guo LW, Reinhard MK, Soper NJ, Philpott GW, Connett J, Fleshman JW (1995) Impact of pneumoperitoneum on trocar site implantation of colon cancer in hamster model. Dis Colon Rectum 38: 1182–1188

Lagadec P, Jeannin JF, Reisser D, Pelletier H, Olsson O (1987) Treatment with endotoxins of peritoneal carcinomatosis induced by colon tumor cells in rats. Invasion Metastasis 7: 83–95

Lee SW, Southall J, Allendorf J, Bessler M, Whelan RL (1998b) Traumatic handling of the tumor independent of pneumoperitoneum increases port-site implantation rate of colon cancer in a murine model. Surg Endosc 12: 828–834

Lee SW, Whelan RL, Southall JC, Bessler M (1998a) Abdominal wound tumor recurrence after open and laparoscopic-assisted splenectomy in a murine model. Dis Colon Rectum 41: 824–831

Marquet RL, Ijzermans JNM, De Bruin RW, Fiers W, Jeekel J (1987) Anti-tumor activity of recombinant mouse tumor necrosis factor (TNF) on colon cancer in rats is promoted recombinant rat interferon gamma; toxicity is reduced indomethacin. Int J Cancer 40: 550–553

Martin MS, Bastien H, Martin F, Viry B (1973) Transplantation of intestinal carcinoma in inbred rats. Biomedicine 19: 555–558

Mathew G, Watson DI, Rofe AM, Baigrie CF, Ellis T, Jamieson GG (1996) Wound metastases following laparoscopic and open surgery for abdominal cancer in a rat model. Br J Surg 83: 1087–1090

Mathew G, Watson DI, Ellis T, De Young N, Rofe AM, Jamieson GG (1997b) The effect of laparoscopy on the movement of tumor cells and metastasis to surgical wounds. Surg Endosc 11: 1163–1166

Mathew G, Watson DI, Rofe AM, Ellis T, Jamieson GG (1997a) Adverse impact of pneumoperitoneum on intraperitoneal implantation and growth of tumor cell suspension in an experimental model. Aust N Z J Surg 67: 289–292

Neuhaus SJ, Watson DI, Ellis T, Rowland R, Rofe AM, Pike GK, Mathew G, Jamieson GG (1998) Wound metastasis after laparoscopy with different insufflation gases. Surgery 123: 579–583

Ottow RT, Steller EP, Sugarbaker PH, Wesley RA, Rosenberg SA (1987) Immunotherapy of intraperitoneal cancer with interleukin 2 and lymphokine-activated killer cells reduces tumor load and prolongs survival in murine models. Cell Immunol 104: 366–376

Paik PS, Misawa T, Chiang M, Towson J, Im S, Ortega A, Beart RW Jr (1998) Abdominal incision tumor implantation following pneumoperitoneum laparoscopic procedure vs. standard open incision in a syngeneic rat model. Dis Colon Rectum 41: 419–422

Prehn RT, Main JM (1957) Immunity to methylcholanthrene-induced sarcomas. J Natl Cancer Inst 18: 769–778

Reisser D, Fady C, Lagadec P, Martin F (1991) Influence of the injection site on the tumorigenicity of a cloned colon tumor cell line in the rat. Bull Cancer 78: 249–252

Sellers GJ, Whelan RL, Allendorf JD, Gleason NR, Donahue J, Laird D, Bessler MD, Treat MR (1998) An in vitro model fails to demonstrate aerosolization of tumor cells. Surg Endosc 12: 436–439

Southall JC, Lee SW, Allendorf JD, Bessler M, Whelan RL (1998) Colon adenocarcinoma and B-16 melanoma grow larger following laparotomy vs. pneumoperitoneum in a murine model. Dis Colon Rectum 41: 564–569

Vaage J, Pepin K (1985) Morphological observations during developing concomitant immunity against a C3H/HC mammary tumor. Cancer Res 45: 659–666

Volz J, Koster S (1996b) The effects of pneumoperitoneum on intraperitoneal tumor implantation in nude mice. Gynaecol Endosc 5: 193–196

Volz J, Koster S, Weiss M, Schmidt R, Urbasckek R, Melchert F, Albrecht M (1996a) Pathophysiology of a pneumoperitoneum in laparoscopy: a swine model. Am J Obstet Gynecol 174: 132–140

Volz J, Koster S, Schaeff B, Paolucci V (1998) Laparoscopic surgery: the effects of insufflation gas on tumor-induced lethality in nude mice. Am J Obstet Gynecol 178: 793–795

Watson DI, Mathew G, Ellis T, Baigrie CF, Rofe AM, Jamieson GG (1997) Gasless laparoscopy may reduce the risk of port-site recurrences following laparoscopic tumor surgery. Arch Surg 132: 166–169

Whelan RL, Sellers GJ, Allendorf JD, Laird D, Bessler MD, Nowygrod R, Treat MR (1996) Trocar site recurrence is unlikely to result from aerosolization of tumor cells. Dis Colon Rectum 39: 7–13

Wu JS, Brasfield EB, Guo LW, Ruiz M, Connett JM, Philpott GW, Jones DB, Fleshman JW (1997) Implantation of colon cancer at trocar sites is increased by low pressure pneumoperitoneum. Surgery 122: 1–7

Wu JS, Guo L-W, Ruiz MB, Pfister SM, Connett JM, Fleshman JW (1998b) Excision of trocar sites reduces tumor implantation in an animal model. Dis Colon Rectum 41: 1107–1111

Wu JS, Jones DB, Guo LW, Brasfield EB, Ruiz MB, Connett JM, Fleshman JW (1998a) Effects of pneumoperitoneum on tumor implantation with decreasing tumor inoculum. Dis Colon Rectum 41:141–46

Wu JS, Pfister SM, Ruiz MB, Connett JM, Fleshman JW (1998c) Local treatment of abdominal wound reduces tumor implantation. J Surg Oncol 69: 9–14

CHAPTER 8

Pathogenesis: Transportation of Tumor Cells in Animal Studies

M.L. Texler, P.J. Hewett

Introduction

"… when the tumor is broken into during an operation the risk of transplantation must be great. In such a case small portions conveyed by the fingers or knife might easily find a suitable position on the raw-surface for renewed growth, hence the so-called recurrence." (Lawrie 1906)

Tumor metastasis is a multi-step and selective process (Thomas 1961). Hematogenous spread of tumor normally involves "selective growth of specialised sub-populations of highly metastatic cells endowed with specific properties that befit them to complete each step of the metastatic process" the so called "metastatic cascade." (Poste and Filder 1980). The transport of tumor cells from the primary tumor across the peritoneal cavity (by peritoneal fluid, instruments, blood or CO_2) enables a tumor cell to bypass many of the steps of haematogenous spread. The mode of this transport (the "vector") has been the subject of animal research.

Research to Date

Small Animal Models

Mice, rats and hamsters have been used in small animal models to compare the effects of laparoscopic versus open surgery (Allendorf et al. 1997; Jones et al. 1995; Mathew et al. 1997). Much of this work has focused on the impact of insufflation and the presence of aerosolization.

Aerosolization and Insufflation or Gasless Techniques

Some in vivo studies have focussed on the "chimney effect" and the impact of CO_2 pneumoperitoneum. If CO_2 insufflation is harmful, a benefit should be seen when a gasless technique is used. No evidence of viable aerosolization has been seen in a rat model

(Whelan et al. 1996). This was supported by the finding that no viable cells were seen in the smoke plume when electro-surgery or the harmonic scalpel were used (Nduka and Darzi 1997). In one study, gasless laparoscopy did not prevent port-site recurrences in a rat model. Although no insufflation was used, direct contact of the port-site with tumor enabled tumor spread to the extraction site (Bouvy et al. 1996a,b). In a contrasting study, gasless laparoscopy may prevent tumor dissemination when compared with CO_2 insufflation. Mathew et al. used a detection system of tumor growth in a recipient rat or the presence of ^{51}Cr labelled cells in a water trap of the exiting CO_2 (Mathew et al. 1997; Watson et al. 1997). Radiolabelled cells were detected within water traps. They also found that recipient rats developed tumors when CO_2 insufflation was used, thus supporting aerosolization of viable tumor cells. The difference in findings between these studies may be due to a dose- and time-related effect as the study by Mathew et al. (1997) used higher concentrations of tumors with longer insufflation times compared with other studies (Bouvy et al. 1996; Hewett et al. 1996, 1999).

Large Animal Models

Pigs are a large animal commonly used for laparoscopic surgery research due to the similarities between their abdominal anatomy and that of humans (Bessler et al. 1996; Reissman et al. 1996).

Tumor Cell Dispersal During Laparoscopy Only

Allardyce et al. (1996, 1997, 1998) designed a pig model using ^{51}Cr labelled HeLa cells. After laparoscopic surgery was carried out, biopsies of various locations were taken and analysed in a γ radiation counter. With their model they could detect ~30 radiolabelled cells per biopsy. Another group developed a model where saline washings taken from trocars and CO_2 filters were analysed (Hewett et al. 1996). A real time model to detect ^{99m}Tc radiolabelled LIM 1215 (an adherent human colonic tumor cell line) movement as it occurs within the pig is the latest model to be developed. This model uses a 25 cm diameter gamma camera placed ventrally to the pig's abdomen during laparoscopy or surgery to detect radiolabelled tumor cell movement. The median sensitivity of this model was 500 ^{99m}Tc radiolabelled LIM 1215 cells (Hewett et al. 1999).

In the Allardyce et al. studies, ports used by the operating surgeon were contaminated with more tumor cells than the port used by the assistant. Postoperative withdrawal of ports was associated with contamination of port-sites. In addition, rostral movement of tumor cells was associated with a head down position of the pig. When more tumor cells were used, higher rates of contamination were seen (Allardyce et al. 1996). Instruments became contaminated with tumor cells when free intraperitoneal tumor cells were present. These instruments subsequently contaminated trocars (Allardyce et al. 1996, 1997, 1998; Hewett et al. 1996). Using a real time radiolabelled model (with an inoculum of 10–20 million radiolabelled LIM 1215 cells in supine pigs), widespread movement of pelvic placed intraperitoneal radiolabelled LIM 1215 cells occurred with and without CO_2 insufflation. When no insufflation was used, the radiolabelled LIM 1215 cells moved from the pelvis and predominantly up the left paracolic gutter. When CO_2 insufflation was used (insufflation entered the umbilical trocar and vented via the left flank trocar at a rate of $1-2 l \cdot min^{-1}$), the radiolabelled cells moved to the right upper quadrant (away from the direct flow of gas) (Fig. 8.1). Instruments, port-sites and trocars became contaminated. When 30 mL of free intraperitoneal blood was introduced

with the LIM 1215 cells, movement was more restricted since the blood coagulum trapped the free radiolabelled cells. Trocar and port-site contamination was greatest when there were periods of desufflation in the presence of free intraperitoneal blood (Table 8.1). However no aerosolization of tumor cells was detected in the 16 animals studied (Hewett et al. 1999).

Aerosolization

Aerosolization of epithelial cells has been seen during CO_2 pneumoperitoneum in a single study in the pig model (Knolmayer et al. 1996). If normal cells are aerosolized, it seems reasonable to expect exfoliated tumor cells to also aerosolize. Another study however did not detect aerosolization when using dry CO_2 in vivo. (Whelan et al. 1996).

In many studies using porcine models, no aerosolization of tumor cells has been seen with laparoscopy only (Allardyce et al. 1997; Hewett et al. 1996, 1999). The aerosolization of tumor cells was observed (in the absence of intraperitoneal manipulation) in only 2/17 pigs, and this was only in the presence of gross contamination of the peritoneal cavity with ~15 million LIM 1215 cells. The use of heated and humidified CO_2 did not have an effect upon aerosolization rates. Tumor cells were also detected at an inactive trocar filter, during CO_2 insufflation, when the abdominal contents were manipulated by endoscopic instruments (Hewett et al. 1996). As a new filter was used for each stage of the laparoscopy, this suggested that tumor cells may be aerosolized either during instrumentation, because no positive filter was detected in this pig prior to this phase or tumor cells present within the trocar from the earlier insufflation phase may have travelled further up the trocar to the filter (since the trocars were not

Table 8.1. Proportion of trocar chambers and port-sites contaminated by radiolabelled LIM 1215 cells based on presence of blood and insufflation (c2-test of total trocar values, d.f. = 2, $P = 0.0026$, c2-test of port-site contamination d.f. = 2, $P = 0.0007$. Hence port-site and trocar chamber contamination is greatest when the peritoneum is desufflated in the presence of free intraperitoneal blood)

Group description	Right trocar	Camera trocar	Left trocar	Totals trocar	Right port-site	Camera port-site	Left port-site	Totals port-site
Cells with insufflation followed by instrumentation	0/3	0/3	1/3	1/9	0/3	0/3	2/3	2/9
Cells and blood without insufflation followed by instrumentation	2/2	2/2	2/2	6/6	2/2	2/2	2/2	6/6
Cells and blood with insufflation followed by instrumentation	0/2	0/2	2/2	2/6	0/2	0/2	0/2	0/6

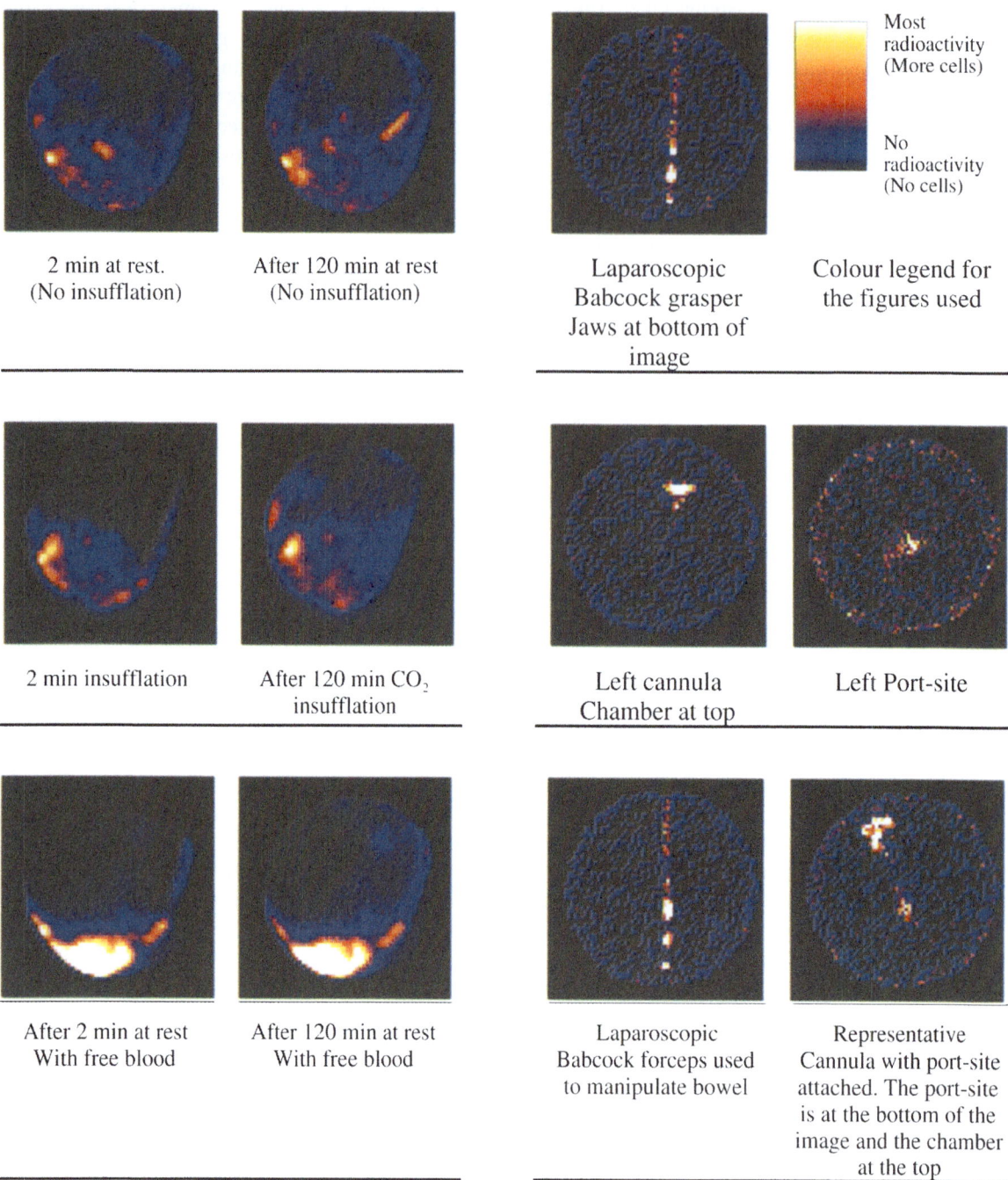

Fig. 8.1. Gamma camera images of pigs (*on left*) and laparoscopic graspers and trocars with port-sites (*on right*). Images of pigs are oriented similarly to a plain abdominal film. A colour legend is shown at the *upper right*. The right flank is on the *left* of the images, the left flank on the *right* of the images. The *top of the images* correspond to the costal margins and the *bottom of the figures* correspond to the pelvis. Radiolabelled cells introduced into the pelvic peritoneal cavity move towards to the upper abdomen regardless of the presence or absence of insufflation. When free blood is present, this movement is slowed

changed at each phase) and been detected. Tumor cells found at the filter on the trocar through which the laparoscopic Babcock forceps was passed may arrive there via direct transport on the tip of the instrument (Texler et al. 1997).

Tumor Cell Dispersal During Laparoscopic Surgery

A real time radiolabelled LIM 1215 model was used to determine tumor cell movement during both open and laparoscopic surgery. An inoculum of 10–

Table 8.2. Rates of contamination of objects used with the various forms of surgery versus tumor model used. The numerator is the number of objects contaminated. The denominator is the number of objects sampled. Dashes represent non applicable objects. A P-value (Fisher's two tailed exact test) comparing disseminated cells and intraluminally placed cells is in the right column

Object	Open disseminated	Laparoscopic disseminated	Open enema	Laparoscopic enema	p value Fisher's
Clip applicator	3/7	4/7	0/4	0/5	0.019
Linear cutter/stapler	4/8	5/7	0/5	0/5	0.028
Transanal stapler	6/8	7/7	5/5	5/5	0.500
Resected bowel	6/6	6/6	5/5	5/5	1.000
Extraction site/wound edge	3/3	6/6	0/1	0/5	0.002
Packs	7/8	3/4	0/5	0/1	0.003
Gloves	7/8	6/6	0/5	0/5	0.002
Laparoscope	–	0/6	–	0/4	1.000
Laparoscopic shears	–	6/7	–	0/5	0.015
Laparoscopic Babcock forceps	–	7/7	–	0/5	0.001
Trocar chambers	–	16/26	–	0/20	<0.001
Port-sites	–	12/24	–	0/20	<0.001

20 million ^{99m}Tc radiolabelled LIM 1215 was used within the supine animal. Either a laparoscopic-assisted four 12 mm-port technique was used (the extraction site was in the left iliac fossa) or an open approach through a midline laparotomy. When radiolabelled LIM 1215 cells were placed intraperitoneally, there was widespread dispersal of tumor cells in both the open and laparoscopic-assisted surgical groups. Instruments, gloves, packs, trocars chambers, wound edges and port-sites became contaminated (Table 8.2 and Fig. 8.2). When radiolabelled LIM 1215 was placed into the colonic lumen, no spillage from the lumen was seen in the current study (Fig. 8.3). This contrasts with the findings of Allardyce et al. (1998), since they detected intra-luminally placed radiolabelled tumor cells at wound edges

(i.e. spillage from the bowel lumen was detected in their study). Allardyce et al. (1998) recorded an average of 788 radiolabelled tumor cells at wound edges after laparoscopic surgery with intraluminally placed tumor cells. They used a total laparoscopic approach whereas we used a laparoscopic-assisted approach.

Cannula Chamber Contamination

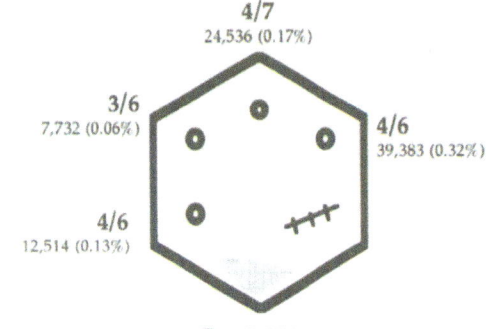

P = 0.928

Portsite Contamination

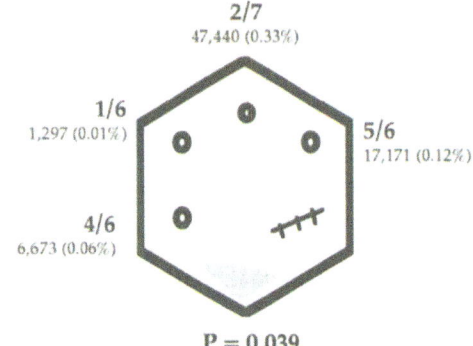

P = 0.039

Fig. 8.2. Summary of incidence of trocar chamber and port-site contamination after laparoscopic-assisted segmental colonic resection with intra-peritoneally placed radiolabelled LIM 1215. The incidence is expressed as the number of positive trocar chambers or port-sites divided by the number of trocar chambers or port-sites sampled. When the incidences of contamination at the left and lower right trocars were grouped together, and the incidences of contamination at the camera and right upper trocars were grouped together, the following c2-value was obtained (p = 0.928). A significant association between proximity to pelvis and incidence of port-site contamination was seen (p = 0.039, c2-test) when the incidences of contamination at the left and lower right trocars were grouped together, and the incidences of contamination at the camera and right upper trocars were grouped together. Median numbers of cells contaminating the trocar chambers or port-sites (with percentage of total cells administered in parentheses) are also shown. There was no association between site of the trocar and the percentage dose contamination at the port-site (p = 0.257, Kruskal-Wallis)

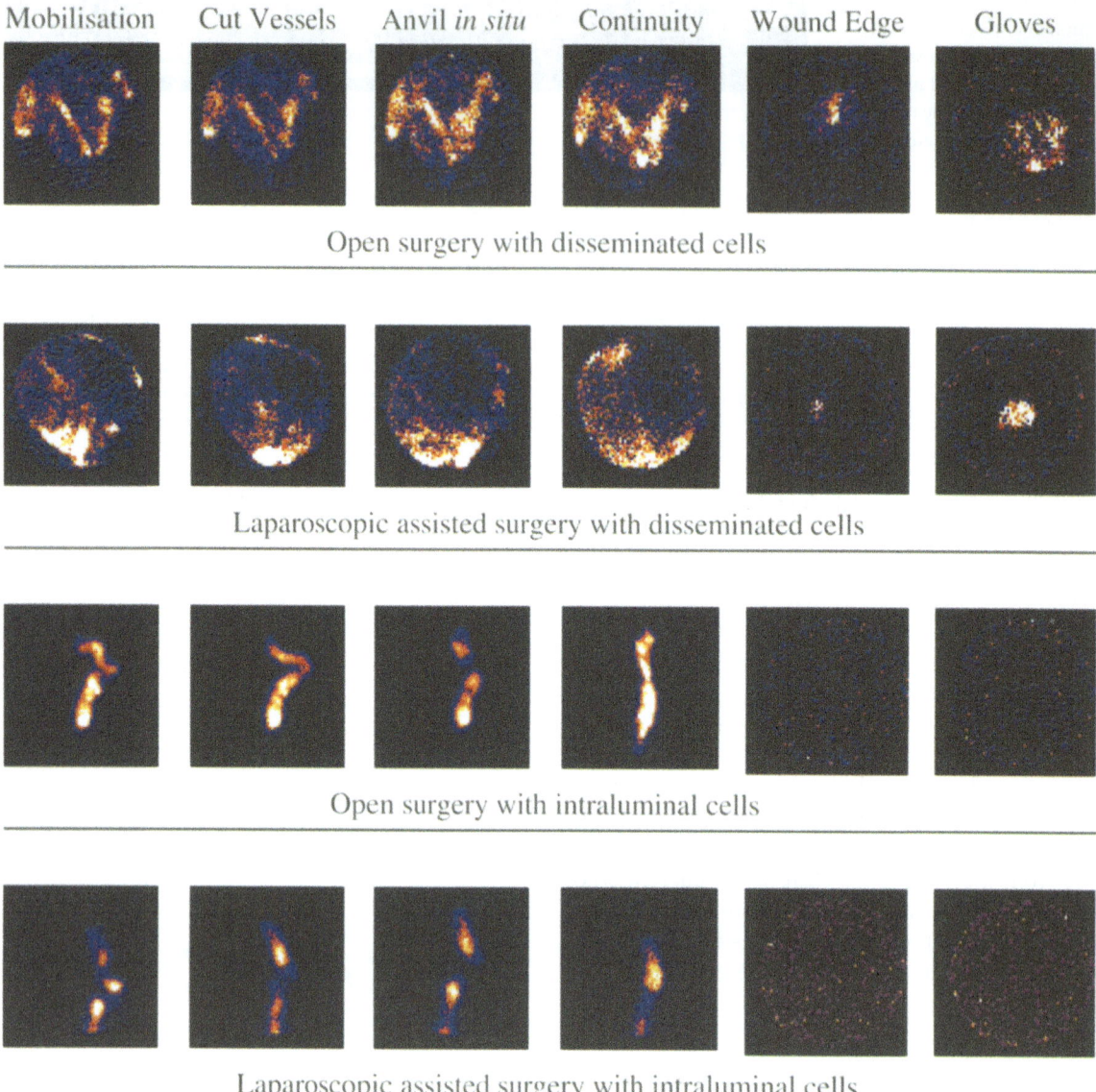

| Mobilisation | Cut Vessels | Anvil *in situ* | Continuity | Wound Edge | Gloves |

Open surgery with disseminated cells

Laparoscopic assisted surgery with disseminated cells

Open surgery with intraluminal cells

Laparoscopic assisted surgery with intraluminal cells

Fig. 8.3. Gamma camera images obtained from open and laparoscopic-assisted segmental colonic resection. (Orientation and colouring of images is the same as Fig. 8.1). Representative steps from the surgery are shown. Cells disperse widely throughout the peritoneal cavity with both open and laparoscopic-assisted surgery, including contamination of gloves and wound edges/extraction sites. With intraluminally placed cells, no extra luminal contamination occurs with either open or laparoscopic-assisted surgery. Note that with laparoscopic surgery with disseminated cells, a laparoscopic grasper can be seen in the upper part of the 2nd image as a linear object

Discussion

The main focus of this chapter was the study of the mode of transport of tumor cells across the peritoneal cavity from "tumor" to port-site, and examination of the factors influencing this movement. Most of the research to date has interpreted results based on the location of tumor cells at the conclu-

sion of surgery. Initial conditions were created, then the surgery was performed. The movement of cells during the intra-operative period was not studied. Hence, the nature of factors affecting this movement were inferred from where tumor cells were located at the end of surgery. This is analogous to watching only the opening and closing scenes of a movie and guessing the intervening storyline (Allardyce et al. 1996, 1997, 1998; Mathew et al. 1997).

Gamma camera ("real time") analysis is a rapid and sensitive form of repeated macro-autoradiography. The advantage of the gamma camera was that repeated measures could be performed on the intact living animal during laparoscopy. Thus, cell movement was analyzed as it occurred. To use the previous analogy; the 'movie' was watched from start to finish, making the storyline more understandable.

Small animal models need to be closely evaluated in the light of the findings from these porcine studies. The low rate of aerosolization witnessed above is in contrast to results from well designed studies indicating that aerosolization may be an issue only in the small animal model (Mathew et al. 1997). It may be that the small volume of the peritoneal cavity in rodents is enough to alter gas flow dynamics to give this picture which cannot be effectively reproduced in the large animal model.

Radiolabelled Cell Models in the Pig

Results have demonstrated that, with the abdomen at rest, radiolabelled LIM 1215 diffused throughout the peritoneal cavity over a 2 h-period. The mechanisms of movement include gravity, as alluded to by Allardyce et al. (1997). This movement may be enhanced by: anatomical factors such as the presence of paracolic gutters acting as channels of movement. Other factors, such as peristalsis of bowel loops, changes in the intra-abdominal pressure by respiration, and capillary action of fluid between loops of bowel, may play an additional role. The major difference in intraperitoneal radiolabelled LIM 1215 movement between the peritoneal cavity at rest and the peritoneal cavity undergoing CO_2 insufflation was the differential rate of movement to the left and right upper quadrants. The true significance of this movement differential is currently unclear. The 1–2 l/min flow of CO_2 gas across the visceral surface may slow down the countercurrent movement of radiolabelled LIM 1215 cells. There was a suggestion that the CO_2 flow from the midline camera trocar to the left iliac fossa trocar may have reduced radiolabelled LIM 1215 movement from the pelvis to the LUQ with preferential movement to the RUQ. When the abdomen was not insufflated, there was preferential movement of labelled LIM 1215 to the LUQ (Fig. 8.1).

When free blood was mixed with radiolabelled LIM 1215 cells in the absence of insufflation, movement was influenced by the same factors listed above. Once again the flow of cells was from the pelvis to the upper abdomen. One possible explanation may be that capillary action was drawing up the blood between loops of the coiled pig caecum. The countercurrent effect may not have been seen because the blood coagulum was stickier than the culture medium used in the non-blood studies (and hence more difficult to move with the insufflating current).

Despite the different methodologies used by Allardyce et al. (1997) and our studies, there was some agreement between the results. Firstly, the mechanical lifting devices used in the absence of insufflation by Allardyce et al. (1997) did not eliminate cell dispersion. This was confirmed by the observation that radiolabelled LIM 1215 cells dispersed widely throughout the peritoneal cavity during the initial period of no insufflation. Secondly, Allardyce et al. (1996) showed that aerosolization was unlikely to be the mechanism for tumor cell dispersion and tumor cell implantation at the port-site. This was supported by the uncommon event of LIM 1215 cells on the filters through which vented CO_2 had travelled.

Contamination of laparoscopic instruments by malignant cells was notable in Hewett et al.'s study and confirmed previous findings that LIM 1215 cells do adhere to laparoscopic instruments used for manipulation and resection of colon (Allardyce et al. 1996, 1997; Hewett et al. 1999). In the real time studies, the left flank ("active") trocar was the main manipulating port. As expected, the left flank trocar showed LIM 1215 contamination in the majority of procedures (Table 8.1). Allardyce et al. (1996) revealed that a greater number and proportion of chromium labelled cells were deposited in the port-site used by the operator and camera operator compared with other port-sites. In Hewett et al.'s study no radiolabelled LIM 1215 cells were identified in the camera trocar when insufflation was used (with or without free blood) but this trocar was kept relatively still during the above procedures. In contrast, there was frequent movement of the camera and camera port during the operative procedure as was the case during Allardyce's study (1996). The passage of an instrument through a trocar, and movement of the trocar within the abdominal wall, seem to be key factors in trocar and port-site contamination. When blood and LIM 1215 cells were combined within the peritoneal cavity without insufflation, all trocars and port-sites were found to be contaminated with LIM 1215 cells the study (Hewett et al. 1999). It would appear that LIM 1215 cells within a blood matrix became more adherent to the port-site, particularly when the trocars and port-sites had been in contact with the peritoneal cavity contents for an extended period of time. This scenario occurs in a clinical setting when desufflation takes place during laparoscopic-assisted colectomies whilst the resected colon is exteriorised.

Segmental Colonic Resection Studies

A study of open and laparoscopic-assisted colonic resection using a real time radiolabelled tumor cell model was developed. As expected, intraperitoneally placed LIM 1215 dispersed widely (throughout the abdominal cavity and onto gloves, instruments and trocars) during both laparoscopic-assisted and open surgery. Port-sites closest to the initial inoculum had higher rates of LIM 1215 contamination (Fig. 8.2). When radiolabelled LIM 1215 were disseminated, the linear stapler used during open surgery was less contaminated than the linear stapler used during laparoscopic surgery (Table 8.2). This may reflect the more complex manoeuvring (and hence greater risk of contamination) involved during laparoscopic-assisted surgery. Conversely, the gloves used during laparoscopic-assisted surgery were less contaminated than the gloves used during open surgery, which reflects the more direct handling of the intraperitoneal contents during open surgery. Wound edge/extraction site contamination with radiolabelled LIM 1215 was detected during both open and laparoscopic-assisted surgeries when radiolabelled LIM 1215 were placed intraperitoneally. This finding agrees with Allardyce et al. (1998). There was no difference in the proportion of radiolabelled LIM 1215 cells found on the wound edges between open and laparoscopic-assisted surgery when radiolabelled LIM 1215 were placed intra-peritoneally. None of the intra-luminally placed radiolabelled LIM 1215 cells were detected on instruments, gloves, wound edges, port-sites or trocars when both open and laparoscopic-assisted surgery was used (Table 8.2). This contrasts with Allardyce et al. (1998) who used a more sensitive cell detection system (best cell resolution ~30 cells). For Hewett et al.'s 1996 study, the median cell resolution was 500 and 4 times more radiolabelled cells than Allardyce et al. (1998) were used. Thus, any spilled radiolabelled LIM 1215 cells from the colonic lumen should have been seen in the real time study. Also, Allardyce et al. used a complete laparoscopic approach (which involves complex intraperitoneal manipulation of the colon), whereas a laparoscopic-assisted technique (with less handling of bowel) was used in the real time study (Allardyce et al. 1996, 1997, 1998). Spillage of intra-luminally placed tumor cells, from the proximal stump, would occur when the anvil is placed. With a total laparoscopic approach, this spillage would be into the peritoneal cavity. When a laparoscopic-assisted approach is used, any spillage would be onto the surrounding skin and wound edges. This spillage was not detected in the current study. This suggests that laparoscopic-assisted colonic resection, cf. total laparoscopic colonic resection, causes less spillage of intraluminal radiolabelled tumor cells.

Conclusions

Tumor cells needed to be exfoliated by some means (trauma from the surgeon) before port-site recurrence occurred. Aerosolization of tumor cells only occurred during grossly contaminated and prolonged surgery, and did not act as a major mode of tumor cell transport. Contamination of surgical instruments and trocars acted as a mode of tumor cell transport. Studies suggest that possibly poor operative technique and not the type of surgery may lead to tumor cell exfoliation. The delivery of cells from the primary tumor to a port-site is clearly a key point in port-site recurrence of malignancy.

Based on the research to date, the proposed mechanisms for the movement of tumor cells from the primary tumor to a port-site during laparoscopic surgery are as follows:

- Laparoscopic instruments need to breach the tumor, liberating cells into the peritoneal cavity and onto laparoscopic instruments
- Tumor cells are carried across the peritoneal cavity by peritoneal fluid currents
- These fluid currents are influenced by physical factors
- Laparoscopic instruments and trocars are vectors of tumor cell transport
- Circumstances where the port-site is brought into prolonged contact with free cells (such as during insufflation) will facilitate port-site contamination
- Presence of free blood in the abdominal cavity might facilitate cell dispersion

References

Allardyce RA, Morreau P, Bagshaw PF (1996) Tumor cell distribution following laparoscopic colectomy in a porcine model. Dis Colon Rectum 39: 47–52

Allardyce RA, Morreau P, Bagshaw PF (1997) Operative factors affecting tumor cell distribution following laparoscopic colectomy in a porcine model. Dis Colon Rectum 40: 939–945

Allardyce RA, Morreau PN, Frizelle FA, Bagshaw PF (1998) Tumor cell wound distribution after colectomy in a porcine model. Aust N Z J Surg 68: 363–366

Allendorf JD, Bessler M, Whelan RL (1997) A murine model of laparoscopic-assisted intervention. Surg Endosc 11: 622–624

Bessler M, Whelan RL, Halverson A, Allendorf JDF, Nowygrod R, Treat MR (1996) Controlled trial of laparoscopic-assisted vs open colon resection in a porcine model. Surg End osc 10: 732–735

Bouvy ND, Marquet RL, Jeekel H, Bonjer HJ (1996a) Impact of gas(less) laparoscopy and laparotomy on peritoneal tumor growth and abdominal wall metastases. Ann Surg 224: 694–700; discussion 700–701

Bouvy ND, Marquet RL, Jeekel H, Bonjer J (1996b) Gasless laparoscopy versus CO_2 pneumoperitoneum in relation to the development of abdominal wall metastases (Abstract). Surg Endosc 10: 210

Hewett PJ, Thomas WM, King G, Eaton M (1996) Intraperitoneal cell movement during abdominal carbon dioxide insufflation and laparoscopy. An in vivo model. Dis Colon Rectum 39: 62–66

Hewett PJ, Texler ML, Anderson D, Chatterton B (1999) In vivo real time analysis of intraperitoneal radio-labelled tumor cell movement during laparoscopy, Dis Colon Rectum [in press]

Jones DB, Guo LW, Reinhard MK, Soper NJ, Philpott GW, Connett J, Fleshman JW (1995) Impact of pneumoperitoneum on trocar site implantation of colon cancer in hamster model. Dis Colon Rectum 38: 1182–1188

Knolmayer TJ, Asbun HJ, Bowyer M (1996) An experimental model of cellular aerosolization during laparoscopic surgery (abstract). Surg Endosc 10: 181

Lawrie H (1906). Cancer contagion and innoculation, B M J 1: 198

Mathew G, Watson DI, Ellis T, De Young N, Rofe AM, Jamieson GG (1997) The effect of laparoscopy of the movement of tumor cells and metastasis to surgical wounds. Surg Endosc 11: 1163–1166

Nduka CC, Darzi A (1997) Port-site recurrence in patients undergoing laparoscopy for gastrointestinal malignancy (letter). Br J Surg 84: 583

Poste G, Fidler IJ (1980) The pathogenesis of cancer metastasis. Nature 283: 139–146

Reissman P, Teoh TA, Skinner K, Burns JW, Wexner SD (1996) Adhesion formation after laparoscopic anterior resection in a porcine model: a pilot study. Surg Laparosc Endosc 6: 136–139

Texler ML, King G, Hewett P (1997) Intraperitoneal tumor cell movement with heated-humidified insufflating CO_2: a porcine model (Abstract) Aust N Z J Surg 67 (Suppl.): A28

Thomas CG (1961) Tumor cell contamination of the surgical wound: experimental and clinical observation. Ann Surg 153: 697–704

Watson DI, Mathew G, Ellis T, Baigrie CF, Rofe AM, Jamieson GG (1997) Gasless laparoscopy may reduce the risk of port-site recurrences following laparoscopic tumor surgery. Arch Surg 132: 166–168; discussion 169

Whelan R, Sellers G, Allendorf J, Laird D, Bessler M, Nowygrod R, Treat M (1996) An in vitro model of pneumoperitoneum fails to demonstrate aerosolization of tumor cells (abstract). Surg Endosc 10: 181

CHAPTER 9

Pathogenesis: Local Effects in the Wound in Animal Studies

C.A. Jacobi, H.J. Bonjer

Introduction

The exact mechanisms of the development of port-site recurrences are not totally understood yet, instrumental manipulation and mechanical tumor cell spillage seem to play the major role in this rare complication. Port-site recurrences have also been reported both in advanced tumor stages and after resection of colon cancer in UICC stage I (Fingerhut 1995; Lauroy et al. 1994). Therefore, changes in the peritoneal environment during laparoscopy might also influence intra- and extraperitoneal tumor growth during laparoscopy and pneumoperitoneum (Bonjer et al. 1998), carbon dioxide has been shown to stimulate tumor cell growth in different animal models (Bouvy et al. 1996, 1998; Jacobi et al. 1997; Jones et al. 1995) and seems to be also partly responsible for metastases mainly in the trocar sites. Furthermore, local ischemia in the port-sites has been reported to cause enhanced tumor growth in animal models (Jacobi et al. 1997; Tseng et al. 1998). It seems that increased necrosis and release of intracellular cytokines as well as the suppression of local immunological (Jacobi et al. 1999) and mesothelial defense (Kopernik et al. 1998) is supporting the adherence and the growth of free intraperitoneal tumor cells. As shown in further experimental studies, changes in the structure of the peritoneum are also caused by insufflation of carbon dioxide (Bloechle et al. 1999). In laparoscopic procedures with either warm or cold carbon dioxide, the number of microvilli decreased, the mesothelial cells were rounded up and intercellular contact was partly disturbed.

The local changes demonstrated during laparoscopic surgery have to be included in the discussion of this technique in cancer patients. Results of experimental models are summarized and discussed in regard to their clinical relevance.

Experimental Tumor Models

Tumor cell suspension models (Fig. 9.1) have been used in rats, mice, hamsters and pigs to evaluate the possible benefits or negative effects of pneumoperitoneum in cancer surgery (Bouvy et al. 1996, 1998; Jacobi et al. 1997a,b, 1998; Jones et al. 1995; Mathew et al. 1997a,b; Reymond et al. 1999). Although these models can be used to simulate intraoperative tumor spillage during laparoscopy, the number of free tumor cells after instrumental manipulation in patients is still unknown. Furthermore, the number of injected cells does certainly influence the development of port-site recurrences and controversial results might be the consequence (Wu et al. 1998). Nevertheless, the influences of carbon dioxide, acidosis and elevated intraperitoneal pressure as well as the effects of open procedures on in vivo tumor cell growth can be investigated in these models. Other models used subcutaneous or retroperitoneal tumor cell injection as well as solid tumor models in the spleen, the liver, the caecum, and renal capsule (Allendorf et al. 1995; Bouvy et al. 1998; Giuffrida et al. 1997; Le Moine et al. 1998; Lee et al. 1998a,b). Instrumental manipulation can be evaluated during open and laparoscopic procedures in these models, but resection of tumor-bearing organs might also lead to changes in immunological (spleen) or renal (kidney) functions. A solid tumor model of a colonic carcinoma does not exist. Furthermore, all models have been established in rodents with different immunological functions and perioperative changes compared to humans. Therefore, results of tumor models may be different from clinical findings in cancer patients.

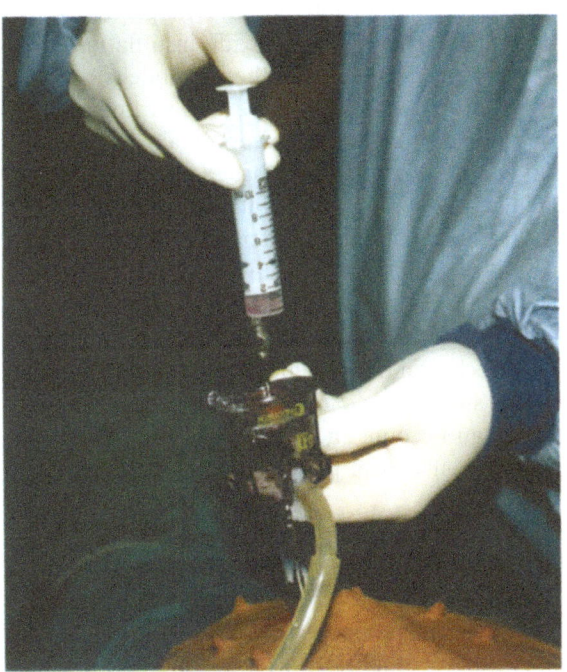

Fig. 9.1. Most experimental models used in port-site recurrences research are cell suspension models, where tumor cells are injected directly into the peritoneal cavity

Chimney Effect and Aerosolization of Tumor Cells

Because of insufflation and exsufflation of gas during laparoscopy, possible aerosolization and movement of tumor cells have been proposed to cause implantation of tumor cells into the trocar incision. Although it seemed logical that this so-called chimney (Fig. 9.2) effect can explain tumor cell movements into abdominal incisions, aerosolization of tumor cells has only been partly proven in some experiments (Knolmayer et al. 1997; Mathew et al. 1997a,b; Tseng et al. 1998). Because all models used tumor cell suspension models, it seems that contamination with cell contaminated fluids was investigated rather than the so-called chimney effect. Other investigations showed that instrumental contamination (Fig. 9.3) seems to be responsible for tumor cell movement within the abdominal cavity rather than the aerosolization of tumor cells by the insufflated gas (Hewett et al. 1996; Thomas et al. 1996). Whelan et al. could nicely demonstrate that aerosol of tumor cells is not likely to form in a high pressure CO_2 environment in several experiments in vitro and in vivo (Whelan et al. 1996). These results were confirmed by Allardyce et al., who found no role of CO_2 insufflation in the aerosolization of tumor cells

in a porcine model (Allardyce et al. 1996). Clinical data about the movements of peritoneal tumor cells and their aerosolization are rare. In a clinical study, Champault found cells in the smoke after coagulation during laparoscopy, but tumor cells were neither analysed nor found in this study (Champault et al. 1997). Instrumental contamination and cells in the peritoneal lavage were found to be important for intraperitoneal tumor spillage while no tumor cells were found in the aerosol in patients with pancreatic cancer and diagnostic laparoscopy (Reymond et al. 1997). Looking at the low incidence of port-site recurrences in recent clinical trials with a large number of patients undergoing laparoscopic colon cancer resection, the role of aerosolization of tumor cells in the development of metastases seems to be of lesser importance (Balli et al. 1999; Fleshman et al. 1996; Franklin et al. 1996; Johnstone et al. 1996; Lacy et al. 1995; Milsom et al. 1998; Volz et al. 1996; Wexner and Cohen 1995; Wexner and Latulippe 1997).

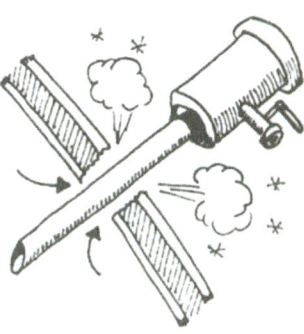

Fig. 9.2. Cellular contaminations at port-sites are most likely explained by contaminated fluids rather than by the so-called chimney effect

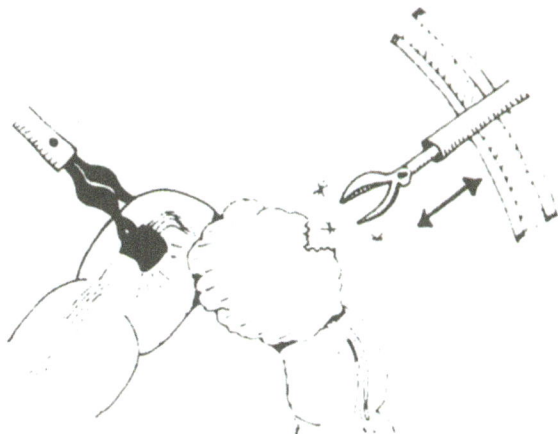

Fig. 9.3. Instrumental contamination seems to be mainly responsible for tumor cells movement within the abdominal cavity during cancer laparoscopy

Influence of Different Gases and Elevated Intraperitoneal Pressure

The gas utilized in laparoscopic surgery has been suggested to influence tumor growth and cause the development of port-site recurrences. Experimental studies about the effect of different insufflation gases have reported conflicting results. Jacobi et al. could demonstrate that carbon dioxide resulted in an increased growth of colonic cancer cells in vitro, ex vivo, and in vivo (Jacobi et al. 1997). These results have been confirmed by other authors (Bouvy et al. 1996, 1998; Dorrance et al. 1996; Jones et al. 1995; Watson et al. 1997; Wu et al. 1997). On the other hand, Neuhaus et al. could not find a significant difference of tumor growth after carbon dioxide insufflation in comparison to the control group (Neuhaus et al. 1998). These differences might be partly explained by using different cell lines, different amounts of intraperitoneal tumor cells, and the tumor cell biology. Beside carbon dioxide, helium has been used as an alternative gas in experimental tumor models and has been shown to have either inhibitory effects or no effects on tumor growth (Jacobi et al. 1997, 1998; Neuhaus et al. 1998) and therefore might be useful for cancer surgery. But, low solubility of helium raised the question whether helium is increasing the effects of gas embolism during laparoscopy and accidental injury of large venous vessels. Previous experimental investigations did not show any significant changes in cardiopulmonary functions after vessel injury during pneumoperitoneum with either carbon dioxide or helium (Jacobi et al. 1999). Therefore, the incidence of gas embolism during laparoscopy and accidental injury of venous vessels seems to be very low. Because of acidosis, possible cardiopulmonary dysfunction and stimulation of tumor cell growth during carbon dioxide insufflation, helium should be used and evaluated in clinical studies.

Nevertheless, it has been demonstrated that increased intraperitoneal pressure is correlated with promotion of subcutaneous and intraperitoneal tumor growth in a rat model (Jacobi et al. 1998). In comparison to these results elevated pressure during incubation of colonic cancer cells in vitro caused suppression of tumor cell growth. Thus, in vivo effects might be explained by perioperative immune depression caused by higher intraperitoneal pressures. In order to avoid elevated pressure and insufflation of gases, gasless laparoscopy has been used in different tumor models (Bouvy et al. 1996, 1998; Mathew et al. 1996, 1997; Watson et al. 1997). Tumor growth was significantly lower after gasless procedures than after carbon dioxide insufflation in all experimental models. But, the rat models that were used for these experiments are hardly comparable to the clinical situation. The abdominal wall of the rat can be lifted without any tissue trauma or local ischemia and almost all operations are feasible with this technique in rodents. In patients, lifting systems are still causing local pressure and tissue trauma at the abdominal wall and technical problems are known to make laparoscopic resections difficult. Thus, technical improvements in lifting systems for gasless surgery have to be realized before this technique can become an alternative minimal invasive procedure in cancer patients.

Local Wound Conditions, Ischemia and Local Necrosis

From experimental work in conventional surgery it is well known that local wound conditions are important for the development of metastases. It has been demonstrated that intracardial, intraperitoneal, and intraluminal injection of tumor cells caused a significant 1000-fold enhancement of growth of tumor cells in colonic anastomosis and laparotomy wounds (Skipper et al. 1989). Wound conditions in trocar sites have not been clearly investigated yet, although it might be that local factors, like ischemia and necrosis with release of growth stimulating factors, do influence local tumor adherence and growth.

Tseng et al. reported that local ischemia caused significant increase of tumor metastases after laparoscopy in rats (Tseng et al. 1998). Colon cancer cells were injected into the peritoneum and a significant higher amount of tumor was observed in the trocar that had previously been crushed using a clamp to induce local ischemia compared to noncrushed sites. Jacobi et al. showed a significant difference between tumor growth at abdominal incisions when electrocautery was used compared to a normal scalpel in a rat cancer model (Jacobi et al. 1997). Both authors pointed out that local ischemia or necrosis might be important for the attachment of tumor cells at port-sites. Furthermore, necrosis and release of intracellular cytokines and other factors might stimulate tumor growth at abdominal incisions in these models. Nevertheless, the exact local ptO_2 and local ischemia at trocar sites have not been investigated. Furthermore, local concentration of cytokines or number of present cells need to be analysed in the future.

Samel et al. investigated bowel microcirculation because it has been thought that elevated intraperitoneal pressure leads to a decrease of celiac and mesenteric blood flow resulting in intravascular stasis and possible thromboembolic complications (Samel et al. 1998). The decrease of blood flow might also cause ischemia which has been discussed to enhance the development of tumor metastases. Microcirculation was measured by intravital epiluminescence-fluorescent-microscopy (IVM) using a peritoneal cavity expander with a cylindrical chamber to exteriorize a segment of the distal jejunum, an optical window and a muzzle for gas insufflation. Pneumoperitoneum was performed with carbon dioxide over 60 min with either 10 mmHg or 15 mmHg. The control group underwent no pneumoperitoneum and was taken to evaluate physiologic mucosal microcirculation. Investigation of mucosal microcirculation was performed before and 60 min after carbon dioxide insufflation. While pneumoperitoneum with an intraperitoneal pressure of 10 mmHg did not impair mucosal microcirculation, a significant decrease was found at a pressure of 15 mmHg. This decrease was associated with mucosal ischemia and necrotic epithelial cells. The blood flow of the liver has also been reported to be significantly decreased during laparoscopy with carbon dioxide at a pressure of 15 mmHg when compared to control group (Gutt et al. 1997). This decrease of blood flow was correlated with a decrease of phagocytotic function of liver macrophages in rats which might be important for the clearance of tumor cells in the portal system in cancer patients.

Local Effects on Mesothelial Cells and Peritoneal Structure

Bloechle et al. demonstrated that different techniques during surgical procedures influence the peritoneal structure and mesothelial cells (Bloechle et al. 1999). A total of 100 patients underwent peritoneal biopsy at the beginning and end of the operation. The patients were either operated by laparotomy ($n=25$), gasless laparoscopy ($n=25$), laparoscopy with warm (38 °C) carbon dioxide ($n=25$), or cold (21 °C) carbon dioxide ($n=25$). Electron microscopic examinations showed that the microvilli stayed intact, mesothelial cells kept their form, intercellular contact was not disturbed, and junctions were closed during gasless and open surgery. In laparoscopic procedures with either warm or cold carbon dioxide, the number of microvilli decreased, the

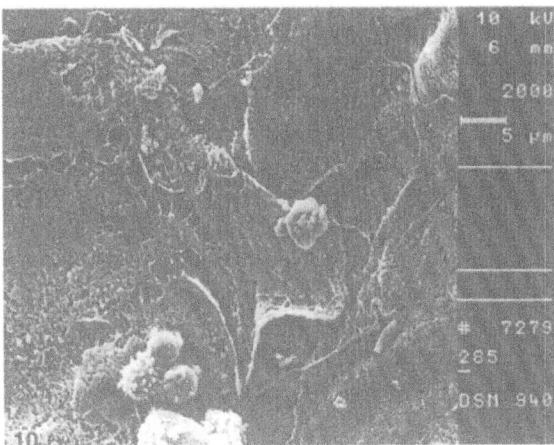

Fig. 9.4. Severe morphological changes in the peritoneal mesothelial layer were observed after CO_2 pneumoperitoneum (reproduced from Bloechle et al. 1999)

mesothelial cells were rounded up and intercellular contact was partly disturbed. While the basal membrane stayed intact, there were denuded areas caused by disconnected mesothelial cells. The authors concluded that carbon dioxide damages the mesothelial cells as well as the cell junctions which might explain tumor cell implantation during and after laparoscopic procedures (Fig. 9.4).

Kopernik et al. could further demonstrate that carbon dioxide pneumoperitoneum leads to a significant decrease of cytokine production and mitochondrial activity of human peritoneal mesothelial cells (Kopernik et al. 1998). Furthermore, disruption of the peritoneal surface seems to increase tumor cell adherence as shown by Goldstein (1993) in a mouse model. Similar results were found by Farrell et al. (1999). After closure of the port-sites in a 2-layer technique (fascia and skin) the incidence of port-site recurrences could be significantly reduced in a colon cancer rat model. Thus, changes of peritoneal structure and local cytokine release of mesothelial cells might also be discussed in the field of port-site recurrences.

Changes of Intra- and Extracellular pH and Calcium Levels in Peritoneal Macrophages or Tumor Cells

One possible mechanism of the promotion of tumor cell growth might be the changes of intracellular calcium and pH levels in tumor cells as well as peritoneal macrophages. It has been demonstrated that stimulation of cell growth is associated with increased intracellular calcium metabolism. Furthermore, significant intracellular acidosis might change the proliferation index of malignant cells. Wildbrett and Jacobi could demonstrate that cells of a colon adenocarcinoma DHD/K12/TRb and peritoneal macrophages showed significant changes of either pH or calcium levels after incubation with the different gases (Wildbrett and Jacobi 1998). While helium did not cause significant changes of intracellular free calcium, carbon dioxide incubation caused a significant increase of calcium levels in tumor cells and macrophages. The increase in tumor cells was significantly higher compared to the peritoneal macrophages. Intracellular pH levels decreased from 7.4 to 6.2 after carbon dioxide incubation and increased from 7.4 to 9.0 in the helium group. The decrease of intracellular pH levels and the increase of free calcium were associated with a significant stimulation of tumor cell growth in the carbon dioxide group over 5 days. The authors hypothesized that stimulation of tumor growth caused by carbon dioxide may be due to a significant increase of cell metabolism and intracellular acidosis.

Kuntz et al. found significant changes of pH levels in the abdominal cavity, blood and subcutaneous tissue after laparoscopy with carbon dioxide compared to helium, xenon, air and N_2O (Kuntz 1998). While levels decreased only slightly in peripheral blood, there were marked decreases in pH levels in the subcutaneous fat tissue as well as in the peritoneal fluids. Furthermore, pH levels were lower after laparoscopy with higher pressures (3, 6 and 9 mm Hg) when compared to the control group (0 mm Hg) which could be explained by local ischemia. Volz et al investigated pathophysiologic features of pneumoperitoneum in a swine model (Volz et al. 1996) and demonstrated a significant correlation between elevated intraperitoneal pressure during carbon dioxide pneumoperitoneum and systemic as well as local acidosis. Local pH levels, which might be important for the development of metastases, were again significantly lower than systemic levels. Unfortunately, neither tumor growth nor development of port-site recurrences were investigated in both studies. Thus, the correlation of increased tumor growth and acidosis still remains theoretical.

Effects on Peritoneal Macrophages and Cytokine Production

The function of peritoneal macrophages and the local immune response have been discussed to be influenced by carbon dioxide pneumoperitoneum and thus could also be due to the development of perioperative metastases (Fig. 9.5). Puttick et al. evaluated cancer cell lysis of peritoneal macrophages after gas incubation with 100% helium or 100% carbon dioxide (Puttick et al. 1998). Carbon dioxide led to a significant decrease of cancer cell lysis while helium had no significant influence on cell lysis. The viability of the cells were not affected by either helium or carbon dioxide incubation. A comparison to air, simulating the situation during laparotomy, was not performed in this experiment. Thus, it remains unclear whether open surgery is causing similar changes in cancer cell lysis.

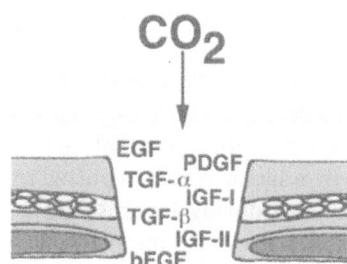

Fig. 9.5. Many cytokines involved in wound repair have been shown to play a role in tumor growth also. The influence of CO_2 and of pressure on cellular cytokine secretion is still unclear

The local immunological defenses against tumor cells after laparoscopic and conventional surgery has been reported by Sietses and Cuesta in 1998. They found a significant suppression of monocyte-mediated cytotoxicity against SW 948 colon cancer cells after laparotomy when compared to laparoscopic procedures. Similar results were found by Lee and coworkers reporting a significant lower apoptotic rate of tumor cells after laparotomy compared to laparoscopy in rats (Lee et al. 1998a). Although the mechanisms of these phenomena remain unclear, it appears that immunological defense against tumor cells may be better preserved in cancer patients undergoing laparoscopic resection than conventional resection.

Beside macrophages, other immunocompetent cells may also be influenced by laparoscopy and carbon dioxide insufflation. Splenic lymphocyte proliferation was significantly lower after laparotomy when compared to either carbon dioxide pneumoperitoneum or control group in mice (Lee et al. 1998b). In a second experiment the authors could demonstrate that immune suppression in this model was not caused by carbon dioxide insufflation but related to abdominal incision length (Lee et al. 1998a). These results are in contrast to the results of Jacobi, who found significant increase of tumor growth after laparotomy and laparoscopy with room air compared to carbon dioxide and control group in a rat model (Jacobi et al. 1997). Furthermore, Watson et al. demonstrated a significant increase in peritoneal tissue macrophage release of superoxide and tumor necrosis factor after laparotomy and laparoscopy with air when compared to control and laparoscopy with CO_2 (Watson et al. 1995). Peritoneal macrophage FITC-candida albicans ingestion was further only decreased after laparoscopy with air and laparotomy. Thus, intraperitoneal air also seems to influence the local immune response.

The direct correlation between tumor growth and systemic immunological changes has been investigated by Jacobi, using a colon adenocarcinoma DHD/K12/TRb model in BD IX rats (Jacobi et al. 1998). Subcutaneous and intraperitoneal tumor growth as well as immunological changes (peripheral leukocyte subpopulations, plasma levels of TNF-α and IL-10) were determined after insufflation with either carbon dioxide or helium and in a control group. Subcutaneous tumor growth was promoted by carbon dioxide (99 ± 55 mg) ($p < 0.01$) compared to helium (40 ± 41 mg) and the control group (36 ± 33 mg). Total intraperitoneal tumor weight was 718 ± 690 mg in the carbon dioxide group compared to helium (549 ± 233 mg) and the control group (521 ± 221 mg). While peripheral leukocyte subpopulations only differed between the laparoscopic groups and the control group, TNF-α plasma levels were significantly decreased and IL-10 plasma levels significantly increased in the carbon dioxide group compared to helium and control group in the postoperative course. Thus, it seems that carbon dioxide pneumoperitoneum actually modulates immunological function of macrophages as confirmed by Puttick (Puttick et al. 1998). Nevertheless, a comparison to conventional laparotomy was not performed in this study.

Cytokine response of peritoneal macrophages after pneumoperitoneum with carbon dioxide has been evaluated by different groups showing controversial results. Puttick et al. reported that spontaneous and stimulated production of TNF-α were significantly suppressed after helium and carbon diox-

ide incubation compared to the control group (Puttick et al. 1998). In contrast to this, Jacobi et al. found a significant increased IL-1β release of peritoneal macrophages after carbon dioxide insufflation compared to helium and control group (Jacobi et al. 1999). It seems that insufflation of carbon dioxide and additional acidosis has different effects on the production and release of intracellular cytokines.

Conclusions

Laparoscopic procedures in cancer patients and the development of port-site recurrences have raised some substantial questions which are in general important for oncological surgery. Although the problem of port-site recurrences is mainly related to the surgeon, the technique, and manipulation of the tumor-bearing organ, some other factors, which are related to laparoscopy itself, have been demonstrated to influence tumor growth. The possible stimulation of tumor cell growth and suppression of local immune defense by carbon dioxide, as shown in many experimental studies, can be avoided by the alternative use of helium. Therefore, helium should be evaluated in prospective randomized clinical trials. New therapeutic strategies, including instillation of cytotoxic and immune modulating agents in combination with laparoscopy and different gases, were reported to strongly inhibit tumor growth in experimental investigations. Nevertheless, perioperative pathophysiological and immunological changes caused by either open or laparoscopic procedures have to be further evaluated to understand the tumor disease under the conditions of operative intervention. The results of these studies may help to create new therapeutic strategies, including nonsurgical treatment.

References

Allardyce R, Morreau P, Bagshaw P (1996) Tumor cell distribution following laparoscopic colectomy in a porcine model. Dis Colon Rectum 39: 47–52

Allendorf JDF, Bessler M, Kayton ML, Osterling SD, Treat MR, Nowygord R, Whelan RL (1995) Increased tumor establishment and growth after laparotomy vs laparoscopy in a murine model. Arch Surg 130: 649–653

Balli JE, Franklin ME, Almeida JA, Glass JL, Kazantsev G, Diaz JA (1999) How to prevent port-site recurrence in laparoscopic colorectal surgery. Surg Endosc 13 (Suppl 1): 4

Bloechle C, Kluth D, Holstein AF, Emmermann A, Strate T, Zornig C, Izbicki JR (1999) A pneumoperitoneum perpetuates severe damage to the ultrastructural integrity of parietal peritoneum in gastric perforation-induced peritonitis in rats. Surg Endosc 13:683–688

Bonjer HJ, Gutt CN, Hubens G, Krahenbuhl L, Kim SH, Bouvy ND, Tseng L, Paolucci V, Whelan R, Jacobi CA (1998) Port-site recurrences in laparoscopic surgery. First workshop on experimental laparoscopic surgery, Frankfurt 1997. Surg Endosc 12: 1102–1103

Bouvy ND, Marquet RL, Jeekel H, Bonjer HJ (1996) Impact of gas(less) laparoscopy and laparotomy on peritoneal tumor growth and abdominal wall metastases. Ann Surg 224 (6): 694–701

Bouvy ND, Giuffrida MC, Tseng LN, Steyerberg EW, Marquet RL, Jeekel H, Bonjer HJ (1998) Effects of carbon dioxide pneumoperitoneum, air pneumoperitoneum, and gasless laparoscopy on body weight and tumor growth. Arch Surg 133 (6): 652–656

Champault G, Taffinder N, Ziol M, Riskalla H, Catheline JMC (1997) Cells are present in the smoke created during laparoscopic surgery. Br J Surg 84: 993–995

Dorrance HR, Oein K, O'Dwyer PJ (1996) Laparoscopy promotes tumor growth in an animal model (Abstract). Surg Endosc 10: 559

Farrell TM, Johnson AB, Metreveli RE, Smith CD, Hunter JG (1999) Fascial closure limits metastasis after pneumoperitoneum. Surg Endosc 13: 33

Fingerhut A (1995) Laparoscopic colectomy. The French experience. In: Jaeger R, Wexner SD (eds) Laparoscopic colorectal surgery. Churchill Livingstone, New York, pp 253–257

Fleshman JW, Nelson H, Peters WR, Kim HC, Larach S, Boorse R, Ambroze W, Leggett P, Bleday R, Stryker S, Christenson B, Wexner S, Senagore A, Rattner D, Sutton J, Fine AP (1996) Early results of laparoscopic surgery for colorectal cancer. Retrospective analysis of 372 patients treated by Clinical Outcomes of Surgical Therapy (COST) Study group. Dis Colon Rectum 39: 53–58

Franklin ME, Rosenthal D, Abrego-Medina D, Glass JL, Norem R, Diaz A (1996) Prospective comparison of open versus laparoscopic colon surgery for carcinoma: five year results. Dis Colon Rectum 39: 35–46

Giuffrida MC, Marquet RL, Kazemier G, Wittich P, Bouvy ND, Bruining HA, Bonjer HJ (1997) Laparoscopic splenectomy and nephrectomy in a rat model. Description of a new technique. Surg Endosc 11: 491–494

Goldstein DS, Lu ML, Hattori T (1993) Inhibition of peritoneal tumor cell implantation: model for laparoscopic cancer surgery. J Endourol 7: 237–241

Gutt CN, Heinz P, Kaps W, Paolucci V (1997) The phagocytosis activity during conventional and laparoscopic operations in the rat. A preliminary study. Surg Endosc 11: 899–901

Hewett PJ, Thomas WM, King G, Eaton M (1996) Intraabdominal cell movement during abdominal carbon dioxide insufflation and laparoscopy. Dis Colon Rectum 39: 7–13

Hofer SOP, Molema G, Hermens RAEC, Wanebo HJ, Reichner JS, Hoekstra HJ (1999) The effect of surgical wounding on tumor development. Eur J Surg Oncol 25:231–243

Jacobi CA, Ordemann J, Böhm B, Zieren HU, Liebenthal C, Volk HD, Müller JM (1997a) The influence of laparotomy and laparoscopy with different gases on tumor growth in a rat model. Surg Endosc 11: 618–621

Jacobi CA, Sabat R, Böhm B, Zieren HU, Volk HD, Müller JM (1997b) Pneumoperitoneum with carbon dioxide stimulates growth of malignant colonic cells. Surgery 121: 72–78

Jacobi CA, Ordemann J, Bohm B, Zieren HU, Sabat R, Muller JM (1997c) Inhibition of peritoneal tumor cell growth and implantation in laparoscopic surgery in a rat model. Am J Surg 174: 359-363

Jacobi CA, Wenger F, Sabat R, Volk T, Ordemann J, Müller JM (1998a) The impact of laparoscopy with carbon dioxide versus helium on immunologic function and tumor growth in a rat tumor model. Dig Surg 15: 110–116

Jacobi CA, Ordemann J, Wenger F, Gutt C, Sabat R, Zieren HU, Müller JM (1998b) The impact of elevated intraabdominal pressure during laparoscopy on tumor growth and trocar metastases in a rat model. Br J Surg 85: 1419–1422

Jacobi CA, Junghans T, Peter F, Ordemann J, Müller JM (1999a) Gas embolism during laparoscopy with CO_2 or helium. Surg Endosc 13: 45

Jacobi CA, Peter FJ, Wenger FA, Ordemann J, Müller JM (1999b) New therapeutic strategies to avoid intra- and extraperitoneal metastases during laparoscopy. Results of a tumor model in the rat. Dig Surg (in press)

Johnstone PAS, Rohde DC, Swartz E, Fetter JE, Wexner SD (1996) Port-site recurrences after laparoscopic and thoracoscopic procedures in malignancy. J Clin Oncol 14: 1950–1956

Jones DB, Guo LW, Reinhard MK, Soper NJ, Philpott GW, Connet J, Fleshman JW (1995) Impact of pneumoperitoneum on trocar site implantation of colon cancer in hamster model. Dis Colon Rectum 38: 1182–1188

Knolmayer TJ, Egan JC, Bowyer MW, Asbun HJ (1997) Aerosolization of tumor cells during carbon dioxide insufflation. Surg Endosc 11: 204

Kopernik G, Avinoach E, Grossmann Y, Levy R, Yulzari R, Rogachev B, Douvdevani A (1998) The effect of a high partial pressure of carbon dioxide environment on metabolism and immune functions of human peritoneal cells – Relevance to carbon dioxide pneumoperitoneum. Am J Obstet Gyecol 179: 1503–1510

Kuntz C (1998) pH Alterations of blood and subcutaneous fat on exposure to different gases (CO_2, helium, air, NO_2, xenon) at different pressures. Data presented at the Second Workshop of Experimental Laparoscopic Surgery 1998, Rotterdam, Netherlands

Lacy AM, Garcia-Valdecasas JC, Taurá P, Bordas JM, Grande L, Fuster J, Cugat E, Visa J (1995) Is laparoscopic colectomy a safe procedure in synchronous colorectal carcinoma? Report of a case. Surg Laparosc Endosc 5:75–76

Lauroy J, Chaumpault G, Risk N, Boutelier P (1994) Metastatic recurrence at trocar site: should digestive cancers still be managed by laparoscopy? Br J Surg 81: 31

Le Moine MC, Navarro F, Burgel JS, Pellegrin A, Khiari AR, Pourquier D, Fabre JM, Domergue J (1998) Experimental assessment of the risk of tumor recurrence after laparoscopic surgery. Surgery 123: 427–431

Lee SW, Whelan RL, Southall JC, Bessler M (1998a) Abdominal wound tumor recurrence after open and laparoscopic-assisted splenectomy in a murine model. Dis Colon Rectum 41: 824–831

Lee SW, Gleason N, Blanco I, Bessler M, Whelan RL (1998b) Tumor cell apoptosis after laparotomy and laparoscopy. Data presented at the Second Workshop of Experimental Laparoscopic Surgery 1998, Rotterdam, Netherlands

Lee SW, Southall JC, Allendorf JD, Bessler M, Whelan RL (1998c) Traumatic handling of the tumor independent of pneumoperitoneum increases port-site implantation rate of colon cancer in a murine model. Surg Endosc 12: 828–834

Lee SW, Southall JC, Bessler M, Whelan RL (1998d) Lymphocyte proliferation in mice following laparotomy performed in a sealed CO_2 chamber is equivalent to that in mice following full laparotomy performed in room air. Data presented of the Second Workshop of Experimental Laparoscopic Surgery 1998, Rotterdam, Netherlands

Lee SW, Southall JC, Bessler M, Whelan RL (1998e) Lymphocyte proliferation following laparotomy and laparoscopy. Data presented at the Second Workshop of Experimental Laparoscopic Surgery 1998, Rotterdam, Netherlands

Mathew G, Watson DI, Rofe AM, Baigrie CF, Ellis T, Jamieson GG (1996) Wound metastases following laparoscopic and open surgery for abdominal cancer in a rat model. Br J Surg 83: 1087–1090

Mathew G, Watson DI, Ellis T, De-Young N, Rofe AM, Jamieson GG (1997a) The effect of laparoscopy on the movement of tumor cells and metastasis to surgical wounds. Surg Endosc 11(12): 1163–1166

Mathew G, Watson DI, Rofe AM, Ellis T, Jamieson GG (1997b) Adverse impact of pneumoperitoneum on intraperitoneal implantation and growth of tumor cell suspension in an experimental model. Aust N Z J Surg 67(5): 289–292

Milsom JW, Böhm B, Hammerhofer KA, Faszio VW, Steiger E, Elson P (1998) A prospective, randomized trial comparing laparoscopic versus conventional techniques in colorectal cancer surgery: a preliminary report. J Am Coll Surg 187: 46–57

Neuhaus SJ, Watson DI, Ellis T, Rowland R, Rofe AM, Pike GK, Mathey G, Jamieson GG (1998) Wound metastasis after laparoscopy with different insufflation gases. Surgery 123: 579–583

Puttick MI, Nduka CC, Yong L, Darzi A (1998) Macrophage function is suppressed by a carbon dioxide pneumoperitoneum. Data presented at the Second Workshop of Experimental Laparoscopic Surgery 1998, Rotterdam, Netherlands

Reymond MA, Wittekind CH, Jung A, Hohenberger W, Kirchner TH, Köckerling F (1997) The incidence of port-site recurrences might be reduced. Surg Endosc 11: 902–906

Reymond MA, Tannapfel A, Schneider C, Scheidbach H, Kover S, Jung A, Reck Th, Lippert H, Kockerling F (1999) Description of an intraperitoneal tumor xenograft model in the pig. Eur J Surg Oncol (in press)

Samel S, Leister I, Müller A, Stojanovic T, Neufang T, Post S, Becker H (1998) Enteral microcirculation in the pneumoperitoneum – a new rat model for intravital microscopy of mucosal capillary perfusion. Data presented at the Second Workshop of Experimental Laparoscopic Surgery 1998, Rotterdam, Netherlands

Sietses C, Cuesta MA (1998) Monocyte response to increased amount of surgical trauma, laparoscopic versus conventional clinical procedures. Data presented at the Second Workshop of Experimental Laparoscopic Surgery 1998, Rotterdam, Netherlands

Skipper D, Jeffrey MJ, Cooper AJ, Alexander P, Taylor I (1989) Enhanced growth of tumor cells in healing colonic anastomoses and laparotomy wounds. Int J Colorect Dis 4: 172–177

Thomas WM, Eaton MC, Hewett PJ (1996) A proposed model for the movements of cells within the abdominal cavity during CO_2 insufflation and laparoscopy. Aust N Z J Surg 66: 105–106

Tseng LN, Berends FJ, Wittich P, Bouvy ND, Marquet RL, Kazemier G, Bonjer HJ (1998) Port-site recurrences. Impact of local tissue trauma and gas leakage. Surg Endosc 12 (12): 1377–1380

Volz J, Köster S, Weis M, Schmidt R, Urbascheck R, Melchert F, Albrecht M (1996) Pathophysiologic features of a pneumoperitoneum at laparoscopy: a swine model. Am J Obstet Gynecol 174: 132–140

Watson DI, Redmond HP, McCarthy J, Burke PE, Hayes DB (1995) Exposure of the peritoneal cavity to air regulates early inflammatory responses to surgery in a murine model. Br J Surg 82: 1060–1065

Watson DI, Mathew G, Ellis T, Baigrie CF, Rofe AM, Jamieson GG (1997) Gasless laparoscopy may reduce the risk of port-site recurrences following laparoscopic tumor surgery. Arch Surg 132: 166–168

Wexner SD, Cohen SM (1995) Port site metastases after laparoscopic colorectal surgery for cure of malignancy. Br J Surg 82: 295–298

Wexner SD, Latulippe J-F (1997) Laparoscopic colorectal surgery and cancer. Swiss Surg 3: 266–273

Whelan RL, Sellers GJ, Allendorf BA, Laird BA, Bessler MD, Nowygrod R, Treat MR (1996) Trocar site recurrence is unlikely to result from aerosolization of tumor cells. Dis Colon Rectum 39: 7–13

Wildbrett P, Jacobi CA (1998) Influence of carbon dioxide and helium on intracellular calcium and pH levels in tumor cells and peritoneal macrophages. Data presented at the Second Workshop of Experimental Laparoscopic Surgery 1998, Rotterdam, Netherlands

Wu JS, Brasfield EB, Guo LW, Ruiz M, Connet JM, Philpott GW, Jones DB, Fleshmann JW (1997) Implantation of colon cancer at trocar sites is increased by low pressure pneumoperitoneum. Surgery 122: 1–7

Wu JS, Jones DB, Guo LW, Brasfield EB, Ruiz M, Connet JM, Fleshmann JW (1998) Effects of pneumoperitoneum on tumor implantation with decreasing tumor inoculum. Dis Colon Rectum 41: 141–146

CHAPTER 10

Pathogenesis: Immunological Aspects of Animal Studies

S.W. Lee, R.L. Whelan

Introduction

The use of laparoscopic techniques for patients with cancer is controversial. Reports of port wound tumor recurrences following laparoscopic oncologic surgery have raised concerns that minimally invasive methods may have an adverse impact on tumor recurrence rates and long term survival. Despite these legitimate concerns, numerous studies have demonstrated that post-operative immune function is better preserved following laparoscopic surgery than after open surgery. Furthermore, at least one animal study has demonstrated an association between laparotomy-associated immunosuppression and increased extra-abdominal tumor growth in the post-operative period. The implications of this association between immmunosuppression and increased tumor growth may be far-reaching. In theory, better preserved immune function following laparoscopic surgery may translate into lower rates of post-operative sepsis and infectious complications as well as lower tumor recurrence rates and improved survival in patients undergoing curative resection of malignancies. Admittedly, the idea that laparoscopic methods may be associated with an oncologic benefit contradicts the widely held belief that laparoscopic techniques place patients at increased risk for abdominal wound tumors.

Unfortunately, although extra-abdominal tumor growth and post-laparotomy immunosuppression have been assessed together, to the authors knowledge, the relationship of post-operative immune function and port-site tumor growth and establishment has not yet been studied or elucidated. Therefore, at this point in time, it is unclear if and how differences in post-operative immune function impact on the establishment and development of abdominal wound tumor recurrences. It is the purpose of this chapter to review what is presently known about immune function after open and laparoscopic surgery and to explore the possible implications of differences in post-operative immune function on the development of abdominal wound tumors.

Laparoscopic surgery is widely held to be less stressful than standard open surgery. The reported clinical benefits of minimally invasive surgery include decreased post-operative pain, earlier ambulation, earlier return to diet, and shorter hospitalization. Numerous investigators have attempted to determine the precise physiologic reasons for these short term clinical benefits. One particularly promising field of investigation is that of post-operative immune function. Numerous human and animal studies have suggested that immune functions appear to be better preserved following laparoscopic procedures than after the equivalent open procedures.

Immune Suppression Following Open Surgery

Cell-mediated functions are thought to defend against bacterial and viral infection and possibly to limit the spread and development of certain tumors. It has been well documented that cell-mediated immunity is suppressed after major open surgical procedures. The extent of suppression roughly correlates with the degree of trauma caused by the operation. For example, major operations, such as colectomy, suppress immune function to a greater degree than do minor operations, such a herniorrhaphy (Lennard et al. 1985) Impairment of the following cell-mediated functions have been found to occur:

1. Lymphocyte and neutrophil chemotaxis
2. Natural killer cell activity
3. Lymphocyte and macrophage interactions and function
4. Delayed type hypersensitivity (DTH) responses (Nielsen et al. 1989; Christou et al. 1982; Hjortso and Kehlet 1986).

As judged by serial DTH testing, decreased immune function is thought to last about 6–9 days after major abdominal surgery in humans (Hammer et al. 1992).

Is cell mediated immune function important post-operatively? Preoperatively, patients found to be anergic have a significantly higher incidence of sepsis and a higher mortality than normal DTH responders (Pietsch et al. 1977). One study of 727 patients, from the pre-laparoscopic era, found a postoperative sepsis rate of 7.5% and a mortality rate of 4.6% in normal DTH responders whereas anergic and relatively anergic patients had a 30% sepsis rate and a 23% mortality (Christou et al. 1981).

Immune function is important to the cancer patient as well. Numerous investigators believe the cell-mediated and natural immune systems are involved in limiting the spread of certain tumors (Burnet 1970; Boon 1992; Herlyn and Koprowski 1988; Prehn and Main 1957; Rosenberg and Lotze 1986; Tonaka et al. 1988; Eilber and Morton 1970). The fact that anergic cancer patients fare worse than normal DTH responders supports this position. There is a significantly higher incidence of normal DTH responders in the population of patients with resectable tumors (55%) than in those patients found to have inoperable tumors (20%) (Trokel et al. 1994). Even more impressive is the correlation of tumor resectability with the ability of a patient to mount a normal response to a 2,4-dinitrochlorobenzene (DNCB) challenge after prior sensitization. In one study 95% of DNCB responders had resectable lesions. In contrast, 93% of the non-responders were found to have inoperable tumors (Trokel et al. 1994).

In summary, intact immune function is an important prognostic indicator in patients undergoing surgery and, furthermore, major open surgery temporarily suppresses cell-mediated immune function. There are two questions that remain to be answered. The first is, does laparoscopic surgery have a similar impact on immune function as open methods? Secondly, what is the clinical importance, if any exists, of the period of relative immunosuppression that occurs after surgery?

Immune Function After Laparoscopic Procedures

Thus far, immune function after laparoscopic surgery has been assessed via a variety of different tests and approaches including the following:

1. DTH testing
2. Lymphocyte proliferation assays
3. Lymphocyte subpopulation studies
4. Lymphocyte, peripheral blood monocyte, and peritoneal macrophage surface marker and cytokine elaboration studies
5. Serum cytokine evaluations
6. Neutrophil and natural killer cell evaluations
7. Evaluation of macrophage, monocyte, and neutrophil chemotaxis and phagocytosis

In most of the human studies a current group of laparoscopic patients are compared to a recent group of open patients. Some studies merely report results for a group of laparoscopic patients alone. Animal studies usually include an open, laparoscopic and an anesthesia control group. What follows is a brief summary of these studies.

DTH Studies

Delayed-type hypersensitivity (DTH) challenges assess cell-mediated immune function via intradermal injections of specific antigens to which the subject has been exposed in the past. A positive response requires that the antigen be processed and presented via an antigen-presenting cell to a specific CD4+ cell which, in turn, proliferates and then elaborates specific cytokines. These cytokines activate vascular endothelial cells at the challenge site which results in a gathering of effector cells and then elimination of host cells that contain the foreign antigen. Fibrinogen also finds its way into the area and is converted to fibrin which results in an area of induration. The indurated area is measured 1–2 days after the challenge: in humans any wheal with dimensions of 0.5 × 0.5 cm or greater is considered a positive response.

In order to assess cell-mediated immune function after surgery via DTH testing it is necessary to perform a preoperative challenge as well as one or several postoperative challenges. The preoperative challenge provides a baseline response to which the postoperative results can be compared for each subject. As stated above, after major open abdominal surgery in humans it has been demonstrated that there is a significant decrease in the size of the DTH response. The assumption inherent in this type of study is that a decrease in the size of the wheal correlates with a decrease in the functional status of the cell-mediated immune system. Since anergy is associated with increased morbidity and mortality, it is further assumed that a patient with smaller postoperative responses is at higher risk for complications.

Animal DTH Studies

In a rat study carried out by the authors, DTH responses after full sham laparotomy, CO_2 pneumoperitoneum, or anesthesia alone were assessed (Trokel et al. 1994). This study compared the methods of exposure alone and did not involve an intra-abdominal procedure. All rats underwent a preoperative and two postoperative DTH challenges (immediately after surgery and on postoperative day 2). The laparotomy group demonstrated significantly smaller postoperative DTH responses than either the control or the pneumoperitoneum groups for both postoperative challenges. There were no significant difference between the insufflation and anesthesia control groups at any time point. In order to determine if the observed DTH differences would persist when an actual intra-abdominal procedure was performed, a second rat DTH study was carried out that compared open and laparoscopic-assisted cecal resection (LAR). Similar results were noted despite the addition of an intra-abdominal procedure (Allendorf et al. 1996).

In an attempt to correlate postoperative immune function with a relevant clinical endpoint, yet another rat study was undertaken to determine if the observed DTH differences would have an impact on the animals' ability to deal with a bacterial infection. In addition to assessing DTH response, resistance to bacterial dermal infection was evaluated by comparing intradermal abscess formation after a standard bacterial challenge with *Staphylococcus aureus*. Again, a total of three DTH and bacterial challenges were administered (preoperative, immediately after surgery, and postoperative day 2). The open group's pustules were significantly larger than both the pneumoperitoneum and control group's for both postoperative challenges. Not surprisingly, the DTH results were similar to those of the previously mentioned studies. An inverse correlation was found between the size of the bacterial pustule and the DTH induration for the first postoperative challenges (Donahue et al. 1997). Comparable results were noted in a rat study that compared postoperative infection using the same model after laparoscopic and open cecectomy (Southall et al. 1997).

Human DTH Studies

Thus far, two non-randomized human DTH studies have been carried out. In both, the DTH challenges were administered once before surgery and twice postoperatively. In Kloosterman et al.'s study, DTH responses following laparoscopic and open cholecystectomy were compared (Kloosterman et al. 1994). DTH challenges were given 1 day before surgery and on postoperative days 1 and 6. A significant drop in the size of the DTH response was noted after the postoperative day 1 challenge in the open group when compared to the preoperative results. No such differences where found when the laparoscopic group responses were compared. Furthermore, no significant differences were noted for the postoperative day 6 challenges.

The second human DTH study compared open and laparoscopic colectomy patients. DTH challenges to a panel of recall antigens were planted preoperatively and read 24 h and 48 h later. Postoperative challenges were carried out immediately following surgery and on postoperative day 3 with those antigens to which the patient had responded on the preoperative challenge. The individual percentual changes (from baseline) for each antigen were averaged for each challenge so that a single value was obtained for each challenge for each patient. This allowed comparison between patients. The open group demonstrated significantly smaller responses to the postoperative day 3 challenge when compared to the open groups preoperative results. The laparoscopic group postoperative day 3 results, on the other hand, were not significantly different from their preoperative responses. The postoperative day 1 results for both groups were not significantly different from the preoperative results using this method of comparison (Whelan et al. 1998). These human results lend some support to the conclusions of a number of the rodent DTH studies mentioned below.

Lymphocyte Proliferation Assays

Lymphocyte proliferation assays (LPA) assess the ability of a subjects lymphocytes to replicate in vitro. The assumption made in this type of study is that a diminished replication rate is the result of suppression of the immune system. LPAs provide no information regarding lymphocyte subpopulations or of cytokine elaboration and, therefore, are a non-specific evaluation. In a non-randomized study of cholecystectomy patients Griffith et al. found that the open group demonstrated significantly lower proliferation rates 24 h after surgery when compared to their preoperative results. No such difference was found for the laparoscopic group (Griffith et al. 1995).

In a murine study, Horgan et al. compared lymphocyte proliferation rates of mice undergoing either air pneumoperitoneum, sham laparotomy, or anesthesia alone (Horgan et al. 1992). They found that proliferation rates after surgery were significantly lower in the laparotomy group when compared to the anesthesia control group. There were no significant differences noted between the pneumoperitoneum group and either the control group or the laparotomy group. A similar LPA study performed at Columbia University confirmed Horgan's findings and also determined the time course of this effect (Southall et al. 1998). Significantly lower lymphocyte proliferation rates were observed after the sham laparotomy on the 3rd, 4th, and 5th postoperative days when the open results were compared to those of the pneumoperitoneum and anesthesia control groups. On the 8th postoperative day there were no significant differences noted between the groups.

Lymphocyte Subpopulation Studies

Several investigators have determined the ratios of a number of different lymphocyte subpopulations following minimally invasive surgery. Vallina and Velasco determined the number of CD4+ (T-helper) and CD8+ (T-suppressor) cells in peripheral blood samples from laparoscopic cholecystectomy patients. A non-significant decrease in the number of T-helper lymphocytes and a non-significant increase in the T-suppressor lymphocytes found at both postoperative timepoints (POD1 and POD 5–7) were noted. However, the ratio of CD4+/CD8+ cells 24 h after surgery was significantly lower (13%) than the preoperative ratio (Vallina and Velasco 1996). Of note, there was no open group for comparison. Historically, other investigators had demonstrated significantly lower CD4+ and significantly higher CD8+ cell counts postoperatively in open cholecystectomy patients (Hansbrough et al. 1984). Vallina concluded, based on this comparison to historical controls, that there is probably less immunosuppression after laparoscopic cholecystectomy than following open surgery. Decker et al. in a non-randomized study of 43 cholecystectomy patients determined the number of circulating T- and B-cells preoperatively and at three different timepoints after surgery. They found no significant differences in the numbers of T- or B-cells within each group or between groups at any time point (Decker et al. 1996).

T Helper Lymphocyte Subpopulation (Th1/Th2) Studies

Recently it has been recognized that there are subsets of CD4+ helper T cells that produce distinct cytokines in response to antigenic stimulation. Naïve T cells, in response to antigenic stimulation, differentiate into either T-helper1 (Th1) or T-helper2 (Th2) subsets with relatively restricted profiles of cytokine production. Decker et al. indirectly studied the T-helper1 (Th1) and T-helper2 (Th2) ratio by following peripheral blood monocyte cytokine production, in vitro, after stimulation. The levels of IL-4 and IFN-gamma were determined; the former is produced by monocytes in response to stimulation from Th2 cells while the latter is produced following Th1 stimulation. The open group monocyte IL-4 levels were significantly higher than the minimally invasive surgery groups 2 h after open cholecystectomy. There were no differences in IL-4 elaboration at either of the remaining postoperative timepoints. Furthermore, there were no differences in the levels of IFN-gamma noted between groups at any timepoint after surgery. They went on to determine the IFN-gamma/IL-4 ratio as an indirect means of looking at the Th1/Th2 cell ratio and found a shift toward a Th2 response at all timepoints. The open group demonstrated a significantly lower ratio (Th2 shift) than the laparoscopic group 2 h after surgery. There were no such differences noted at the other timepoints (Decker et al. 1996).

The same authors, via yet another indirect method, assessed Th1/Th2 balance by determining and comparing the level of CD23 expression on circulating B-cells and HLA-DR expression on peripheral blood monocytes. Significant HLA-DR and CD23 differences between the open and laparoscopic groups were noted at 2 h and 24 h postoperatively. The HLA-DR/CD23 ratio was shifted toward the Th2 side at all timepoints; only at 2 h was the difference between these ratios significant (Decker et al. 1996).

Monocyte Function and Antigen Expression

Monocytes play a very important role in both innate and cell-mediated immune functions. Best known as effector cells, they phagocytoze infected or altered cells and are also the principal source of TNF and IL-1 following T-cell stimulation. In addition, they also play an important role in the presentation of antigen to T-cells and, thus, are also involved in the afferent arm of cell-mediated immune responses. Not surprisingly, there are numerous ways to assess monocytes.

Monocyte HLA-DR Levels

Only those monocytes or other antigen presenting cells (APC's) that express Class II MHC molecules are capable of presenting antigen to CD4+ helper T lymphocytes. The percentage of the circulating monocytes that express HLA-DR has been shown to correlate with short term outcome after major elective surgery and trauma (Hershman et al. 1990; Faist et al. 1988; Appel et al. 1989). Significantly higher HLA-DR levels have been found after open surgery or trauma in patients who underwent an uneventful recovery when compared to the values determined for patients that became septic or died (Hershman et al. 1990). There was no difference found when the laparoscopic patient data was analyzed. In contrast, a second non-randomized study of cholecystectomy patients by Decker et al. demonstrated significantly lower HLA-DR levels in both the open and laparoscopic groups 2 h and 24 h after surgery. The open group demonstrated a greater drop in HLA-DR expression than the laparoscopic group although it is not stated whether the difference between groups was significant (Decker et al. 1996).

Monocyte TNF and Superoxide Anion Release

Redmond et al. in a prospective and randomized human study of cholecystectomy patients studied in vitro monocyte production of TNF and superoxide anion release (Redmond et al. 1994). TNF is the principal pro-inflammatory cytokine released in response to gram-negative bacterial infection. Superoxide anion aids in the killing of foreign pathogens by monocytes. On the first and third post-operative days the open patient's circulating blood monocytes released significantly more TNF than the laparoscopic groups monocytes. Similarly, the open group monocytes released more superoxide anion than the monocytes from the laparoscopic group. An animal study by the same group that compared laparotomy to CO_2 pneumoperitoneum, found similar results with regards to monocyte release of superoxide anion and TNF (Sandoval et al. 1996). These results indicate that the open groups monocytes and neutrophils have been primed and activated to a greater degree than those of the laparoscopic group. This data suggests that the open patients might be better prepared or "armed" to deal with a bacterial infection. Therefore, these differences could be viewed as beneficial to the open patients. However, excess production of these mediators may result in a cycle of repeated activation that may be detrimental. Furthermore, the authors point out that activated neutrophils and monocytes can cause dysfunction in the lungs, liver, and kidneys.

Monocyte Phagocytosis and Cytotoxicity

Watson et al. (1995) in a murine study compared sham laparotomy to a brief CO_2 pneumoperitoneum. The ability of isolated monocytes to phagocytize *Candida albicans* was assessed 24 h after the intervention. Uptake of candida by the laparotomy group monocytes was significantly less than that of the control or the CO_2 pneumoperitoneum groups monocytes. In the same study, peritoneal and circulating monocyte expression of the MAC-1(CD11b) receptor was also assessed. This receptor plays an important role in monocyte recognition of complement-coated pathogens and other opsonized particles prior to phagocytosis. Significantly lower expression was noted in the laparotomy group animals when compared to the control or CO_2 pneumoperitoneum group results.

Neutrophil Function

Redmond et al. in the study mentioned above, investigated both neutrophil chemotaxis and neutrophil elaboration of superoxide anion 1 and 3 days after open or laparoscopic cholecystectomy. Significantly increased chemotaxis was noted in the open group 24 h after surgery when compared to the laparoscopic group results. Likewise, PMN production of O_2 was significantly greater after open surgery than after the laparoscopic equivalent on both postoperative days 1 and 3 (Redmond et al. 1994). The clinical importance of these differences is not entirely clear. As per the discussion in the monocyte section above, increased release of O_2 acts to prime and activate PMN's for the elimination of bacteria which might be construed as being beneficial to the open patients. Similarly, at first glance, improved chemotaxis would appear to be an advantage for the open surgery patients. Although the authors admit that these and other of their findings "may be beneficial" they also suggest that such PMN stimulation may result in over activation and cause local or pulmonary tissue injury.

Natural Killer Cell Activity

In the limited number of studies performed to date, no significant differences in natural killer (NK) cell activity have been noted in either animals or humans (Griffith et al. 1995; Sandoval et al. 1996).

Mechanism of Postoperative Immunosuppression

What is it about laparotomy and procedures performed using open technique that causes temporary suppression of the immune system? The two most widely held hypotheses are:

1. The degree of immunosuppression is a function of the incision length
2. That peritoneal exposure to air causes postoperative immunosuppression

In a rat DTH study, the relationship of the length of the abdominal incision to postoperative immune function was investigated. Five groups were compared:

1. Sham full laparotomy
2. Mini-laparotomy (half the xiphoid to pubis distance)
3. Open cecal resection (via full laparotomy)
4. LAR
5. Anesthesia control

Significantly smaller DTH responses were observed in the full laparotomy and open cecal resection groups when compared to the LAR group and anesthesia control responses. Of note, the mini-laparotomy group DTH responses were not significantly different from the control group. Therefore, immunosuppression was found only with the full laparotomy and not with the mini-laparotomy (Sandoval et al. 1996). These results lend support to the hypothesis that the immunosuppression is related to the overall length of the abdominal incision.

Watson et al. compared sham laparotomy to CO_2 pneumoperitoneum, air pneumoperitoneum and anesthesia alone. They followed monocyte and neutrophil release of superoxide anion or TNF as well as monocyte phagocytosis and several other parameters. Both the laparotomy group and the air pneumoperitoneum group demonstrated significantly greater superoxide anion release and TNF release from monocytes than the anesthesia or CO_2 pneumoperitoneum groups. Similarly, monocyte phagocytosis was decreased after both laparotomy and air pneumoperitoneum but not after CO_2 insufflation or anesthesia alone. The authors point out that if the incision alone was the problem then the air insufflation group should not have demonstrated the im-

munosuppressive changes it did. The authors conclude that there is a factor in air, most likely small amounts of lipopolysaccharide (LPS), that causes immunosuppression upon exposure to the peritoneal cavity. They further believe that the LPS in the air results in translocation of gut bacteria-derived LPS across the bowel wall which is directly responsible for the observed immunosuppression (Watson et al. 1995).

Lee et al. in a recent murine study that compared lymphocyte proliferation rates, tested Watson et al.'s hypothesis by comparing a full laparotomy performed in a sealed CO_2 chamber to full laparotomy carried out in room air. The two laparotomy groups were compared to an anesthesia control and a CO_2 insufflation group. Lymphocyte proliferation was assessed on postoperative day 2 in all groups. Significantly lower proliferation rates were found for both laparotomy groups when compared to the results of the anesthesia control and the CO_2 insufflation group (Lee et al. 1998). These results suggest that laparotomy and not the presence of air in the abdomen is the cause of the immunosuppression. The DTH study mentioned (Sandoval et al. 1996) above also refutes the hypothesis that peritoneal air exposure is the critical factor in bringing about immunosuppression since the peritoneal cavities of animals in both the small and the large incision laparotomy groups were exposed to air yet significantly decreased DTH responses were seen only in the full laparotomy group.

It is important to note that different immune parameters were assessed in the above studies. Therefore, it is difficult to directly compare the results or to draw a final conclusion. In all likelihood, both the incision and air exposure probably cause different immune system alterations. Further study is needed in this area to better elucidate why and how the immune system is affected after surgery.

Relationship Between Postoperative Immunosuppression and Tumor Growth

A number of different investigators have found that distant tumor metastases are more likely to become established and will grow more rapidly after laparotomy than after anesthesia alone (Eggermont et al. 1988; Goshima et al. 1989; Ratajczak et al. 1992). A more recent murine study, carried out at Columbia University, also assessed tumor growth after surgery. This study compared tumor growth after full sham laparotomy, after CO_2 pneumoperitoneum, and after anesthesia alone. This study demonstrated that extra-abdominal tumors are more likely to become established and that tumors will grow more rapidly after sham laparotomy than after pneumoperitoneum or anesthesia alone (Allendorf et al. 1995). Importantly, despite the fact that the pneumoperitoneum group had significantly smaller tumors than the open group, the pneumoperitoneum groups tumors were still significantly larger than the anesthesia control groups lesions. Similar results were noted when open cecal resection was compared to laparoscopic-assisted cecal resection in a later study (Allendorf et al. 1998).

In an attempt to determine if there was any relationship between cell-mediated immunosuppression and increased tumor growth after laparotomy, the initial Columbia tumor study, described above, was repeated in athymic mice which have no T-lymphocytes. Tumor growth following sham laparotomy and CO_2 pneumoperitoneum was compared. Interestingly, the differences in tumor growth between these two groups that had been previously noted in immunocompetent mice, were lost in the athymic mice. These results suggested that the increased tumor growth seen after laparotomy in the immunocompetent mice was, in part, related to the cell-mediated immunosuppression that had been documented to occur after laparotomy. Therefore, there appeared to be an association between immunosuppression and increased tumor growth following laparotomy (Allendorf et al. 1999). It is important to note that in all of the tumor studies mentioned above extra-abdominal tumor growth was assessed.

Immune Function and Port-site Tumors

The preceding sections of this chapter, hopefully, have made the point that surgery, in general, causes immunosuppression and that less immunosuppression occurs following laparoscopic procedures than after the equivalent open surgical procedures. Furthermore, in several animal studies, these differences in immune function were found to correlate with an important clinical endpoint, namely, susceptibility to infection. In other animal studies that assessed tumor growth and establishment after surgery, significantly increased tumor growth and establishment rates were noted in animals undergoing open surgery when compared to laparoscopic animals. In yet another study that utilized athymic mice (which have no T-cells), the previously observed differences in tumor growth between open and laparo-

scopic groups were lost. This implied that the cell-mediated immunosuppression documented to occur after open surgery, in part, accounted for the accelerated tumor growth observed in the open animals.

It is important to note that in all of the animal studies mentioned above tumor growth at an extra-abdominal site (intradermally on the back of the rodents) was assessed. It has not been demonstrated that similar differences in tumor growth occur for intra-abdominal tumors or abdominal wound tumors. Therefore, no definitive or authoritative statements can be made regarding the impact of immune function differences on the probability of port wound tumor formation. In theory, improved systemic immune function should either have a positive impact (lower incidence of tumors) or no effect on port wound tumor formation.

Some critics argue that if immune function is better preserved after laparoscopic procedures then port wound tumors should not form. However, this is an unreasonable oversimplification when one considers the myriad of factors that contribute to the formation of a tumor metastasis. Two other important variables that should be considered are the tumor cell burden (number of tumor viable cells in the wound) and the biology of the tumor. A large number of viable tumor cells implanted in a port wound may overwhelm the ability of the immune system to prevent the metastasis from forming. Stated in a slightly different way, poor technique, which is the most likely means by which tumor cells become separated from the primary, cannot be compensated for by the modest immune benefit associated with laparoscopic methods. Similarly, a small inoculum for an aggressive tumor cell line may have a higher rate of establishment when compared to a much larger innoculum for a less virulent tumor. Therefore, it is important to try and place in perspective the relative importance of the factors that may contribute to the development of a tumor metastasis. In summary, it is wholly possible that a port wound tumor may form in the face of better preserved immune function.

Local Versus Systemic Immune Function

The majority of the human and animal studies reviewed above suggest that in general, open surgery is associated with greater immunosuppression than minimally invasive access methods. However, there are some notable exceptions and some results that are difficult to interpret. Different readers may come up with very different interpretations or explanations for a given set of experimental results. Is a stimulated macrophage a good thing or a bad thing to have in the abdomen on the first several days following surgery? Is it always better to have a result similar to that of the anesthesia control group? Might not some postoperative immune function changes be useful or serve a function? How certain are we that increased expression of a certain antigen by a lymphocyte or an effector cell correlates well with either a specific immune activity or, more importantly, to a meaningful clinical endpoint?

Further, a distinction can and should be made between systemic immune function and intra-abdominal or intra-peritoneal immune function (so-called local immune function). DTH challenges and tests that utilize peripheral blood mononuclear cells assess the systemic immune response. In contradistinction, experiments that isolate and study peritoneal macrophages are evaluating intra-peritoneal immune function. Minimally invasive methods may have different effects locally and sytemically. Furthermore, different elements or aspects of the minimally invasive procedure may be responsible for either the local or the systemic alterations. For example, systemic suppression of cell mediated immune responses may be a function of the length of the incision whereas the local intra-abdominal effects may reflect the impact of the CO_2 pneumoperitoneum.

Conclusions

The "take home" message of all this is that there is no simple pat answer to the question 'Is laparoscopy better for the immune system than open surgery'? There are a multitude of different effects at numerous levels of the immune system which can be interpreted in numerous ways. It has also become painfully clear that the division and assignment of immune system activities into either cell-mediated, humoral, or native (i.e. non-specific) categories is a vast oversimplification that has little relevance given our current understanding of the immune system. Further studies will be needed in order to better work out the import of subtle differences in immune parameters and to better explain just where along the complex intertwined immune system pathways surgical trauma exerts itself. Despite the limitations alluded to above, evaluation of the impact of surgery of all types on immune function remains a promising field of study. Armed with a better understanding, it may prove possible via alterations in our surgical methods or via pharmacologic means to limit the detrimental immune system changes that occur after both open and laparoscopic surgery.

References

Allendorf JDF, Bessler M, Kayton M, Oesterling SD, Treat MR, Nowygrod R, Whelan RL (1995) Increased tumor establishment and growth after laparoscopy and laparotomy in a murine model: Arch Surg 130(6): 649–653

Allendorf JD, Bessler M, Whelan RL, Trokel M, Laird DA, Terry MB, Treat MR (1996) Better preservation of immune function after laparoscopic-assisted vs. open bowel resection in a murine model. Dis Colon Rectum 10: 67–72

Allendorf JD, Bessler M, Horvath KD, Marvin MR, Laird DA, Whelan RL (1998) Increased tumor establishment and growth after open versus laparoscopic bowel resection in mice. Surg Endosc 12: 1035–1038

Allendorf JD, Bessler M, Horvath KD, Marvin MR, Laird DA, Whelan RL (1999) Increased tumor establishment and growth after open versus laparoscopic surgery in mice may be related to differences in postoperative T-cell function. Surg Endosc 13: 233–235

Appel SH, Wellhausen SR, Montgomery R, DeWeese RC, Polk HC (1989) Experimental and clinical significance of endotoxin independent HLA-DR expression on monocytes. J Surg Res 47: 44–48

Boon T (1992) Toward a genetic analysis of human tumor rejection antigens. Adv Cancer Res 58: 177–210

Burnet FM (1970) The concept of immunological surveillance. Progr Exp Tumor Res 13: 1–27

Christou NV, Meakins JL, MacLean LD (1981) The predictive role of delayed hypersensitivity in preoperative patients. Surg Obstet Gynecol 152: 297–301

Christou NV, Superina R, Broadhead M, Meakins JL (1982) Postoperative depression of host resistance: determinants and effect of peripheral protein-sparing therapy. Surgery 92: 786–792

Decker D, Schondorf M, Bidlingmaier F, Hirner A, von Ruecker AA (1996) Surgical stress induces a shift in the type-1/type-2 T-helper cell balance, suggesting down regulation of cell mediated and up-regulation of antibody-mediated immunity commensurate to the trauma. Surgery 119: 316–325

Donahue JP, Whelan RL, Wickens J, Buxton E, Allendorf JDF, Southall JC, Lee SW, Bessler M (1997) Susceptibility to dermal bacterial infection is greater after laparotomy vs laparoscopy in a murine model. Surg Endosc 11: 195

Eggermont AM, Steller EP, Marquet RL, Jeekel J, Sugarbaker PH (1988) Local regional promotion of tumor growth after abdominal surgery is dominant over immuno therapy with interleukin-2 and lymphokine activated killer cells. Cancer Detect Prevent 12: 421–429

Eilber FR, Morton DL (1970) Impaired immunologic reactivity and recurrence following cancer surgery. Cancer 25: 362–367

Faist E, Mewes A, Strasser T, Walz A, Alkan S, Baker C, Ertel W, Heberer G (1988) Alteration of monocy te function following major injury. Arch Surg 123: 287–292

Goshima H, Saji S, Furata T, Taneumura H, Takao H, Kida H, Takahasi H (1989) Experimental study on preventative effects of lung metastases using LAK cells induced from various lymphocytes - special references to enhancement of lung metastasis after laparotomy stress. J Jpn Surg Soc 90: 1245–1250

Griffith JP, Everitt NJ, Lancaster F, Boylston A, Richards SJ, Scott CS, Benson EA, Sue-Ling HM, McMahon MJ (1995) Influence of laparoscopic and conventional cholecystectomy upon cell-mediated immunity. Br J Surg 82: 677–680

Hammer JH, Nielsen HJ, Moesgaard F, et al, (1992) Duration of postoperative immunosuppression assessed by repeated delayed type hypersensitivity skin tests. Eur Surg Res 24: 133–137

Hansbrough JF, Bender EM, Zapata-Sirvent R, Anderson J (1984) Altered helper and suppressor lymphocyte populations in surgical populations in surgical patients: a measure of postoperative immunosuppression. Am J Surg 148: 303–307

Herlyn M, Koprowski H (1988) Melanoma antigens: immunological and biological characterization and clinical significance. Ann Rev Immunol 6: 283–308

Hershman MJ, Cheadle WG, Wellhausen SR, Davidson PF, Polk HC (1990) Monocyte HLA-DR antigen expression characterizes clinical outcome in the trauma patient. Br J Surg 77: 204–207

Hjortso NC, Kehlet H (1986) Influence of surgery, age, and serum albumin on delayed hypersensitivity. Acta Chir Scand 152: 175–179

Horgan PG, Fitzpatrick M, Couse NF, Gorey TF, Fitzpatrick JM (1992) Laparoscopy is less immunotraumatic than laparotomy. Minim Invasive Ther 1: 241–244

Kloosterman T, von Blomberg ME, Borgstein P, Cuesta MA, Scheper RJ, Meijer S (1994) Unimpaired immune functions after laparoscopic cholecystectomy. Surgery 115: 424–428

Lee SW, Southall JC, Bessler M, Whelan RL (1998) Lymphocyte proliferation in mice following full laparotomy performed in a sealed CO_2 chamber is equivalent to that in mice following full laparotomy performed in room air (Abstract). Surg Endosc 12: 4

Lennard TWJ, Shenton BK, Borzotta A, Donnelly PK, White M, Gerrie LM, Proud G, Raylor RM (1985) The influence of surgical operations on components of the human immune system. Br J Surg 72: 771–776

Nielsen HJ, Moesgaard F, Kehlet H (1989a) Ranitidine for prevention of postoperative suppression of delayed hypersensitivity. Am J Surg 157: 291–294

Pietsch JB, Meakins JL, MacLean LD (1977) The delayed hypersensitivity response: application in clinical surgery. Surgery 82: 349–355

Prehn RT, Main MJ (1957) Immunity to methylcholanthrene-induced sarcomas. J Natl Cancer Inst 18: 769–778

Ratajczak HV, Lange RW, Sothern RB, Hagen KL, Vescei P, Wu J, Halberg F, Thomas PT (1992) Surgical influence on murine immunity and tumor growth: relationship of body temperature and hormones with splenocytes. Proc Soc Exp Biol Med 199: 432–440

Redmond HP, Watson WG, Houghton T, Condron C, Watson RGK, Boucher-Hayes D (1994) Immune function in patients undergoing open vs laparoscopic cholecystectomy. Arch Surg 129: 1240–1242

Rosenberg SA, Lotze MT (1986) Cancer immunotherapy using interleukin-2 and interleukin-2 activated lymphocytes. Annu Rev Immunol 4: 681–709

Sandoval BA, Robinson AV, Sulaiman TT, Shenk RR, Stellato TA (1996) Open versus laparoscopic surgery: a comparison of natural antitumoral cellular immunity in a small model. Am Surg 62: 625–631

Southall JC, Lee SW, Donahue JP, Bessler MD, Whelan RL (1997) Susceptibility to dermal bacterial infection is greater after open than laparoscopic cecal resection in a murine model. Dis Colon Rectum 40: 40–41

Southall JC, Lee SW, Bessler M, Whelan RL (1998) Time course of differences in lymphocyte proliferation after laparotomy vs. insufflation (Abstract). Surg Endosc 12: 485

Tonaka K, Yoshioka T, Bieberich C, Jay G (1988) The role of the major histocompatability complex class 1 antigens in tumor growth and metastasis. Annu Rev Immunol 6: 359–380

Trokel MJ, Bessler M, Treat MR, Whelan RL, Nowygrod R (1994) Preservation of immune response after laparoscopy. Surg Endosc 8(12): 1385–1388

Vallina VL, Velasco JM (1996) The influence of laparoscopy on lymphocyte subpopulations in the surgical patient. Surg Endosc 10: 481–484

Watson RWG, Redmond HP, McCarthy J, Burke PE, Hayes DB (1995) Exposure of the peritoneal cavity to air regulates early inflammatory responses to surgery in a murine model. Br J Surg 82: 1060–1065

Whelan RL, Franklin M, Donahue J (1998) Postoperative cell mediated immune response is better preserved after laparoscopic versus open colectomy in humans: a preliminary study (Abstract). Surg Endosc 12: 4

Pathogenesis: Free Viable Cancer Cells and Cancer Cell Liberation in Clinical Studies

P. Buchmann, D. Christen, L. Stocchi, H. Nelson

Introduction

The traditional pathways of tumor cell transportation involve blood vessels and lymphatic vessels causing hematogenous and lymphatogenous metastases, respectively. Since close lymphatic connections between the abdominal viscera and the abdominal wall are scarce, it appears unlikely that port-site recurrences are due to lymphatic spread of cells originating from visceral cancers. However, hematogenous dissemination of cancer cells to sites of active cellular proliferation seems more prevalent. Cancer cells were detected, employing monoclonal antibodies for tumor-associated antigens (Juhl et al. 1994; Lindemann et al. 1992) in bone marrow of up to 40% of patients with digestive cancers. Murthy et al. (1989) demonstrated that tumor cells injected intravenously can cause tumor formation at the site of the laparotomy. Fresh wounds provide blood clots with a variety of tissue-specific growth factors creating a favorable environment for tumor cell growth (Murthy et al. 1989; Gutmann et al.1995). On the other hand, high vascularization that is part of wound healing might play a protective role, also referred to as "metastatic inefficiency".

Direct implantation of tumor cells, which are present in the peritoneal cavity, in abdominal wounds appears the most likely mode of tumor cell transportation. Reports of tumor recurrence at the extraction site after laparoscopic cholecystectomy in patients with unexpected gallbladder cancer provide convincing evidence of direct tumor implantation (Drouard et al. 1991). Surprisingly, tumor recurrence at port-sites has also been reported after laparoscopic removal of gallbladders with cancers which were limited to the mucosa. Perforation of the gallbladder during dissection and removal did not occur in these cases. Intraluminal spread of gallbladder cancer cells contaminating the peritoneal cavity or trocar sites via the cystic duct appears most likely in these cases (Texler et al. 1998). This is in analogy to intraluminal spreading of cancer cells in colonic cancer contaminating staple lines or anastomoses which has been recognized as a source of anastomotic recurrence. This phenomenon could provide the explanation of port-site recurrence which occurred after colectomy, without opening the bowel, for Dukes' A cancers.

In addition to shedding of tumor cells during extraction of tumors through narrow incisions in the abdominal wall and intraluminal spreading of tumor cells, viable cancer cells floating in the peritoneal cavity play a role in the pathogenesis of port-site recurrences. This is illustrated by a case report by Ugarte (1995) on a patient who had a laparoscopic cholecystectomy 3 months prior to a right hemicolectomy for cancer. During laparoscopic cholecystectomy, the right colon had not been manipulated. Several months after right hemicolectomy, a port-site recurrence was noted. The only feasible explanation was implantation of free viable colon cancer cells in a port-site at the time of laparoscopic cholecystectomy.

Predictive Value of Exfoliated Cells

Viable tumor cells have repeatedly been demonstrated as present within the peritoneal cavity (Fig. 11.1) as well as in the bowel lumen, mesorectum and in uninvolved mucosa during surgery (Skipper et al. 1987). Furthermore, tumor cells have been observed on circular staplers, in cases where the surgical doughnuts did not show any evidence of malignancy (Gertsch et al. 1992). However, while peritoneal cytology is a standardized accepted criterion for TNM staging for ovarian and endometrial tumors (1997), although recently advocated (Schott et al. 1998) it has never been definitely proven to be a prognostic indicator in colorectal cancer. In particular, investigators are still evaluating the hypothesis that the presence of exfoliated tumor cells could be

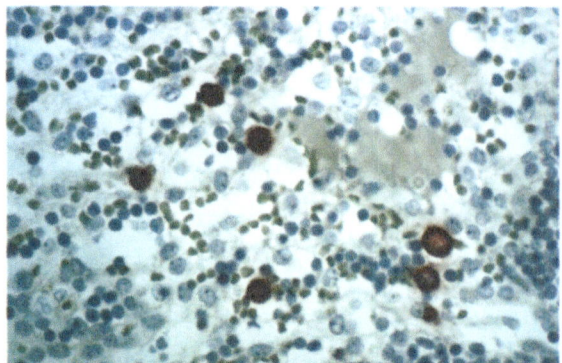

Fig. 11.1. Mononuclear antibody Ber-Ep4 staining showing exfoliated colorectal cancer cells in the peritoneal fluid. Courtesy of R. Steinert and P. Stosiek, Academic Hospital Cottbus, Germany

predictive of local recurrence, including the abdominal wall. A fundamental requirement for implantation is that exfoliated cells be viable. Therefore, initial studies have been focused on assessing whether spilled cells are alive and not simply necrotic debris. Viable exfoliated cells with inherent metastatic potential have repeatedly been demonstrated, both by their ability to incorporate tritiated thymidine (Fermor et al. 1986), and to form cell colonies in vitro (Skipper et al. 1987). It may be that the variable results according to positive cytologies relate to variable methodologies of tumor cell retrieval. A subsequent issue has regarded the accuracy of different retrieval methodologies. Several variables affect the retrieval of malignant cells, including tumor stage, timing of retrieval and the technique adopted. Furthermore, several modalities have been adopted to detect exfoliated tumor cells, including conventional cytology, immunocytochemistry and a more complex approach involving the use of magnetic fields, to perform magnetic cell sorting using antibody-labeled magnetic beads. Peritoneal brushing techniques have not demonstrated any advantage over traditional cytology (Murphy et al. 1993). Free malignant cells have generally been analyzed both in pre-resection and in post-resection washings. In fact, an increased retrieval rate after resection would support the hypothesis that cells could be dispersed into the abdominal cavity as a result of surgical manipulation, falling into the peritoneum from disrupted blood or lymphatic vessels, or directly from the resection margin or the bowel lumen.

While the presence of pre-resection positive cells in the washing has been frequently associated with a more advanced disease, it is not clear that retrieval of tumor cells after completion of surgical resection

is associated with a worse prognosis. Free malignant cells have been found in 3.7%–15% of pre-resection washings and 13.3%–26.7% in post-resection washings using conventional cytologic techniques (Martin and Goellner 1986; Murphy et al. 1993; Horattas et al. 1997). It is therefore apparent that the positive retrieval rate for cancer is also variable within patients analyzed with traditional methods. In fact, differentiation of viable cells from fibroblasts, mesothelial and inflammatory cells can be difficult and subject at least in part to the personal judgement of the examiner (Zuna et al. 1989). In addition, it has been reported that positive retrievals can also result from benign cells originating from the fallopian tubes or foci of endometriosis (Zuna and Mitchell 1988).

Alternative tests have been introduced to overcome these limitations. Some authors have advocated immunocytochemistry, although other studies have not been able to confirm its benefits. Leather and colleagues have analyzed peritoneal washings taken from 35 patients with colorectal cancer pre- and postresection. Analysis has been performed with conventional cytology and a panel of ten different monoclonal antibodies. Yields from pre- and postoperative washings were increased from 11.4% and 14.3% to 31.4% and 31.4%, respectively (Leather et al. 1994). In another series of 30 patients whose peritoneal fluid was analyzed in a similar fashion, both cytology and monoclonal antibodies identified abnormal cells in 7 cases each, but only 2 patients had identical results from the 2 techniques (Ambrose et al. 1989). The use of magnetic fields to sort cells (magnetic activated cell sorter, MACS) has been proposed as a more accurate detection technique (Wong et al. 1995). In a study on 26 patients with stage II–IV disease, free malignant cells were identified in 11 cases (42.3%). None of the patients were positive in the pre-resection peritoneal washing only and the presence of free tumor cells was associated with advanced disease (Wong et al. 1996). Most recently, DNA analyses on supernatants of peritoneal fluid with the polymerase chain reaction has been proposed as an adjunctive method which could be useful to confirm malignancy when tumor cells are not detected and could therefore improve accuracy further (Yamashita et al. 1998).

Although the adoption of more sophisticated techniques has been associated with an increasing yield of positive cells, more complex techniques are not as widely available as traditional cytologic examination and could not be widely applied in most laboratories. In addition, the central issue remains on whether this information is clinically relevant and useful.

Correlation with Local Recurrence and Survival

At least four studies using conventional cytologic examination have failed to show any malignant cells released in the peritoneum from tumors resected with curative intent (Martin and Goellner 1986; Murphy et al. 1993; Horattas et al. 1997; Kim et al. 1998). In other words, only advanced, metastatic or recurrent disease were associated with intraperitoneal tumor shedding. Few studies have been able to analyze peritoneal washings related to survival following surgery. Horattas and colleagues analyzed 50 patients with a 2-year follow-up and found 5 patients with a positive peritoneal cytology before resection of colorectal cancer. All of them had advanced (stage IV) disease or poorly differentiated carcinoma and died much earlier than patients with negative washings, typically between 4 and 10 months after surgery. No conversions from negative pre-resection to positive post-resection washings were noted (Horattas et al. 1997). This would support the contention that malignant cells are released in the peritoneum as a result of an advanced disease and not spilled during surgical manipulation of the large bowel. As a further support to this theory, Kim and colleagues analyzed the presence of malignant cells in the peritoneal fluid pre- and post-resection of 19 patients who underwent laparoscopic resection of colorectal cancer compared with 19 open counterparts, using conventional cytology plus immunocytochemistry (Ber-EP4 antibody). Although the accuracy of this specific modality had been previously validated by a pilot study, no malignant cells were demonstrated in the peritoneal fluid at any time of retrieval in either groups (Kim et al. 1998).

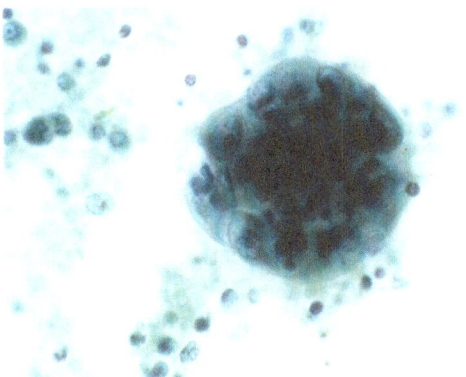

Fig. 11.2. Papanicolaou's staining of exfoliated cells of a colorectal carcinoma. Courtesy of the Institute of Cytology, University Hospital, Zurich, Switzerland

Buchmann et al. (1997) studied peritoneal washings by Papanicolaou staining (Fig. 11.2) and monoclonal antibodies (Fig. 11.1) for colonic cancer cells in patients having either open or laparoscopic resections of colorectal cancers. At the initiation of surgery, 8% of all patients had positive washings when excluding those patients with peritoneal carcinomatosis. After mobilization of the affected bowel segment, 3% of the laparoscopically operated patients had positive washings while 11% of the conventionally operated patients had positive washings. At the final phase of surgery, all washings were negative. Underlining the unclear value of peritoneal washings is the occurrence of a port-site recurrence in one patient who had negative washings during removal of a pT3N2M1 rectal cancer.

Hase and colleagues (1998) have observed 140 patients for a minimum of 8-year follow-up or until death after performing intraoperative peritoneal lavage cytology at laparotomy and at the end of resection, adopting various cytologic techniques. Seven characteristics were found to be associated with increased probability of exfoliating malignant cells, including macroscopic peritoneal dissemination, liver metastases, more than 20 ml of ascites, ulcerated tumors with indefinite borders, invasion of serosal surface or beyond, annular or semiannular shape and moderate or marked lymphatic invasion. In the subset of 88 patients undergoing resection with curative intent, only circumferential involvement was found to be associated with more likely positive cytology. All three patients with positive post-resection cytology suffered tumor recurrence after surgery. However, while two of them had a positive peritoneal lavage also at laparotomy, only one became positive after completion of colonic resection. In addition to this, six patients with positive pre-resection cytology became negative post-resection. The reason for these findings is unclear. Further, the recurrence rate was comparable to that of patients with negative cytology (33.3% vs 32.9%, respectively). Therefore, it is reasonable to believe that data from this study is not sufficiently compelling to support the hypothesis of positive cytology occurring as a result of surgical manipulation.

This same group analyzed the data to examine for a relationship between cytology, results and T-stage. There was no correlation between positive cytology and T-stage. When curative resection was performed and tumors did not involve the serosa, 10.3% were still positive. Circumferential involvement of the lumen was found to be predictive of positive cytology among the cases resected with curative intent, with 16.4% of patients with annular or semiannular tumors vs. none of the patients with two-thirds or less of the circumference involved (Hase et al 1998).

Several investigators have proposed different methods to reduce the number of exfoliated cells, supporting the concept that this measure would in turn lead to a decreased recurrence rate, among which the so-called no touch technique is probably the best known. However, when this technique was tested in a prospective randomized fashion and evaluated in large retrospective series, no significant benefit was demonstrated (Wiggers et al. 1988; Slanetz et al. 1998).

Despite advancements in detection techniques, there is still scarce evidence that a positive peritoneal washing can be predictive of recurrence, either at the abdominal wall or elsewhere. Further studies are warranted to select the most accurate methodology and assess a sound correlation between positivity and prognosis. In the absence of any proven benefit, peritoneal washings are not currently warranted as standard of care.

References

Alexander RJT, Jaques BC, Mitchell KG (1993) Laparoscopically assisted colectomy and wound recurrence. Lancet 341: 249–250

Ambrose NS, MacDonald F, Young J, Thompson H, Keighley MR (1989) Monoclonal antibody and cytological detection of free malignant cells in the peritoneal cavity during resection of colorectal cancer – can monoclonal antibodies do better? Eur J Surg Oncol 15: 99–102

Buchmann P, Christen D, Buschta G, Sartoretti Ch (1997) Intraperitoneal tumor cell spread during colorectal cancer surgery: follow up of the comparison of laparoscopic versus open surgery. Langenbecks Arch Chir Suppl Kongressbd 114: 1122–1124

Buchmann P, Christen D, Buschta G (1999a) Intraperitoneal tumor spread during surgery for colorectal cancer (submitted)

Buchmann P, Buschta G, Christen D (1999b) Intraperitoneal free tumor cells in colorectal cancer. Surgery - port-site recurrences and outcome. Langenbeck Arch Chir (in press)

Cook TA, Dehn TCB (1996) Port-site recurrences in patients undergoing laparoscopy for gastrointestinal malignancy. Br J Surg 83: 1419–1420

Drouard F, Delamarre J, Capron JP (1991) Cutaneous seeding of gallbladder cancer after laparoscopic cholecystectomy. N Engl J Med 325: 1316

Fermor B, Umpleby HC, Lever JV, Symes MO, Williamson RCN (1986) Proliferative and metastatic potential of exfoliated colorectal cancer cells. J Natl Cancer Inst 76: 347–349

Fusco MA, Paluzzi MW (1993) Abdominal wall recurrence after laparoscopic-assisted colectomy for adenocarinoma of the colon. Report of a case. Dis Colon Rectum 36: 858–861

Gertsch P, Baer HU, Kraft R, Maddern GJ, Altermatt HJ (1992) Malignant cells are collected on circular staplers. Dis Colon Rectum 35: 238–241

Gutman M, Fidler IJ (1995) Biology of human colon cancer metastasis. World J Surg 19: 226–234

Hase K, Ueno H, Kuranaga N, Utsunomiya K, Kanabe S, Mochizuki W (1998) Intraperitoneal exfoliated cancer cells in patients with colorectal cancer. Dis Colon Rectum 41: 1134–1140

Horattas MC, Evasovich MR, Topham N (1997) Colorectal carcinoma and the relationship of peritoneal cytology. Am J Surg 174: 334–337

Johnstone PA, Rohde DC, Swartz SE, Fetter JE, Wexner SD (1996) Port-site recurrences after laparoscopic and thoracoscopic procedures in malignancy. J Clin Oncol 14: 1950–1956

Juhl H, Stritzel M, Wroblewski A, Henne-Bruns D, Kremer B, Schmiegel W, Neumaier M, Wagener C, Schreiber HW, Kalthoff H (1994) Immunocytological detection of micrometastatic cells: comparative evaluation of findings in the peritoneal cavity and the bone marrow of gastric, colorectal and pancreatic cancer patients. Int J Cancer 57: 330–335

Kim SH, Milsom JW, Gramlich TL, Toddy SM, Shore GI, Okuda J, Fazio VW (1998) Does laparoscopic vs. conventional surgery increase exfoliated cancer cells in the peritoneal cavity during resection of colorectal cancer? Dis Colon Rectum 41: 971–978

Leather AJ, Kocjan G, Savage F, Hu W, Yiu CY, Boulos PB, Northover JM, Philips RK (1994) Detection of free malignant cells in the peritoneal cavity before and after resection of colorectal cancer. Dis Colon Rectum 37: 814–819

Lindemann F, Schlimok G, Dirschedl P, Witte J, Riethmuller G (1992) Prognostic significance of micrometastatic tumor cells in bone marrow of colorectal cancer patients. Lancet 340: 685–689

Martin JK Jr, Goellner JR (1986) Abdominal fluid cytology in patients with gastrointestinal malignant lesions. Mayo Clin Proc 61: 467–471

Murphy PD, Wadhera V, Griffin SM, Burgess P, Farrell D, Tylor I, Hair T, Clague MB, Griffith CD (1993) Free peritoneal tumor cell identification in patients with gastric and colorectal cancer. J R Coll Surg Edinb 38: 28–32

Murthy SM, Goldschmidt RA, Rao LN, Ammirati M, Buchmann T, Scanlon EF (1989) The influence of surgical trauma on experimental metastasis. Cancer 64: 2035–2044

Nieveen van Dijkum EJ, de Wit LT, Oberdorp H, Gouma DJ (1996) Port-site recurrences following diagnostic laparoscopy. Br J Surg 83: 1793–1794

Schaeff B, Paolucci V, Henze A (1999) Electron microscopic study on mesothelial cells after laparoscopic operations. Surg Endosc 13: S 24

Schott A, Vogel I, Krueger U, Kalthoff H, Schreiber HW, Schmiegel W, Henne-Bruns D, Kremer B, Juhl H (1998) Isolated tumor cells are frequently detectable in the peritoneal cavity of gastric and colorectal cancer patients and serve as a new prognostic marker. Ann Surg 227: 372–379

Skipper D, Cooper AJ, Marston JE, Taylor I (1987) Exfoliate d cells and in vitro growth in colorectal cancer. Br J Surg 74: 1049–1052

Slanetz CA Jr (1998) Effect of no touch isolation on survival and recurrence in curative resections for colorectal cancer. Ann Surg Oncol 5: 390–398

Stockdale AD, Pocock TJ (1985) Abdominal wall metastasis following laparoscopy: a case report. Eur J Surg Oncol 11: 373–375

Texler ML, King G, Hewett PJ (1998) From inside out. Microperforation of the gallbladder during laparoscopic surgery may liberate mucosal cells. Surg Endosc 12: 1297–1299

Uras C, Altinkaya E, Yardimci H, Goksel S, Yavuz N, Kaptanoglu L, Akcal T (1996) Peritoneal cytology in the determination of free tumor cells within the abdomen in colon cancer. Surg Oncol 5: 259–263

Ugarte F (1995) Laparoscopic cholecystectomy port seeding from a colon carcinoma. Am Surg 61: 820–821

Walsh DCA, Wattchow DA, Wilson TG (1993) Subcutaneous metastases after laparoscopic resection of malignancy. Aust N Z J Surg 63: 5635

Wiggers T, Jeekel J, Arends JW, Brinkhorst AP, Kluck HM, Luyk CI, Munting CD, Povel JA, Rfutten AP, Volovics A (1988) No-touch isolation technique in colon cancer: a controlled prospective trial. Br J Surg 75: 409–415

Wong LS, Bateman WJ, Morris AG, Fraser IA (1995) Detection of circulating tumor cells with the magnetic activated cell sorter. Br J Surg 82: 1333–1337

Wong LS, Morris AG, Fraser IA (1996) The exfoliation of free malignant cells in the peritoneal cavity during resection of colorectal cancer. Surg Oncol 5: 115–121

Yamashita K, Kuba T, Shinoda H, Takahashi E, Okayasu I (1998) Detection of K-ras point mutations to cytologic examination. Am J Clin Pathol 109: 704–711

Zuna RE, Mitchell ML (1988) Cytologic findings in peritoneal washings associated with benign gynecologic disease. Acta Cytol 32: 139–147

Zuna RE, Mitchell ML, Muliack KA, Weijchert WM (1989) Cytohistologic correlation of peritoneal washing cytology in gynecologic disease. Acta Cytol 33: 327–336

CHAPTER 12

Pathogenesis: Transportation of Tumor Cells in Clinical Studies

M. Pross, K. Ridwelski, M.A. Reymond

Introduction

The exact mechanisms responsible for the development of port-site recurrences within the abdominal wall are still unclear. Such abdominal wall recurrences can occur or not in close proximity with the tumor. In any case, it has to be assumed that, for a port-site recurrence to develop, tumor cells must be present within the abdominal cavity (or disseminated during surgery by various mechanisms), and transported into the site of recurrence (hereafter the port-site), where these cells finally find conditions for growth.

Different patterns of spread may be important. In theory, one possible mechanism responsible for the development of abdominal wall recurrences could be hematogenous or lymphatic dissemination. Besides the most common locations of distant metastases, such as liver and lungs, micrometastatic dissemination to areas with active cellular proliferation such as the bone marrow has been shown for a variety of malignancies, including colorectal cancer. When monoclonal antibodies specific for tumor associated antigens and cytokeratins were tested, up to 40% of the patients examined had positive cells in the bone marrow (Lindemann 1992). Similarly, there is experimental evidence that tumor cells injected intravenously can result in tumor formation at the site of laparotomy (Murthy 1989). However, in the absence of clear anatomic connections to the abdominal wall, this mechanism is of unlikely significance.

A second possible mechanism may be direct tumor implantation during the procedure, including during extraction of the surgical specimen. In support of this, a number of investigators have focused their efforts on measuring tumor cell numbers, that is the number of viable malignant cells that can be retrieved from the abdominal cavity at the time of surgery. Results from these studies have been contradictory and, to date, a clear correlation between positive cytology and recurrence has not been convincingly demonstrated.

One alternative hypothesis is that malignant cells can be released from the tumor bed as a result of surgical manipulation with subsequent implantation in the abdominal wall, among other sites of local recurrence.

This chapter focuses on data obtained in the human patient concerning the mechanisms by which tumor cells can be transported into the port-site.

Mechanisms Involved in the Transport of Tumor Cells

Based on the aforementioned clinical data, we decided in autumn 1995 to study the relative importance of the various mechanisms mentioned above in the transport of tumor cells. This study was designed to assess, quantitatively and qualitatively, the contamination with tumor cells of the peritoneal cavity, of the surgical instruments and of the CO_2 pneumoperitoneum during a staging laparoscopy for pancreatic cancer. Staging laparoscopy for pancreatic cancer is an excellent model for investigating such questions because over 90% of such cancers carry a mutation of the codons 12 or 13 of the k-ras gene (Jiang et al. 1989), thus permitting detection of a small number of cancer cells.

Intraoperative samples were obtained from 12 patients who underwent a staging laparoscopy for pancreatic cancer at the Universities of Erlangen, Würzburg, Regensburg and Ulm at the beginning of 1996. Diagnosis of pancreatic adenocarcinoma was based on histopathological analysis in all cases. Positive and negative control cell lines – with or without k-ras mutations – were supplied. Peritoneal washings were sampled at the beginning of the procedure. The carbon dioxide used during the procedure was collected using a trocar into a Bülau bottle filled with phosphate buffered saline (PBS) solution. This solution was pH-controlled and gently heated to preserve the viability of the cells. At the end of the procedure, trocars and instruments were rinsed separately.

Analysis of the samples was performed using conventional cytology, as well as molecular amplification methods, to confirm the results and to increase sensitivity. After vital staining with trypan blue, the viability of the cells was assessed by conventional microscopy. After Giemsa staining, the samples were analyzed by a senior pathologist who was blinded to the sample origin. A cell counting was performed af-

ter fixation and adapted to the initial sample volume. DNA was extracted according to the usual protocols. Then, the ubiquitous human ß-globin gene was amplified by polymerase chain reaction (PCR). This allowed us to assess the presence of small numbers of human cells, for example in the pneumoperitoneum. Then, a second, non-radioactive method involving PCR amplification of k-ras first exon sequences (157 bp) was performed to specifically detect the presence of tumor cells. A dilution analysis with the mutant control cell line showed that the PCR allowed us to detect less than 10 cells in PBS (Fig. 12.1). Then, to

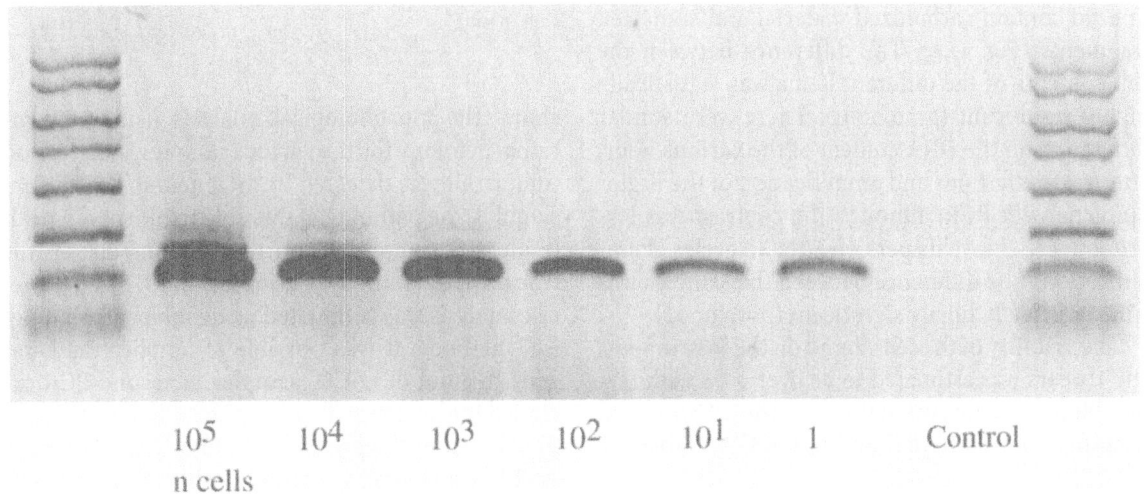

10^5 10^4 10^3 10^2 10^1 1   Control

n cells

Fig. 12.1. Polymerase chain reaction (35 cycles) of the k-ras gene, with serial dilutions in phosphate-buffered saline solution (PBS), showing that the method is able to detect the presence of less than 10 cells

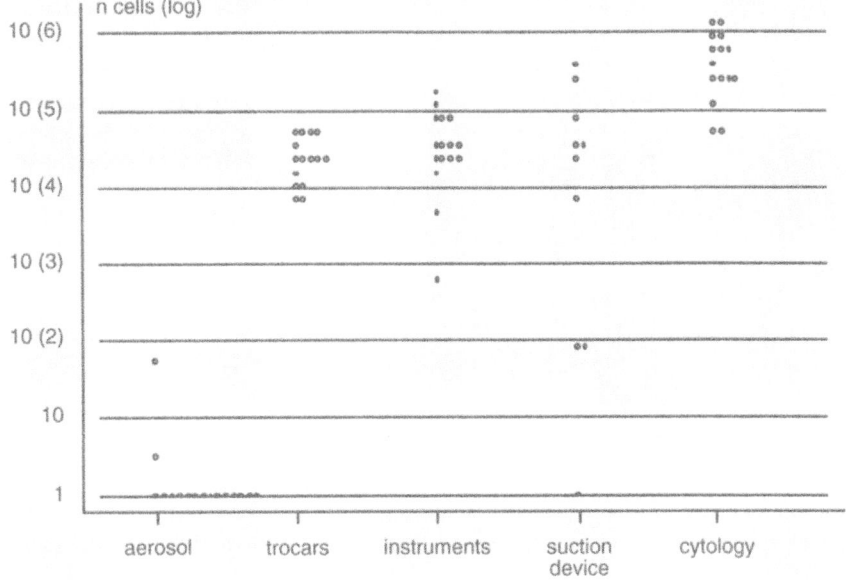

Fig. 12.2. Quantitative results of conventional cytology, showing significant differences between the relative cell content of the different items (Kruskal-Wallis test, $p < 0.0001$)

further increase sensitivity, a second 40-cycle PCR was performed with the products of the first 40-cycle PCR. In spite of this second amplification, the negative controls remained negative. Finally, the PCR products were digested to allow the detection of restriction fragment length polymorphism (RFLP), i.e., the presence of mutations in codons 12 and/or 13 of the k-ras gene.

Figure 12.2 shows the cellular characteristics of the various samples. The peritoneal washing contained the most cells ($5.3 \times 10^5 \pm 4.1 \times 10^5$ cells) (Fig. 12.3), although the suction device ($7.7 \times 10^4 \pm 1.2 \times 10^5$), instruments ($4.9 \times 10^4 \pm 4.6 \times 10^4$) and trocars ($2.9 \times 10^4 \pm 1.8 \times 10^4$) also bore many cells. The CO_2 contained almost no nucleated cells (3.4 ± 12.4), but did contain carbonized material and some cell fragments (Fig. 12.4). The difference between the cell contents of the different items was statistically highly significant ($p = 0.0001$). There were similar differences in the DNA content of the various items after serial dilutions and amplification of the ß-globin gene with PCR, although the contrast was less pronounced due to dispersion after 40 cycles of amplification. The difference between the samples was still statistically highly significant ($p = 0.0002$).

The viability of the cells found on the instruments and trocars was estimated to be over 90% with trypan blue and conventional microscopy. Using vital staining, no cells were found in the CO_2. Table 12.1

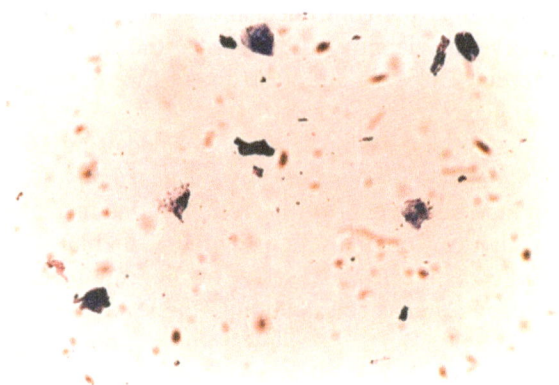

Fig. 12.4. Example of cytology of CO_2-pneumoperitoneum, showing the presence of cell fragments, carbonized fragments and very rare nucleated cells (*upper left*) (original magnification, ×100)

shows the morphological analysis using conventional cytology for the various samples. Whereas no tumor cell was detected in the pneumoperitoneum samples, the pathologist was able to morphologically identify tumor cells on the instruments, on the trocars and within the peritoneal fluid. A more precise analysis was conducted using molecular biological methods. It was possible to amplify the k-ras gene in 6 out of 12 CO_2 samples. A second PCR excluded the presence of DNA in the other 6 CO_2 samples, and thus the presence of tumor cells (Fig. 12.5). An RFLP analysis of 4 of the 6 positive PCR products was possible and showed the presence of tumor cells (Fig. 12.6). The remaining 2 CO_2 samples contained insufficient DNA for RFLP analysis.

Table 12.1. Cytological analysis of peritoneal washing, instruments and CO_2-pneumoperitoneum during staging laparoscopy for pancreatic cancer

Patient	Peritoneum	Instruments	Trocars	Suction device	CO_2
1	+ N	+ N	+ N	+ N	–
2	+ S	++ T	+ S	+ S	–
3	+ T	+ S	(+) S	(+) N	(+) N
4	++ S	X	+ N	X	–
5	++ T	++ N	+ N	X	–
6	+ N	+ N	+ N	(+) N	(+) N
7	+ N	+ S	+ N	X	–
8	++ T	+ N	+ S	X	–
9	+ N	+ N	+ N	++ S	(+) N
10	++ T	+ N	+ T	(+) N	–
11	+ N	+ S	(+) N	(+) N	–
12	+ N	+ N	+ N	X	–

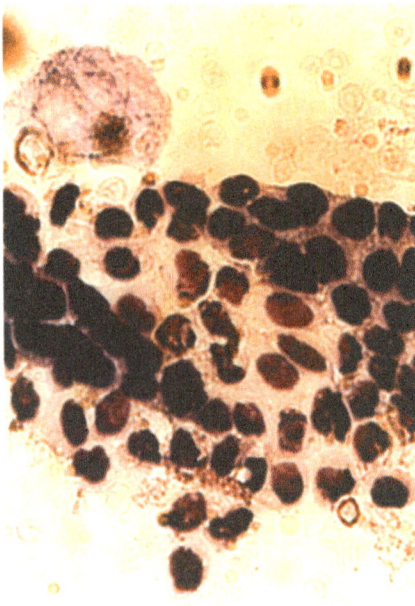

Fig. 12.3. Example of cytology of the peritoneal cavity, showing the highest cellular content and the presence of tumor cells (original magnification, ×100)

–, no cells; N, normal cells; (+), isolated cells; S, suspect cells; +, cells; T, tumor cells; ++, many cells; X, no sample

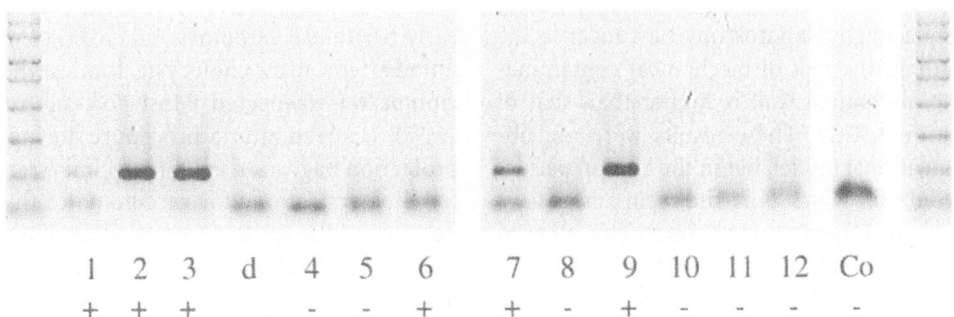

Fig. 12.5. Second k-ras PCR (40 cycles, after dilution of 1:1000), with the products of a first PCR (40 cycles) showing the absence of any gene amplification in 6 out of 12 aerosol samples. Thus, it can reasonably be assumed that these CO_2 samples contained no nucleated cells. *d*, control cholecystectomy

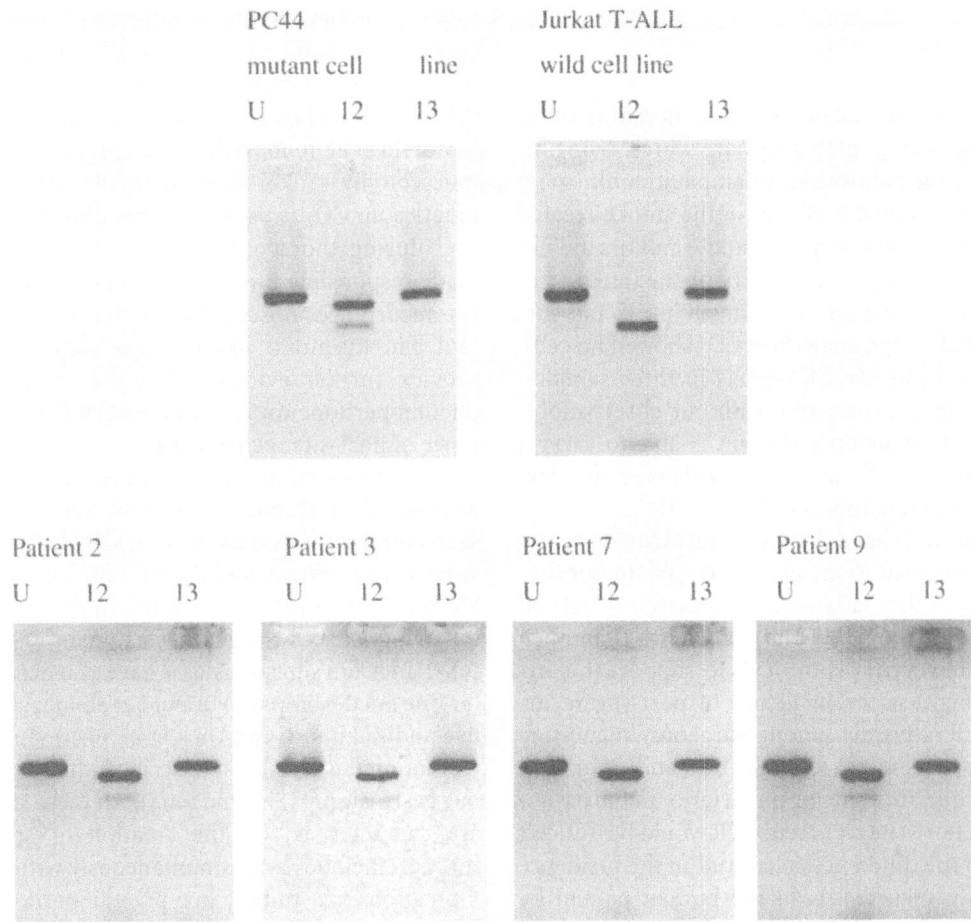

Fig. 12.6. Restriction analysis of the 4 aerosols from which the k-ras gene could be amplified, showing the presence of a mutant gene. Thus, very low levels of free-floating tumor cells could be detected in these 4 CO_2 samples. *12*, restricted with *Mv*AI (codon 12); *13*, restricted with *Hph*I (codon 13); –, uncut PCR product

In summary, these observations showed very clearly that, during a staging laparoscopy for cancer in the human patient, the risk of mechanical contamination of the abdominal wall is higher than that of seeding through CO_2. These results were not obtained in an animal model, but in the human patient in a procedure for which port-site recurrences have been described (Jorgensen et al. 1995). This allowed us to suggest that the incidence of port-site recurrences might be reduced if proper surgical technique is applied, an hypothesis that has been widely confirmed in the meantime (Johnstone et al. 1996). For example, in 191 laparoscopic colectomies for cancer, involving the anchoring of trocars with sutures, the bagging of specimens, washing of devices and the suturing of peritoneum, Franklin et al. observed no port-site recurrences (Franklin et al. 1996).

Data From the Literature

Data obtained in human patients concerning cellular seeding during laparoscopy are scarce. Using filters placed on the trocars, Champault et al. (1997) observed the presence of cells in the smoke created during laparoscopic surgery, but the authors did not further characterize the viability or the integrity of these cells. In another study involving 25 patients (Bonjer et al. 1997), analysis of CO_2 showed no cells, but revealed positive CEA-levels in three samples. These results are consistent with our observations, namely that pneumoperitoneum is able to carry a few mesothelial cells, and perhaps also very low levels of free-floating tumor cells.

It has been claimed that port-site recurrences are essentially related to the use of CO_2 pneumoperitoneum – and that laparoscopy is therefore related with a higher rate of wound recurrence than open surgery. However, it is difficult to support this hypothesis because the incidence of port-site recurrences differs greatly among surgeons, suggesting that differences in patient selection and/or operating technique are of major importance in the pathogenesis of port-site recurrences. It would be difficult to explain the differences observed in the incidence of port-site recurrences in the human patient by constant factors such as pneumoperitoneum. In the meantime, it is widely accepted that the incidence of port-site recurrences is a surgeon-related variable, dependent on experience and expertise (Johnstone et al. 1996).

A recent overall review of port-site recurrences covering responses with answers from 443 hospitals in Germany reported 109 port-site recurrences or early peritoneal carcinosis, 76 (70%) of which were found after routine cholecystectomies where no carcinoma was suspected. Most port-site recurrences (63%) occurred after a procedure during which no protection bag was used for specimen retrieval. After cholecystectomy for carcinoma of the gallbladder, 56% of the recurrences developed in the extraction port (Schaeff et al. 1998). Such observations underscore the role of mechanical inoculation of tumor cells into the abdominal wall, either because the surgeon was unaware of the presence of cancer, or because he failed to protect the wound during extraction of the resected specimen.

A number of port-site recurrences have been reported after thoracoscopy for cancer. Two recent studies involved 21 (Downey et al. 1996) and 15 cases of recurrences following thoracoscopy (Egan et al. 1997). On reviewing the literature, we found further cases of port-site recurrences after thoracoscopy (Collard and Reymond 1996; Downey et al. 1996; Boutin and Rey 1993; Fry et al. 1995; Buhr et al. 1995; Sartorelli et al. 1996; Wille et al. 1997), and also after thoracotomy (Yokoi et al. 1996). In usual clinical practice no CO_2 is used for expanding the thoracic wall during thoracoscopy. Thus, CO_2 can not be made responsible for the occurrence of most port-site recurrences observed after thoracoscopy (Collard and Ryemond 1996). These clinical findings provide further evidence that the presence of a pneumoperitoneum is not necessary for the occurrence of port-site recurrences.

Many other comparable local recurrences in the abdominal or thoracic wall have been described: such complications have been reported after mediastinoscopy (Sullivan and Passamonte 1982; Rate and Solin 1989; Egan et al. 1997) and in drainage tracts following cancer surgery (Chapman 1989; Solin 1983). Incision site metastases have also occurred after fine needle biopsy (Voravud et al. 1992; Nankhonya and Zakhour 1991; Dick et al. 1974). Tumor implantation has also been described after percutaneous gastrostomy (Sharma 1994). All these situations are characterized by the creation of a channel through the body wall simultaneously with the manipulation of a tumor, but pneumoperitoneum is used only in laparoscopy.

In advanced tumor stages, malignant cells are usually already present within the abdominal cavity at the beginning of the procedure. During open and laparoscopic colorectal resections, tumor cells can be found within the peritoneal cavity even at early tumor stages. The quantity of cells does not seem to be influenced by the type of procedure or the time of sampling (Buchmann et al. 1996). In our own study, undertaken during staging laparoscopies for pancreatic cancer, peritoneal cytology identified tumor cells in half of the cases (Reymond et al. 1997). The presence of free-floating tumor cells within the abdominal cavity is a condition for the later occurrence of port-site recurrences. Contamination of the port-site with peritoneal fluid containing tumor cells is then likely to occur (Fig. 12.7). Very interestingly, port-site recurrences have also been observed after excision of trocar sites. Thus, it has to be as-

sumed that contamination also happens after the end of the surgical procedure (Wu et al. 1998). This explains why most port-site recurrences were observed at advanced tumor stages and when the port-site was not closed at the end of the procedure.

In summary, in a clinical setting, laparoscopy using CO_2 at pressures between 10 and 15 mm Hg has no relevant effect on the level of free-floating tumor cells, even though low levels of tumor cells can be detected in some aerosols. Mechanical inoculation of the abdominal wall by the surgical specimen or an instrument is significantly more likely to occur (Fig. 12.8). This must be the case in thoracoscopy and mediastinoscopy, where no CO_2 is used (Collard and Reymond 1996). These facts imply that a good operative technique and proper indications can prevent the occurrence of most port-site recurrences (Kökkerling et al. 1997), as confirmed by experimental studies and clinical results obtained by experienced laparoscopic surgeons.

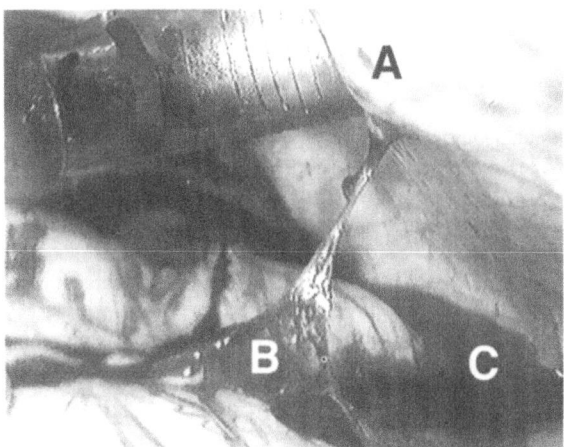

Fig. 12.7. In the presence of peritoneal fluid containing tumor cells (e.g., at advanced tumor stages), contamination of the port-site (*A*) is very likely to occur during the procedure or after the extraction of the trocars. *C*, blood; *B*, tumor

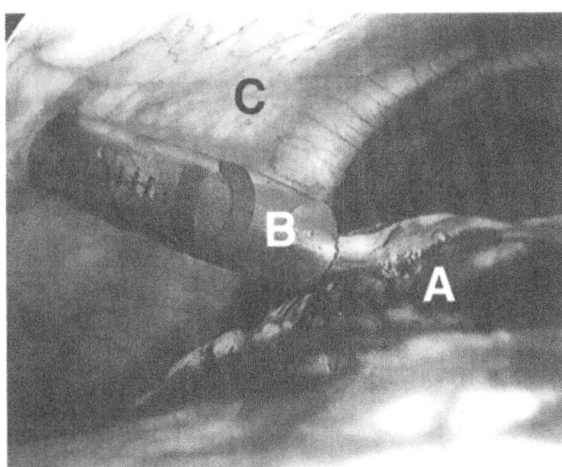

Fig. 12.8. In advanced tumor stages (here, during a staging laparoscopy for Hodgkin's lymphoma) trocars (*B*) can come in contact with the tumor mass (*A*), e.g., because of sudden intraperitoneal pressure loss after suction. *C*, abdominal wall

References

Bonjer J, Dam JH van, Romjin M, Eijck CHJ van (1997) Port-site recurrences: role of aerosolization of tumor cells. Surg Endosc 11:192

Boutin C, Rey F (1993) Thoracoscopy in pleural malignant mesothelioma: a prospective study of 188 consecutive patients. Part 1: Diagnosis. Cancer 72:389–393

Buchmann P, Christen D, Moll C, Flury R (1996) [Intraperitoneal tumor cell spread during colorectal cancer surgery: a comparison of laparoscopic versus open surgery.] Langenbecks Arch Chir 381 [SII]:573–576

Buhr J, Hurtgen M, Kelm C, Schwemmle K (1995) Tumor dissemination after thoracoscopic resection for lung cancer. J Thorac Cardiovasc Surg 110:855–856

Champault G, Taffinder N, Ziol M, Riskalla H, Catheline JMC (1997) Cells are present in the smoke created during laparoscopic surgery. Br J Surg 84:993–995

Chapman WC (1989) Tumor seeding from percutaneous biliary catheter tract. Ann Surg 209:1989

Collard JM, Reymond MA (1996) Video-assisted thoracic surgery (V.A.T.S.) for cancer: risk of parietal seeding and of early local recurrence. Int Surg 81:343–346

Dick R, Heard BE, Hinson KEW (1974) Aspiration needle biopsy of thoracic lesions: an assessment of 227 biopsies. Br J Dis Chest 68:86–93

Downey RJ, McCormack P, LoCicero III J, and the Video-Assisted Thoracic Surgery Study Group (1996) Dissemination of malignancies following video-assisted thoracic surgery. J Cardiovasc Surg 111:954–960

Egan C, Knolmayer TJ, Bowyer MW, Asbun HJ (1997) Port-site recurrences: a current review of the literature. Surg Endosc 11:196

Franklin ME, Rosenthal D, Abrego-Medina D, Dorman JP, Glass JL, Norem R, Diaz A (1996) Prospective comparison of open vs. laparoscopic colon surgery for carcinoma. Dis Colon Rectum 39:S35–S46

Fry WA, Sidiqqui A, Pensler JM (1995) Thoracoscopic implantation of cancer with a fatal outcome. Ann Thorac Surg 59:42–45

Jiang W, Kahn SM, Guillem JG, Lu SH, Weinstein IB (1989) Rapid detection of ras oncogenes in human tumors; applications to colon, esophageal, and gastric cancer. Oncogene 4:923–928

Johnstone PAS, Rohde DC, Swartz SE, Fetter JE, Wexner SD (1996) Port-site recurrences after laparoscopic and thoracoscopic procedures in malignancy. J Clin Oncol 14:1950–1956

Jorgensen JO, McCall JL, Morris DL (1995) Port-site seeding after laparoscopic ultrasonographic staging of pancreatic carcinoma [letter]. Surgery 117:118–119

Köckerling F, Reymond MA, Schneider C, Hohenberger W (1997) Mistakes and hazards in oncological laparoscopic surgery. Chirurg 68:215–224

Lindemann F, Schlimok G, Dirschedl P, Witte J, Riethmuller G (1992) Prognostic significance of micrometastatic tumour cells in bone marrow of colorectal cancer patients. Lancet 340: 685–689

Murthy SM, Goldschmidt RA, Rao LN, Ammirati M, Buchmann T, Scanlon EF (1989) The influence of surgical trauma on experimental metastasis. Cancer 64: 2035–2044

Nankhonya JM, Zakhour HD (1991) Malignant seeding of needle aspiration tract: a rare complication. Br J Dermatol 1243:285–286

Rate WR, Solin LJ (1989) Mediastinoscopy incision site metastasis: implications for radiotherapeutic treatment. Cancer 63:68–69

Reymond MA, Wittekind C, Jung A, Hohenberger W, Kirchner T, Köckerling F (1997) The incidence of port-site recurrences might be reduced. Surg Endosc 11:902–906

Sartorelli KH, Partrick D, Meagher DP Jr (1996) Port-site recurrence after thoracoscopic resection of pulmonary metastasis owing to osteogenic sarcoma. J Pediatr Surg 31:1443–1444

Schaeff B, Paolucci V, Thomopoulos J (1998) Port-site recurrences after laparoscopic surgery. A review. Dig Surg 15:124–134

Sharma P (1994) Metastatic implantation of an oral squamous-cell carcinoma at a percutaneous endoscopic gastrostomy site. Surg Endosc 8:1232–1235

Solin L (1983) Subcutaneous seeding of pancreatic carcinoma along a transhepatic biliary catheter tract. Br J Radiol 56:83–84

Sullivan WD, Passamonte PM (1982) Mediastinoscopy incision site metastasis: response to radiation therapy. South Med J 72:1428

Voravud N, Shin DM, Dekmezian RH, Dimery I, Lee JS, Hong TW (1992) Implantation metastasis of carcinoma after percutaneous fine-needle aspiration biopsy. Chest 43:1533–1540

Wille GA, Gregory R, Guernsey JM (1997) Tumor implantation at port-site of video-assisted thoracoscopic resection of pulmonary metastasis. West J Med 166:65–66

Wu JS, Guo LW, Ruiz MB, Pfister SM, Connett JM, Fleshman JW (1998) Excision of trocar sites reduces tumor implantation in an animal model. Dis Colon Rectum 41: 1107–1111

Yokoi K, Miyazawa N, Imura G (1996) Isolated incisional recurrence after curative resection for primary lung cancer. Ann Thorac Surg 61:1236–1237

CHAPTER 13

Pathogenesis: Immunological Aspects of Clinical Studies

D. Mutter, M. Aprahamian

Introduction

The risk of port-site recurrence after laparoscopic management of digestive cancer is a serious cause of concern for digestive surgeons. Among the various factors affecting tumor port-site seeding and growth, the immune changes induced by the laparoscopic procedure may play a major role. These changes in cell-mediated immunity have mainly been investigated in experimental studies, and information on the immunological status in patients is limited, restricted to a small number of acute phase protein, cytokine and hormone serological assays in few clinical studies, sometimes linked to investigations on systemic immune status.

All surgical procedures are affected by an immune system involvement resulting from tissue trauma, as well as from a transient modulation of the homeostasis linked to anesthesia. Indeed, any injury to the human body affects several physiological systems such as the cardiovascular, endocrine or immune systems. These alterations are proportional to the extent of the injury. Therefore, it can be expected that the use of minimally invasive surgery results in a minimized physiological response. The evaluation of this body response to surgical injury must be at first carried out in experimental models, but has to be confirmed in human practice.

At this step of the investigations two major drawbacks arise which are usually encountered in clinical research. The first of these is the reduced ability to accurately evaluate the immune function in human beings. Because of the fact that for ethical reasons postoperative patients cannot undergo unduly aggressive tests, the main factors evaluated were the systemic evidence of the immune reaction. Depending on the availability of human laboratory assays, these investigated factors measure particularly the acute phase protein response, as reflected both by serum concentrations of C-reactive proteins and by some cytokines, such as interleukin-1 and interleukin-6. Other systemic markers can be encountered such as histamine or corticosteroid concentrations. Evaluation of some white blood cells and their subpopulations can be also found. An analysis of the literature uncovers other kinds of measurements, whose ability to translate the body's response to surgical procedures and their real impact on the postoperative course is difficult to assess.

The second drawback encountered in clinical testing of laparoscopic repercussions on cell-mediated immunity results from the fact that the port-site seeding is probably also linked to local peritoneal factors which are difficult to evaluate in humans. In fact, investigations on peritoneal leukocyte and macrophage changes after a surgical procedure cannot be performed in humans since delayed sampling of peritoneal cells is impossible for obvious ethical reasons.

This review analyzes the changes in each of the different cell immunity markers found in the literature concerning laparoscopy, in order of the frequency at which they have been studied. It attempts to evaluate their impact on the postoperative course. All reports concerning nonimmunological stress responses (ACTH, cortisol, catecholamines, epinephrine, norepinephrine, etc.) are excluded from this review, as are those dealing with metabolic changes (albumin, transferrin, glucose, growth hormone, TSH, insulin, etc.).

The Acute Phase Proteins

The acute phase protein response to minimally invasive surgery is the most well-investigated parameter found in the literature. It reflects the extent of the surgical injury and appears to be an early event, beginning a few hours after an operation, peaking between 1 or 2 days postoperatively and sometimes lasting more than a week (Vittimberga et al. 1998). The acute phase proteins which have been investigated the most are, by order of magnitude, interleukin-6, C-reactive protein and interleukin-1.

Interleukin-6

This cytokine, currently abbreviated as IL-6, is known to be one of the major mediators of the acute phase protein response, after C-reactive protein. It is also the most frequently investigated in literature evaluating laparoscopy (over 12 clinical studies). IL-6 constitutes a part of the nonspecific, or inflammatory, response of the immune system. It acts as a defense mechanism, counteracting a body aggression such as a surgical trauma (Vittimberga et al. 1998). IL-6 is secreted by macrophages and is present early after tissue injury (Van der Velpen et al. 1994) As an acute phase protein effector, systemic IL-6 reaches the liver where it up-regulates the hepatic component of the acute phase response (Vittimberga et al. 1998). Therefore, it is considered as a detector of the severity of tissue injury (Baigrie et al. 1992). Comparing its serum concentration in conventional and laparoscopic surgery could give clear insight into the physiological response to surgical trauma.

The aim of most of the studies (Table 13.1) was to reproduce a comparative evaluation of the level of IL-6 after surgery, considering laparoscopy as a potentially less aggressive procedure. Most of these studies collect data from cholecystectomies since it is the most widely performed procedure in addition to being well standardized. Unfortunately, the majority of these studies were carried out in very small cohorts (less than 20 patients per group), affecting the accuracy and reliability of these evaluations. Moreover, even if the distribution of the patients' ages was not significantly different in these studies, the wide range of the patients' ages (ranging from 25 to 77 years) in most of the studies (except those of Jakeways et al. 1994; Fukushima et al. 1996, and Hill et al. 1995) suggested the existence of a widely different metabolic and immunological status.

In four out of seven studies comparing the impact of the surgical approach used to perform a cholecystectomy on IL-6 concentrations, a significantly lower increase of the IL-6 level was observed on the first postoperative day when laparoscopy was carried out (Cho et al. 1994; Kloosterman et al. 1994; Glaser et al. 1995; Maruszynski and Pojda 1995). This result was essentially interpreted as the expression of a lesser body injury with laparoscopic procedures. Nevertheless, these observations must be carefully interpreted: five out of these seven studies were performed during the first period of laparoscopic development (i.e., before 1995). Moreover, the surgical technique applied, the selection of patients and the operative duration were not specified in three of these trials. It must be emphasized that the lengthening of the operative procedure in itself has to be considered as an injury. This effect of the duration was already noted in 1993 by MacMahon et al. who pointed out in their study the correlation between IL-6 increase and the duration of the procedure. Such a time-related effect on IL-6 concentration was also observed by Suzuki et al. (1994), comparing laparoscopic "major" (no more information) surgery

Table 13.1. Comparative evaluation of postoperative IL-6 concentrations. In the result columns, the values are presented as "laparoscopic procedure/open procedure", except for the age which is expressed as minimum to maximum

Study	Operation	+CO_2	Patient number	Age (years)	Serum IL-6 (in pg/ml)	P value	Duration (in min)
MacMahon et al. (1993)	Cholecystectomy	Yes	10/10	25–70	110/140	NS	65/46
Cho et al. (1994)	Cholecystectomy	Yes	16/8	ND	51/124	**	ND
Jakeway et al. (1994)	Cholecystectomy	Yes	14/10	44–55	52/61	NS	ND
Kloosterman et al. (1994)	Cholecystectomy	Yes	8/8	26–66	165%/470%[a]	**	72/37
Suzuki et al. (1994)	Cholecystectomy[b]	Yes	17/12	ND	21/186	**	ND
Vander Velpen et al. (1994)	Cholecystectomy	Yes	14/10	27–74	800%/580%[a]	NS	ND
Fukushima et al. (1995)	Colectomy	No	17/12	>60	29/20	NS	ND
Glaser et al. (1995)	Cholecystectomy	Yes	40/18	30–70	8/18	*	73/74
Hill et al. (1995)	Hernia repair	No	14/20	50–60	13/15	NS	58/38
Maruszynski and Pojda (1995)	Cholecystectomy	Yes	11/14	37–71	12/49	***	ND
Hewitt et al. (1998)	Colectomy	Yes	8/8	38–77	42/74	NS	165/107

NS, not significant; ND, not determined

* $p < 0.05$, ** $p < 0.01$, *** $p < 0.001$

[a] Results expressed as an increase in the preoperative basal concentrations

[b] Comparison was made with "major open surgery"

to cholecystectomy and by Fukushima et al. (1996), comparing gas-less laparoscopic assisted colectomy to an open procedure. This last study, working without CO_2, stressed the lack of impact of the CO_2 pneumoperitoneum on the general systemic immune response (Fukushima et al. 1996). This finding was confirmed by the study of Hill et al. (1995) that showed the same change in the IL-6 response after laparoscopic hernia repair and after Lichtenstein and Bassini techniques: the use of a mesh and of an open procedure did not affect the IL-6 systemic response.

No other significant difference could be observed between laparoscopic cholecystectomy and mini-laparotomy (MacMahon et al. 1993). Cho et al. (1994) reported that a restricted elevation of the IL-6 level was not observed in a group of laparoscopically operated patients who underwent an endoscopic retrograde cholangiopancreatography (ERCP) before removal of the gallbladder. One may conclude that the lower IL-6 response gained by laparoscopy can be nullified by the previous ERCP (Cho et al. 1994). This observation would mean that body injuries may be added one to another, and that ERCP should be considered as significantly increasing the body injury linked to cholecystectomy.

On the other hand, IL-6 was found to be nonsignificantly affected in six studies (three on cholecystectomies, two on colectomies and one on inguinal hernia repair) out of 11 (see Table 13.1). It must be emphasized that the operation (as specified in three studies) lasted significantly longer when a laparoscopic procedure was applied. This concurs with the previous reports on the existing correlation between operation duration and IL-6 concentrations (MacMahon et al. 1993).

In conclusion, IL-6 is a sensitive marker of the host defense mechanism. Its major modification is linked to the duration in time of the surgical procedure. It is a poor reflection of tissue damage. Despite all of these aspects, it must be pointed out that no consensus exists about its exact immunologic (Davies and Hagen 1997) or metabolic (Gàl et al. 1994) role The small number of patients involved in all of the series added to the wide variation in the individual IL-6 values (15–634 pg/ml in Cho et al. 1994), renders its significance questionable. Finally, if IL-6 is primarily responsible for the synthesis of the acute phase proteins such as C-reactive protein (Vittimberga et al. 1998) its role in the immune host defense as a cytokine released by activated macrophages cannot be excluded (Davies and Hagen1997; Hill and Hill 1998). Indeed, it acts as a B cell stimula-tory and a T cell differentiation factor. The temporal relationship of IL-6 appearance within the cytokine cascade suggests a strong relationship to antecedent IL-1 and TNF-α stimulation (Davies and Hagen 1997). A clear understanding of its beneficial or detrimental role will demand more randomized, standardized and well-documented clinical trials.

C-Reactive Protein

C-reactive protein, currently abbreviated as CRP, is the most well-known acute phase protein. It is one of the key acute phase markers and constitutes a reliable overall screening test for acute phase reactants (Vittimberga et al. 1998). Conversely to IL-6, which exhibits an early preoperative rise and reaches its maximal values around 24 h after surgery, CRP serum concentration increases only 12 h after an operation and peaks on the second postoperative day (Baigrie et al. 1992).

It has been slightly less clinically investigated than IL-6 in the literature: only ten clinical trials are available (Table 13.2). CRP usually exhibited a ten-fold rise 24 h after a conventional surgical injury, reaching almost 100 mg/l in value (Baiugrie et al. 1992). Apart from the trial of Hill et al. (1995) devoted to inguinal hernia repair in which body injury can be considered as reduced, CRP serum concentrations reported in the literature correspond well to this average postsurgical value as detailed in the Table. As a matter of fact, the acute phase protein response measured by C-reactive protein is less affected by laparoscopy than by open conventional surgery: CRP values are always lower with laparoscopy than with open surgery, showing a significantly lower increase in six out of ten clinical investigations. It should be noted that, in the study of MacMahon et al. (1993) the open cholecystectomy procedure consisted of a "mini" laparotomy and that no information was available about the procedure used in the last study, for which no significant difference was observed (Gàl et al. 1994).

As summarized in Table 13.2, the CRP mean values found in these different studies are not always correlated to the level of the IL-6 cytokine (MacMahon et al. 1993; Cho et al. 1994; Jakeway et al. 1994; Fukushima et al. 1996; Hill et al. 1995). This corroborated our observation of the unreliability of IL-6 as an acute-phase protein marker.

In conclusion, CRP is a sensitive marker of the acute phase protein response. Its modification is linked to the extent of the surgical injury. All of the

Table 13.2. Comparative evaluation of postoperative CRP concentrations. In the result columns, the values are presented as "laparoscopic procedure/open procedure", except for the age which is expressed as minimum to maximum

Study	Operation	Number of patients	Age (years)	Serum CRP (in mg/l)	Probability	Duration (in min)
Mealy et al. (1992)	Cholecystectomy	10/11	37–62	16/76	**	84/81
MacMahon et al. (1993)	Cholecystectomy	10/10	25–70	60/90	NS	65/46
Cho et al. (1994)	Cholecystectomy	16/8	ND	24/104	***	ND
Gàl et al. (1994)	Cholecystectomy	14/14	ND	53/84	NS	ND
Jakeway et al. (1994)	Cholecystectomy	14/10	44–55	17/49	*	ND
Redmond et al. (1994)	Cholecystectomy	22/22	40–59	53/69	NS	69/83
Bolufer et al. (1995)	Various[a]	26/18	47–69	49/95	*	110/105
Halevy et al. (1995)	Cholecystectomy	17/13	30–70	27/127	***	ND
Fukushima et al. (1995)	Colectomy	17/12	>60	60/100	*	ND
Hill et al. (1995)	Inguinal hernia	14/20	50–60	12/23	NS	ND

ND, not determined; NS, not significant

* $p < 0.05$, ** $p < 0.01$, *** $p < 0.001$

[a] Mainly constituted of cholecystectomies (17 laparoscopy versus 8 open surgery), followed by hernia repairs (5 laparoscopy versus 6 open surgery)

clinical investigations available in the literature are in agreement with the opinion that laparoscopy induces a less acute phase protein response and can be considered as less aggressive for the body.

The Other Cytokines

The other mediators of the immune response, such as some cytokines, have been clinically investigated far less than IL-6. Some of them, such as IL-1 or TNF-α, are sometimes considered as acute-phase proteins (Vittimberga et al. 1998) but there is no consensus on the meaning of their systemic level today (Davies and Hagen 1997; Hill and Hill 1998). Our opinion is that they can be considered as serum markers of the systemic immune status after surgery, as suggested previously for IL-6.

Interleukin-1β

Interleukin-1β, currently abbreviated as IL-1β, is the circulating isoform of IL-114 and exhibits an early and transient peak after surgery (between 2 and 4 h after the beginning of the operation) when no postoperative complication was observed. IL-1β precedes and directs the release of the well-investigated IL-6, which directs in turn the release of CRP at the level of the liver (Vittimberga et al. 1998; Davies and Hagen 1997; Hill and Hill 1998). Consequently, IL-1β can be considered as the earliest marker of the immune response to operative injury (Davies and Hagen 1997).

Unfortunately, this early immune status marker has been poorly investigated. Only one study (Glaser et al. 1995) in the existing literature deals with IL-1β after open and laparoscopic surgery. After a strong and significantly higher perioperative peak during open surgery, no significant difference can be found between open and laparoscopic surgery from the first postoperative day onwards. An experimental observation on Lewis rats by our group (unpublished data) concerning IL-1β values corroborates the results of Glaser showing no significant difference between IL-1β serum concentrations from anesthetic control, CO_2 pneumoperitoneum and laparotomy experimental groups one day after procedures. To confirm these initial findings, it would be extremely helpful to schedule clinical prospective trials investigating IL-1β concentrations after laparotomy and laparoscopy. Indeed, in one clinical report, investigating the immune status after laparoscopic cholecystectomy, in the absence of open surgery control, there was no increase in IL-1β (Yoshida et al. 1995) while in another (Evrard et al. 1997) a strong decrease in the IL-1β serum level was observed. However, we must keep in mind that the serum concentration of a cytokine reflects its systemic release at a given moment only, and may provide erroneous information on real cell-mediated immunity after surgery.

Tumor Necrosis Factor-α

The tumor necrosis factor-α cytokine, currently abbreviated as TNF-α, is released by immune cells

The Immune Cells

Table 13.3. Comparative evaluation of total white blood cells. Results are expressed as means ($\times 10^3$ cells/ml). In all studies, total white blood cells were less increased after laparoscopic procedure

Study	Laparoscopy	Laparotomy	P value
Kloosterman et al. (1994)	4.5	8.0	*
Bolufer et al. (1995)	4.2	6.3	***
Halevy et al. (1995)	10.6	14.0	***
Maruszynski et al. (1995)	5.9	6.4	NS
Walker et al. (1999)	7.7	7.9	NS

* $p < 0.05$, ** $p < 0.01$, *** $p < 0.001$

changes are significant in three of these studies (Kloosterman et al. 1994; Bolufer et al. 1995; Halevy et al. 1995). For Kloosterman et al. (1994) the transient increase in granulocyte number observed after open cholecystectomy was missing after laparoscopic cholecystectomy. This was confirmed by two other trials (Maruszynski and Podja 1995; Bolufer et al. 1995). For Halevy at al (1995) however, the total amount of leukocytes was significantly increased after both procedures, but this increase was significantly greater after open surgery. Walker et al. (1999) found, after cholecystectomy, a transient increase in the number of white blood cells after both procedures, but without any significant difference between laparoscopy or mini-laparotomy. Conversely, Hewitt et al. (1998) found a decreased num-

ber of cells with both procedures, without any significant difference between laparoscopy and open surgery.

It appears that the majority of these findings showing a lower white blood cell response to surgical aggression comply with the reduction of the acute phase protein response and support the argument attesting to lesser body injury by laparoscopic procedures.

The total number of lymphocytes appears to be decreased in both procedures for Hewitt et al. (1998) without any difference between them. Lymphocytes were also found to be affected by Christaldi et al. (1997) and by Walker et al. (1999), but with a more important and more lasting reduction after laparotomy. Comparison of the lymphocytes subsets, however, may be helpful to develop a clear understanding of the phenomenon.

Leukocyte Subpopulation Changes

Changes in leukocyte subpopulations, which reflect in part the type of immunosuppression induced by laparoscopic and conventional surgery, have been investigated in only five studies. These results are summarized in Table 13.4.

Among them, the results of two studies examining almost all lymphocyte subpopulations are of great interest, as they highlighted an ubiquitous be-

Table 13.4. Changes in white blood cell subpopulations after laparoscopic surgery versus open surgery. Results are expressed as the level of significance between laparoscopy and open surgery. For all populations there was a slight advantage for laparoscopic surgery

White blood cell populations		Vallina et al. (1996)	Christaldi et al. (1997)	Brune et al. (1998)	Hewitt et al. (1998)	Walker et al. (1999)
Total lymphocytes		+		NS	++	
T cells	CD2					+
	CD3		++	NS	NS	++
	CD4	++	++		NS	+
	CD8	+	++			+
	CD25			NS		NS
NK cells	CD11					+
	CD16		++		NS	+
	CD56					+
	CD57					+
B cells	CD19		NS		NS	NS
Monocytes	CD14			NS	NS	
Activation markers	CD71					++
	HLA-DR			NS	+	+

NS, not significant
+ $p < 0.05$, ++ $p < 0.01$

havior of these particular subclasses of immune cells (Walker et al. 1999; Cristaldi et al. 1997). Indeed, the Pan-T (CD3+), T helper (CD4+) and T suppressor (CD8+) subclasses of T lymphocytes decreased significantly less (and only transiently) after laparoscopy than after laparotomy in both studies. These findings were confirmed by those of Vallina and Velasco (1996), who observed a strong decrease in both T helper and T suppressor lymphocytes after laparotomy versus no change in these subclasses after laparoscopy (with significant differences between the two procedures). T helper and T suppressor lymphocytes also remained unaffected by laparoscopy in the work of Champault et al. (1996) but these two subclasses of T lymphocytes followed the same pattern of changes after laparotomy and laparoscopy in a study by Hewitt et al. (1998) without any significant difference.

The NK cell (CD16+) counts remained low during the whole postoperative month following laparotomy, and were unaffected by laparoscopy in the study by Cristaldi et al. (1997). This NK cell subtype, like the other ones (CD11+, CD56+, CD57+), was slightly depressed after laparoscopy in the study by Walker et al. (1999) but was significantly more depressed after laparotomy.

In the three studies (Hewitt et al. 1998; Walker et al. 1999; Cristaldi et al. 1997) investigating B lymphocytes (Pan B, CD19+), this subclass remained unaffected regardless of the surgical procedure. The same observation was made for CD14+ monocytes (Hewitt et al. 1998; Brune et al. 1998).

In conclusion, it can be considered that, apart from monocytes and B lymphocytes which are never affected by any procedure, all other kinds of lymphocyte subclasses are either unaffected or only slightly and transiently depressed after laparoscopy. On the contrary, these two subclasses of lymphocytes (i.e., NK cells and T lymphocytes) are significantly reduced after open surgical procedures in comparison to laparoscopy. This fact may have an impact on host cell defense against the systemic metastatic spread of a tumor.

Changes in Immune Cell Functions

The impact of laparoscopic surgery on immune cells has not only been evaluated for changes in the number of these cells. The immune cell functions were also investigated in human beings. Some of these investigations were devoted to neutrophil functions (MacMahon et al. 1993; Gàl et al. 1994; Carey et al.

1994). A granulocyte marker, the polymorphonuclear leukocyte elastase (or PNM elastase) constitutes one of the major neutrophil enzymes. This marker is increased significantly after open surgery compared to laparoscopy (MacMahon et al. 1993; Gàl et al. 1994). Moreover, in this latter study, increase in PNM elastase persists only after laparotomy. PNM elastase was also significantly increased in a study by Suzuki et al. (1994) after open surgery, but the authors compared this leukocyte marker under very different circumstances (laparoscopic cholecystectomy as opposed to major abdominal surgery).

Another clinical trial analyzed the effect of laparoscopic surgery on neutrophil activation by their release of an antimicrobial oxidant; the activity was significantly depressed after open surgery (Carey et al. 1994): functionally, the granulocytes are less affected by laparoscopy. Quantitatively, more granulocytes are detected after conventional laparotomy, as reflected both by the cell counts (Maruszynski et al. 1995; Hewitt et al. 1998; Bolufer et al. 1995; Walker et al. 1999; Cristaldi et al. 1997; Vallina and Velasco 1996; Brune et al. 1998) and by PNM elastase concentrations (MacMahon et al. 1993; Gàl et al. 1994; Carey et al. 1994). This observation complies well with the general assumption of a lesser cell-mediated immunity injury by laparoscopic surgery (Vittimberga et al. 1998).

Basically, the delayed type hypersensitivity (DTH) is associated with T cell-related immunological functions. However, DTH responsiveness is a complex immune pathway involving several subclasses of T lymphocytes, acting in a cascade of interactive events (Vittimberga et al. 1998). Consequently, a single T cell disturbance is able to affect the whole DTH response. DTH has been shown to be significantly depressed by laparotomy (Little et al. 1993). Several experimental studies showed that laparoscopic procedure allowed a better maintenance of the DTH response than laparotomy, but the specific component(s) of the cascade responsible for this failure were not determined (Vittimberga et al. 1998). DTH also seems less affected in humans after laparoscopy (Kloosterman et al. 1994; Walker et al. 1999; Brune et al. 1998, Griffith et al. 1995). In the studies by Kloosterman et al. and Brune et al., it was directly associated to changes in the number of HLA-DR monocytes (a kind of immune cell which is required in the process of exogenous antigen presentation to T helper cells), showing that patients remain immunocompetent after laparoscopy. This was found true as well by Walker et al. (1999) who also found after laparoscopy an increased number of CD71+ cells, another activation marker, which is also involved in exogenous antigenic presentation. These studies (Brune et al. 1998; Walker et al. 1999) identified two subclasses of T lymphocytes, involved in the cascade leading to DTH, which are unaffected after laparoscopy and depressed after laparotomy. Thus, the DTH alteration after laparotomy appears to be clearly multifactorial.

The association of DTH response failure with the alteration of polymorphonuclear functions after laparotomy, corroborated by numerous alterations in Pan-T, T helper, T suppressor and NK cell subsets, strongly suggests that host defenses are more depressed after laparotomy than after laparoscopy.

Other Host Defense Mechanisms

Several other mechanisms are involved in host defense (Vittimberga et al. 1998; Davies and Hagen 1997). Among these are some molecules released by stimulated mast cells, monocytes or macrophages (Vittimberga et al. 1998; Davies and Hagen 1997; Hill and Hill 1998; Yoshida et al. 1995).

Histamine

Peripheral histamine may be involved in the systemic immune response to surgical body aggression defense (Vittimberga et al. 1998). Produced by mast cells in reaction to several stimuli, histamine affects cardiovascular, digestive, pulmonary and immune systems. It is involved in the inflammatory response and alters the functions of granulocytes, T lymphocytes and macrophages (Vittimberga et al. 1998). In spite of its great impact on the inflammatory response, the histamine response to laparoscopic injury has been poorly investigated. Only one clinical trial (Nies et al. 1997) was devoted to these parameter changes. This work investigating the plasma levels of histamine in 40 patients after laparoscopic and open cholecystectomy revealed significantly greater intra- and postoperative concentrations in patients undergoing laparoscopic management of their cholecystitis. This finding suggests a subsequent impairment in immune cell functions during and after laparoscopy. Up to now, however, there is no evidence of such an impairment (Kloosterman et al. 1994; Suzuki et al. 1994; Bolufer et al. 1995; Walker et al. 1999; Cristaldi et al. 1997; Vallina et al. 1996) and additional studies will be required to reach a clear understanding of the significance of histamine rise after laparoscopy.

Production of Reactive Oxygen Species

Some of the reactive oxygen species (also called free radicals), such as hydroxyl radical or superoxide anion may be produced in most types of inflammatory tissue injury (Davies and Hagen 1997) and are coming predominantly from leukocytes (Vittimberga et al. 1998; Davies and Hagen 1997). Only a few clinical investigations have been devoted to this aspect of peripheral leukocyte functions (Redmond et al. 1994; Collet et al. 1995). The study of Redmond et al. (1994) analyzed superoxide anion release from both monocytes and polymorphonuclear neutrophils after open and laparoscopic cholecystectomy. On the first postoperative day, open cholecystectomy was associated with a significantly increased release of superoxide anion from both kinds of cells. Conversely, Collet et al. (1995) found no difference in the release of superoxide anion from polymorphonuclear neutrophils after open laparotomy and laparoscopy in an experimental study in pigs. The highly reactive oxygen species is generated by systemic endotoxin and/or INF-(and is considered a sign of an acute inflammation phenomenon (Vittimberga et al. 1998; Davies and Hagen 1997; Szabo 1996). It may also be generated by macrophages, but their involvement has not yet been demonstrated as far as open or laparoscopic surgery are concerned.

The results of the study of Redmond et al. (1994) strongly suggest the occurrence of an acute, but transient inflammatory response after open laparotomy. It would be of great interest to include further investigations on this parameter of inflammation during prospective trials on immune status after laparoscopy.

Nitric oxide, Inducible NO Synthase and Peroxynitrite

The inducible nitric oxide synthase (currently abbreviated as iNOS) directs, under physiopathological stimulation, the release of nitric oxide (currently abbreviated as NO) (Davies and Hagen 1997; Moncada et al. 1991; Szabo 1996). This very famous molecule, the discovery of which was recently rewarded by a Nobel prize, is implicated in a wide variety of physiological and physiopathological situations. Basically, it can be considered that "physiological" NO is released under (almost) constant constitutive NO synthase expression and that "physiopathological" NO is produced in drastic proportions under iNOS control. Among the cells able to express iNOS are polymorphonuclear leukocytes, monocytes and macrophages (in fact white cells able to produce superoxide anion) (Davies and Hagen 1997; Walker et al. 1999). When this very labile molecule is produced in excess, it combines with superoxide anion, generating peroxynitrite anion, a very toxic product. This phenomenon is involved in several pathological situations such as inflammation or shock (Davies and hagen 1997; Szabo 1996).

No clinical information is available yet on iNOS activation status in white blood cells and peritoneal immune cells after laparotomy and laparoscopy. As NO and superoxide anion are produced in similar situations by the same stimulation pathway (bacterial endotoxin and/or cytokines) (Davies and Hagen 1997; Szabo 1996; Moncada et al. 1991), it can be expected that NO follows the same pattern of release as does superoxide anion in monocytes, leukocytes and macrophages. Conclusive data are obviously needed to elucidate the involvement of these numerous reactive oxygen species in the immune response to surgical body injury.

Conclusion

Most of the comparative clinical investigations on systemic cell-mediated immunity status after open surgery and laparoscopy concluded that there is a lower alteration after laparoscopy. Indeed the acute phase protein response appears to be minimized by this procedure and the serum concentrations of cytokines involved in the immune process are better preserved. In the same way, the immune cell populations are less affected (or not affected at all) by laparoscopy. But it also appears, from some studies, that the duration of the laparoscopic procedure has a direct consequence on the level of immunity depression, suggesting that the CO_2 pneumoperitoneum-induced acidosis plays a key role. Obviously, more reliable, well-done prospective studies are needed to assess accurately the immune effect of laparoscopy, allowing for an unequivocal and safe development of this exciting procedure.

References

Baigrie RJ, Lamont PM, Kwiatkowski D, Dallman MJ, Morris PJ (1992) Systemic cytokine response after major surgery. Br J Surg 79:757–760

Bolufer JM, Delgado F, Blanes F, Martinez-Abad M, Canos JI, Martin J, Oliver MJ (1995) Injury in laparoscopic surgery. Surg Laparosc Endosc 5:318–323

Brune IB, Wilke W, Hensler T, Feussner H, Holzmann B, Siewert JR (1998) Normal T lymphocyte and monocyte function after minimally invasive surgery. Surg Endosc 12:1020–1024

Carey PD, Wakefield CH, Thayeb A, Monson JRT, Darzi A, Guillou PJ (1994) Effects of minimally invasive surgery on hypochlorous acid production by neutrophils. Br J Surg 81:557–560

Champault G, Bron M, Catheline JM, Mercadier A (1996) La coelio-chirurgie influence-t-elle l'immunité? J Chir (Paris) 133:51–53

Cho JM, La Porta AJ, Clark JR, Schofield MJ, Hammond SL, Malory PL (1994) Response of serum cytokines in patients undergoing laparoscopic cholecystectomy. Surg Endosc 8:1380–1384

Collet D, Vitale GC, Reynolds M, Klar E, Cheadle WG (1995) Peritoneal host defenses are less impaired by laparoscopy than by open operation. Surg Endosc 9:1059–1064

Cristaldi M, Rovati M, Elli M, Gerl inzani S, Lesma A, Balzarotti L, Taschieri AM (1997) Lymphocytic subpopulation changes after open and laparoscopic cholecystectomy: a prospective and comparative study on 38 patients. Surg Laparosc Endosc 7:255–261

Davies MG, Hagen PO (1997) Systemic inflammatory response syndrome. Br J Surg 84:920–935

Evrard S, Falkenrodt A, Park A, Tassetti V, Mutter D, Marescaux J (1997) Influence of CO_2 pneumoperitoneum on systemic and peritoneal cell-mediated immunity. World J Surg 21:353–357

Fukushima R, Kawamura YJ, Saito H, Saito Y, Hashigushi Y, Sawada T, Muto T (1996) Interleukin-6 and stress hormone responses after uncomplicated gasless laparoscopic-assisted and open sigmoid colectomy. Dis Colon Rectum 39:S29–S34

Gàl I, Lantos L, Röth E (1994) Changes of PMN-elastase and C-reactive protein following traditional and laparoscopic cholecystectomy. Surg Endosc 8:552 (Abstract)

Glaser F, Sannwald GA, Buhr HJ, Kuntz C, Mayer H, Klee F, Herfarth C (1995) General stress response to conventional and laparoscopic cholecystectomy. Ann Surg 221:372–380

Griffith JP, Everitt NJ, Lancaster F, Boylston A, Richards SJ, Scott CS, Benson EA, Sue-Ling HM, McMahon MJ (1995) Influence of laparoscopic and conventional cholecystectomy upon cell-mediated immunity. Br J Surg 82:677–680

Halevy A, Lin G, Gold-Deutsch R, Lavi R, Negri M, Evans S, Cotariu D, Sackier JM (1995) Comparison of serum C-reactive protein concentrations for laparoscopic versus open cholecystectomy. Surg Endosc 9:280–282

Hewitt PM, Ip SM, Kwok SPY, Somers SS, Li K, Leung KL, Lau WY, Li AKC (1998) Laparoscopic-assisted vs. open surgery for colorectal cancer. Comparative study of immune effects. Dis Colon Rectum 41:901–908

Hill AG, Hill GL (1998) Metabolic response to severe injury. Br J Surg 85:884–890

Hill ADK, Banwell PE, Darzi A, Menzies-Gow N, Monson JRT, Guillou PJ (1995) Inflammatory markers following laparoscopic and open hernia repair. Surg Endosc 9:695–698

Jakeway MSR, Mitchell V, Hashim IA, Chadwick SJD, Shenkin A, Green CJ, Carli F (1994) Metabolic and inflammatory responses after open or laparoscopic cholecystectomy. Br J Surg 81:127–131

Kloosterman T, Blomberg BME von, Borgstein P, Cuesta MA, Scheper RJ, Meijer S (1994) Unimpaired immune functions after laparoscopic cholecystectomy. Surgery 115:424–428

Kobayashi E, Yoshida T, Yamauchi H, Yoshida T, Suminaga Y, Miyata M (1995) Immune function in patients undergoing open vs laparoscopic cholecystectomy. Arch Surg 130:676 (Letter)

Little MB, Regan M, Keane RM, Bouchier-Hayes D (1993) Perioperative immune modulation. Surgery 114:87–91

MacMahon AJ, O'Dwyer PJ, Cruikshank AM, McMillan DC, O'Reilly DS, Lowe GD, Rumley A, Logan RW, Baxter JN (1993) Comparison of metabolic responses to laparoscopic and minilaparotomy cholecystectomy. Br J Surg 80:1255–1258

Maruszynski M, Pojda Z (1995) Interleukin 6 (IL-6) levels in monitoring of surgical trauma. A comparison of serum IL-6 concentrations in patients treated by cholecystectomy via laparotomy or laparoscopy. Surg Endosc 9:882–885

Mealy K, Gàllagher H, Barry M, Lennon F, Traynor O, Hyland J (1992) Physiological and metabolic responses to open en laparoscopic cholecystectomy. Br J Surg 79:1061–1064

Moncada S, Palmer MJ, Higgs EA (1991) Nitric oxide: physiology, pathophysiology and pharmacology. Pharm Rev 43:109–142

Nies C, Krack W, Lorenz W, Kaufmann T, Sitter H, Celik I, Rothmund M (1997) Histamine release in conventional versus minimally invasive surgery: results of a randomised trial in acute cholecystitis. Inflamm Res 46:S83–S84

Redmond HP, Watson WG, Houghton T, Condron C, Watson RGK, Bouchier-Hayes D (1994) Immune function in patients undergoing open vs laparoscopic cholecystectomy. Arch Surg 129:1240–1246

Suzuki M, Oka M, Tangoku A, Hazama S, Hisaka K, Hiraki S, Suzuki T (1994) Interleukin-6 and granulocytic elastase levels following laparoscopic cholecystectomy. Surg Endosc 8:447 (Abstract)

Szabo C (1996) The pathophysiological role of peroxynitrite in shock, inflammation and ischemia-reperfusion injury. Shock 6:79–88

Vallina VL, Velasco JM (1996) The influence of laparoscopy on lymphocyte subpopulations in the surgical patient. Surg Endosc 10:481–484

Vander Velpen G, Penninckx F, Kerremans R, Van Damme J, Arnout J (1994) Interleukin-6 and coagulation-fibrinolysis fluctuations after laparoscopic and conventional cholecystectomy. Surg Endosc 8:1216–1220

Vittimberga FJ, Foley DP, Meyers WC, Callery MP (1998) Laparoscopic surgery an the systemic immune response. Ann Surg 227:326–334

Walker CBJ, Bruce DM, Heys SD, Gough DB, Binnie NR, Eremin O (1999) Minimal modulation of lymphocyte and natural killer cell subsets following minimal access surgery. Am J Surg 177:48–54

Yoshida T, Kobayashi E, Suminaga Y, Yamauchi H, Yoshida T, Miyata M (1995) Laparoscopic cholecystectomy minimally impairs postoperative cardiorespiratory and muscle performance. Arch Surg 130:676–677

CHAPTER 14

Mechanical Means For Prevention of Trocar Site Cancer Implantation

M.E. Franklin Jr., J.A. Díaz-E, J. Balli

Introduction

Trocar site implantation has been the Achilles' heel of laparoscopic colon surgery for carcinoma (Cooperman et al. 1991; Jacobs et al. 1991; Phillips et al. 1992). Shortly after the first colon resection was reported, other reports began to appear regarding tumor implantation in trocar and extraction sites (Alexander et al. 1993; Fusco and Paluzzi 1993; Cirocco et al. 1994). Numerous theories and research studies have been proposed and performed in an effort to define the rate, mechanism and the impact of this phenomenon (Bessler et al. 1994; Hewett et al. 1996; Franklin et al. 1996). Although port-site recurrences have been reported in gynecological literature as well as after laparoscopic cholecystectomy (Dobronte et al. 1978; Siriwardena et al. 1993), the effect was to effectively halt many surgeons from performing or even investigating laparoscopic colon resection for cancer. A survey in 1994 of surgeons currently performing this latter procedure in the USA revealed an overall rate of trocar implantation of approximately 1.9% (Ramos et al. 1994). In the meantime, a number larger series by individual experienced laparoscopic surgeons have shown a rate of between 0 and 1% or less (Franklin et al. 1996; Plasencia et al. 1994).

Experimental Data

The exact mechanisms contributing to trocar site implantation have been the subject of numerous reports. The clinical data available so far appear to stress the role of the surgeon as a risk factor (Johnstone et al. 1996).

For this reason, we looked for possible surgical measures that might prevent port-site recurrences (Reymond et al. 1997a) and for a suitable animal model that would permit the assessment of such measures. Different animals have been used for experimental trials in cancer laparoscopy, in particular hamsters (Jones et al. 1995), mice (Dorrance et al. 1996) and rats (Berguer and Gutt 1994; Bouvy et al. 1996). All of these animals are small and do not appear to be optimal for assessing the quality of surgical technique during laparoscopy. To improve the accuracy of such an experimental study, we therefore adapted an intraperitoneal tumor model in the pig (Reymond et al. 1999).

We then decided to investigate the influence of the quality of surgical technique on the incidence of port-site recurrences following oncological laparoscopy. In an experimental, prospective, randomized, single-blind study we compared two groups of animals: in one group, preventive measures were taken, in the second group standardized surgical mistakes were deliberately made in accordance with a protocol (Schneider et al. 1999).

Three experienced laparoscopic surgeons were randomly assigned to six animals, three in each group. The type of procedures (with or without preventive measures) was also randomized. Any deviations from the respective surgical protocol were recorded by an independent observer. The endpoint of the study was the presence or absence of port-site recurrence as assessed by immunohistochemistry. The pathologist was blinded to the type of procedure performed.

Eighteen randomly selected non-syngeneic German domestic pigs were used for this trial. They were aged 6–8 weeks with a mean weight of 33.0 kg. After induction of anesthesia according to standard protocols, the abdominal wall was disinfected with 10% povidone-iodine solution and sterile drapes were used. After insufflating the abdomen with CO_2 through a Veress needle, the first 12 mm trocar (Ethicon, Norderstedt, Germany) was inserted above the umbilicus and a pneumoperitoneum of 12 mm Hg created. After inserting a second 12-mm trocar in the right lower quadrant, 10^7 freshly prepared HeLa cells were injected into the abdominal cavity through the umbilical trocar, under video control.

Two further 12 mm trocars were inserted into the lower abdomen, one of them being positioned in the left lower quadrant at the proximal end of a 40 mm line marking the future position of the minilaparotomy. A classical laparoscopic, short sigmoid resection was then performed with extraperitoneal purse string suture, extra-abdominal insertion of a 21-mm or 25-mm stapler head (Ethicon Endosurgery, Norderstedt, Germany) and intracorporeal anastomosis using transanal double stapling. During the immediate postoperative period, the animals were monitored. When awake, they were allowed to drink milk. Beginning on postoperative day 1, they were allowed free access to normal food and water.

Tissue samples free of necrosis or hemorrhage were obtained from port-sites and anastomoses in all animals. After embeddingg with paraffin, slides were incubated with a mouse anti-human pancytokeratin monoclonal antibody primary antibody (Clone MNF 116, Dako Diagnostik, Hamburg, Germany).

Results

No intraoperative complications occurred and no conversion was necessary. All animals survived the procedure. The mean operating time was 69 min in the control group, and somewhat longer in the group in which preventive measures were applied. During the procedure, the observer recorded the following protocol deviations in the prevention group: in two animals, a gas leak was observed at trocar positions 1 and 2 caused by overlong skin incision; in one of these animals, dislodgment of the surgical drape additionally caused contamination of the minilaparotomy wound when the stapling head was inserted.

All animals survived the period under observation, and were killed after 28 days. All port-sites and minilaparotomy wounds were excised. Table 14.1 shows the results of the histopathological analysis of the port-sites. In the group with standardized surgical mistakes, 23 recurrences were noted (Fig. 14.1, Table 14.2) compared with five in the group in which preventive measures were applied. Interestingly, two of these five recurrences in the prevention group occurred in an animal and at a location for which a protocol deviation had been documented during the procedure. These differences achieved statistical significance ($p = 0.002$). Figure 14.2 shows the macroscopic appearance of such a port-site recurrence. No peritoneal carcinosis nor anastomotic recurrences were observed.

Table 14.1. Details of the operative procedure, showing standardized surgical mistakes in the control group and the application of preventive measures in the prevention group

Operative procedure	Preventive measure animals	Control animals
Length of trocar incision (mm)	15	20
Finition of trocar surfaces	Profile (rough)	Smooth
Trocar fixation	Yes	No
Dislodgment of trocar numbers 1 and 2	No	Twice
Gas leak	No	Yes
Disinfection of instruments with povidone-iodine solution	Yes	No
Drape protection of the minilaparotomy	Yes	No
Peritoneal closure	Yes	No
CO_2 exsufflation through trocars	Yes	No
Rinsing of minilaparotomy and trocar sites with povidone-iodine solution	Yes	No

Table 14.2. Histopathological analysis of port-sites after autopsy: number of port-site recurrences

Port-site	Control animals ($n=9$)	Preventive measure animals ($n=9$)
Trocar 1 (RLQ)	7	2[a]
Trocar 2 (RUQ)	6	2[a]
Trocar 3 (LLQ)	5	0
Minilaparotomy (LUQ)	5	1
Total	23	5

[a] One recurrence in animal 12, in which a protocol violation was recorded

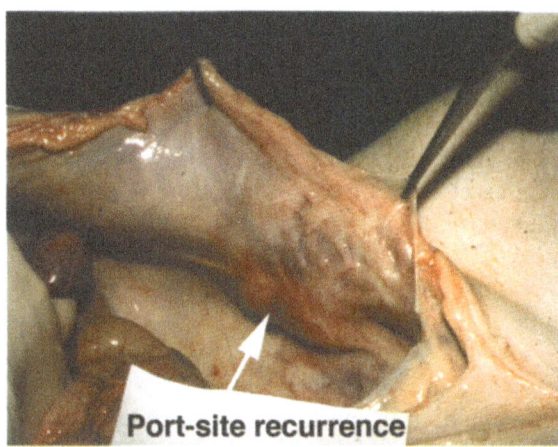

Fig. 14.1. Macroscopic appearance of a port-site recurrence in the pig tumor xenograft model (Reymond et al. 1999)

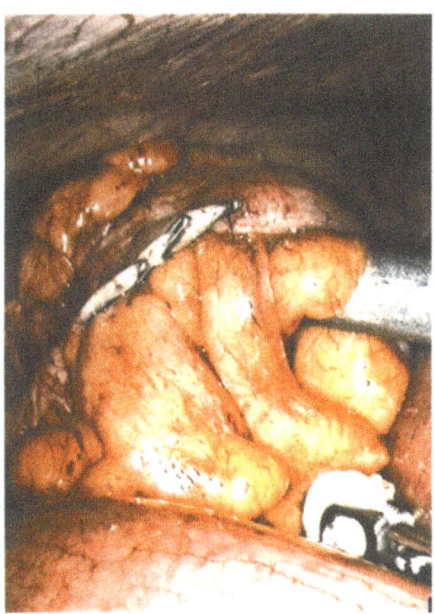

Fig. 14.2. Indirect tumor handling (e.g., with swabs) prevents accidental tumor perforation with sharp instruments (e.g., Babcock forceps). Small tumors should be localized by clips, India ink or intraoperative coloscopy

These results suggest that the quality of the surgical technique has a major influence on the incidence of port-site recurrences in the animal model, which is in good agreement with clinical observations showing large differences in the incidence of port-site recurrences among different surgeons. Following standardized surgical mistakes, tumor recurrence was observed at most port-sites. By employing a meticulous surgical technique in combination with protective measures, we were able to reduce the incidence of port-site recurrences dramatically. This experimental finding is further supported by the observation that two out of five recurrences in the prevention group occurred at a port-site at which a protocol violation took place. After excluding these two events the risk of developing port-site recurrences was reduced by a factor of 7.7 by the strict application of all the proposed protective measures.

It might be asked why the protective measures were unable to prevent all port-site recurrences. This might be explained by the use of a sensitive xenograft model, in which all the animals developed recurrences at at least one port-site in the absence of preventive measures after intraperitoneal injection of a high dose of tumor cells. In this respect, the model does not completely reflect the clinical situation, in which port-site recurrences do not occur in all patients in the absence of the proposed protective

measures. Useful stage- and surgeon-related clinical data on the incidence of port-site recurrence are still not available at present.

Clinical Consequences

It is felt by most experienced laparoscopic colon surgeons that most of the predominant mechanisms of tumor implantation are preventable. Thus, mechanical and technical considerations appear extremely important in prevention of this disastrous complication. Certainly, the stage of the disease at the time of the surgery plays also an essential role. Theoretically, stage A or B tumors should have a very low chance of implantation unless surgical oncological principles are violated, such as opening the specimen in the wound (Fingerhut 1995).

Identification of the Mechanisms of Contamination

There are several categories of mechanical means of trocar site implantation, including the following, that we would like to detail:

- Specimen handling
- Instrument contamination
- Trocar mechanisms
- Specimen removal
- Peritoneal fluid seeding

Specimen Handling and Retrieval

The subject of avoiding handling of the tumor is not new. Decades ago, Gallagher and Turnbull reported improved results utilizing "a no touch" technique which is nothing more than common sense and has carried through to modern surgery in the 1990s (Turnbull et al. 1967). Never was this more true than with laparoscopic surgery where chipping, manipulation and instrumentation of the tumor can occur unintentionally. In initial experiences with laparoscopic colon resection, the tumor was often handled excessively resulting in instrument contamination and seeding of the peritoneal cavity and peritoneal fluid with excessive numbers of tumor cells which ultimately may have contributed to a large number of trocar site implants seen in many early series (Fig. 14.2).

Closure of the ends of a resected segment of bowel has long been practiced to prevent unintentional contamination of the peritoneal cavity by luminal con-

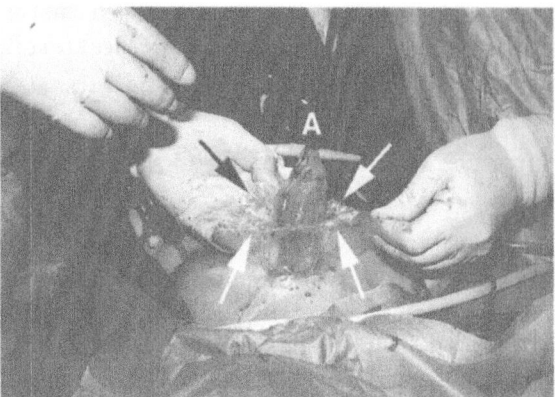

Fig. 14.3. The wound can be protected using self-made, unexpensive protectors

tents and exfoliated cells. Laparoscopically, this can be accomplished as well by stapling the colon, ligating the bowel after resection, or closure immediately after resection with a suturing device or an endoloop. Intraoperative colonoscopy with intraluminal washing by a cytotoxic agent can also be used to reduce or eliminate viable tumor cells before division of the colon.

Extraction of the specimen presents a particularly difficult and cumbersome part of laparoscopic colon surgery for cancer and every effort should be used to prevent contamination during this portion of the procedure. The most efficient method depends on the type of procedure, as well as the extraction site. Protecting the wound (Fig. 14.3) or isolating the specimen by placing the specimen in a non-permeable bag seems to be the best way to isolate specimens which are totally resected intracorporeally. A wound protector may be the most efficient method of protecting the wound for specimens which are still connected to the proximal or distal colon, such as in a right hemicolectomy where an extracorporeal anastomosis is to be performed or a sigmoid colon resection where a laparoscopically assisted procedure is planned. In both instances, all major vascular attachments must be controlled and divided prior to exteriorization of the specimen as part of an oncologically sound resection. It is also very important to avoid tearing of the specimen during extraction, as well as potential contamination of the wound by opening the specimen on the abdominal wall (Fingerhut 1995).

Instrument Contamination

Next to the tumor itself instruments which are used to perform laparoscopic colon resection are by far the most contaminated and the greatest source of

potential contamination of trocar sites (Fielding et al. 1997; Allardyce et al. 1996). The mechanism thoughtto be responsible is that of a contaminated instrument inoculating the trocar which is then pulled unprotected through the wound. A second mechanism is pulling the trocar out and allowing a contaminated instrument laden with tumor cells to pass unprotected through the abdominal wall. Obviously, multiple oncological principles have been violated in these instances and the results are inevitable.

Avoiding direct handling of the tumor will lessen contamination of the instruments. In addition, avoiding peritoneal fluid contamination by the instruments and the trocar will also lessen the chance of trocar inoculation. We have adopted not only a no-tumor handling technique, but have also taken the precaution of cleaning instruments with a Betadine solution or at least dipping the instruments in a Betadine solution between each introduction back into the abdominal cavity (Fig. 14.4).

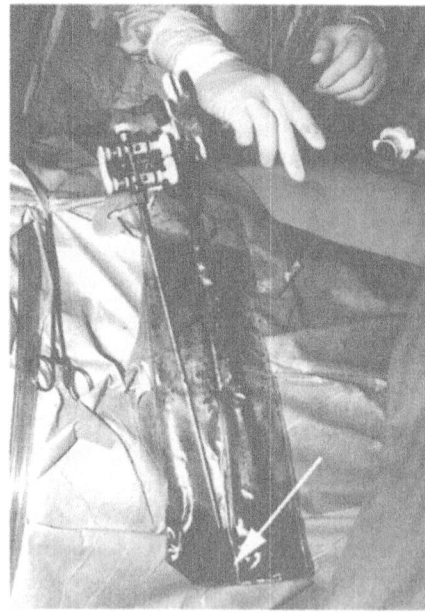

Fig. 14.4. The instruments are contaminated with tumor cells. Thus, they should be dipped into a cytotoxic solution (e.g., Betadine) when they are not in use

Trocar Mechanisms

Four separate mechanisms of trocar site tumor implantation have been postulated. These include:

- Direct inoculation from tumor cells being placed directly on the trocar and the trocar being inadvertently removed during the procedure.

- The so-called chimney effect whereby CO_2-laden cells can potentially contaminate the trocar site by a continuous CO_2 leak.
- An indirect effect where tumor cells irrigate a trocar site when the abdomen is deflated and fluid in the peritoneal cavity flows directly into the trocar wound site (Mathew et al. 1997, Targarona et al. 1998) (Fig. 14.5).
- The tissue trauma effect where excessive tissue trauma at the primary operative trocar creates excessive tissue damage followed by an increase in tumor growth factor and healing response, which encourages potential tumor cell implantation in a fertile environment (Allardyce et al. 1997; Allendorf et al. 1995; Wexner and Cohen 1995).

These mechanisms are all correctable and probably preventable with simple mechanical means.

First, all trocars should be sutured or otherwise transfixed to prevent inadvertent removal. Trocar dislodgment is probably the most common cause of trocar inoculation of remote site trocar implantation. Suturing the trocar to the skin (Fig. 14.5) is probably the most secure and simplest way of securing trocars, but other methods such as a balloon on the peritoneal side, adhesive banding and mechanical deployment devices similar to dry wall anchors have all been used and are effective.

Second, the "chimney effect" implies a significant Co_2 leak around a given trocar site. This mechanism

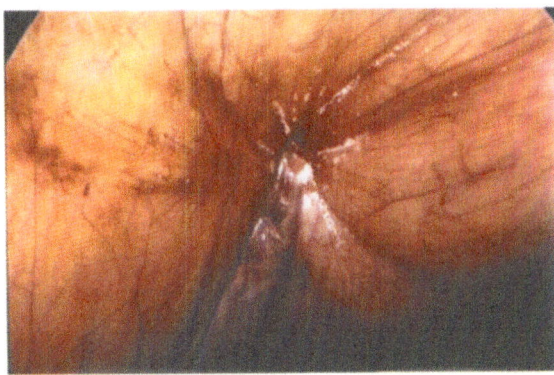

Fig. 14.6. The peritoneum should be closed carefully to prevent implantation of tumor cells into the port-sites after the end of the surgical procedure

can be nullified by initially being sure the skin incision is snug and that undue trauma is not present when placing the trocar. If Co_2 leakage is present, this can be controlled by a towel clip or sutures in the skin or more commonly, in our practice, by placing a transfascial suture with a suture passer and holding the suture securely with a hemostat during the procedure. This same suture can also close the trocar site at the conclusion of the procedure.

Third, tumor-laden fluid "backwashing" into a trocar site can be prevented or at least lessened by four separate steps:

a) Suction all free fluid out of the abdominal cavity prior to trocar removal
b) Dilute fluid by irrigation and removal of as much fluid as possible
c) Close trocar sites at the peritoneal level as soon as the trocar is removed by preplacing sutures with an appropriate (e.g., Carter-Thomason) suture passer (Fig. 14.6)
d) Deflate the abdominal cavity prior to trocar removal, which prevents Co_2 and potentially tumor-laden fluid from flowing through the open trocar site.

Fourth, mechanical damage at trocar sites, particularly involving the primary working port, is a strong potential etiology of port-site recurrence. Therefore, trauma to the area should be minimized as much as possible. The trauma can be minimized by two main means:

a) Assure that the port is placed at a right angle to the peritoneal side of the trocar site and not at an oblique angle, which of necessity will require stretching or tearing of the trocar site on the peritoneal side as the trocar is used during the procedure.

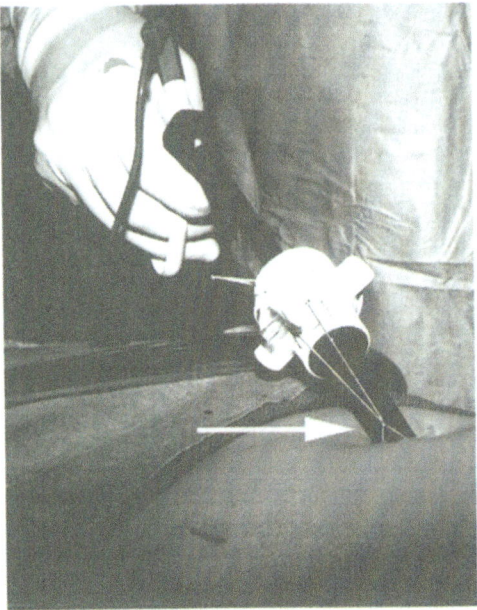

Fig. 14.5. Trocar dislodgment is a severe incident in laparoscopic cancer surgery. Thus, trocars should be secured with skin sutures. Alternatively, balloon trocars can be used

b) Avoid false passage of the trocar and if the trocar is inadvertently removed, be sure replacement is through the initial hole and not through a separate hole adjacent to the first site.

Peritoneal Fluid

Peritoneal fluid has been shown to contain viable tumor cells with the amount of tumor cells increasing in direct proportion to the stage of the cancer. Viable tumor cells have been retrieved from peritoneal fluid aspirate even in stage I and stage II cancers (Wexner and Cohen 1995, Buchmann et al. 1996). Therefore, maneuvers for lessening the likelihood of fluid entering an open port wound are important in preventing port-site recurrence. The simplest way to accomplish this is to remove all fluid or at least dilute the fluid to a point that port-site implantation is highly unlikely. Irrigation of the peritoneal cavity with cytotoxic agents can also lessen the likelihood of implantation and is covered in another portion of this book. Irrigation of the port-site with saline or cytotoxic agents may also lessen the likelihood of implantation and is similarly addressed in other portions of the book. It is suspected that such a contamination can occur after the end of the procedure if the peritoneal wound has not been closed properly (Wu et al. 1998). Closure of the port-site at the peritoneal level with either a purse string device or a device such as a Carter-Thomason suture passer offers protection from potential tumor-laden fluid passing unimpeded into the port-site (Fig. 14.6).

Conclusion

Port-site recurrence and implantation are rare problems and are the Achilles' heel of laparoscopic colon resection for cancer. They are probably preventable by a number of means, particularly mechanically oriented techniques. The mechanical means of port-site implantation prevention involves primarily a reinforcement of good technical maneuvers and common sense, which have been the mainstay of excellent results and low port-site implantation rates noted by skilled laparoscopic surgeons. Surgeons themselves can be instrumental in preventing port-site implantation in almost all patients with the rare exception of patients with a heavy tumor load or carcinomatosis.

References

Alexander R, Jaques B, Mitchell K (1993) Laparoscopic assisted colectomy and wound recurrence. Lancet 341:249–250

Allardyce RA, Morreau P, Bagshaw P (1996) Tumor cell distribution following laparoscopic colectomy in a porcine model. Dis Colon Rectum 39:S47–S52

Allardyce RA, Morreau P, Bagshaw PF (1997) Operative factors affecting tumor cell distribution following laparoscopic colectomy in a porcine model. Dis Colon Rectum 40:939–945

Allendorf JD, Bessler M, Kayton ML, Whelan RL, Treat MR, Nowygrod R (1995) Tumor growth factor after laparotomy or laparoscopy, a preliminary study; Surg Endosc 9:44–52

Berguer R, Gutt CN (1994) Laparoscopic colon surgery in a rat model. A preliminary report. Surg Endosc 8:1195–1197

Bessler M, Whelan RL, Halverson A, Treat MR, Nowygrod R (1994) Is immune function better preserved after laparoscopic versus open colon resection? Surg Endosc 8:881–883

Bouvy ND, Marquet RL, Hamming JF (1996) Laparoscopic surgery in the rat. Beneficial effect on body weight and tumor take. Surg Endosc 10:490–494

Buchmann P, Christen D, Moll C, Flury R, Sartoretti C (1996) Tumor cells in peritoneal irrigation fluid in conventional and laparoscopic surgery for colorectal carcinoma. Swiss Surg 4:S45–S49

Cirocco W, Schwarzman A, Golub R (1994) Abdominal wall recurrence after laparoscopic colectomy for colon cancer. Surgery 116:842–846

Cooperman AM, Katz V, Zimmon D (1991) Laparoscopic colon resection: a case report. J Laparosc Surg 1:221–224

Dobronte Z, Wittmann T, Karacsony G (1978) Rapid development of malignant metastasis in the abdominal wall after laparoscopy. Endoscopy 10:127–130

Dorrance HR, Oein K, O'Dwyer PJ (1996) Laparoscopy promotes tumor growth in an animal model. Surg Endosc 10:559(Abstract)

Fielding G, Lumley J, Nathanson L, Hewitt P, Rhodes M, Sitz R (1997) Laparoscopic colectomy. Surg Endosc 11:745–749

Fingerhut A (1995) Laparoscopic colectomy: the French experience. In: Jager R, Wexner S (eds) Laparoscopic colorectal surgery. Churchill Livingstone, New York, pp 253–257

Franklin ME, Rosenthal D, Abrego D, Dorman JP, Norem R, Glass JL, Díaz-EJA (1996) Prospective comparison of open vs. laparoscopic colon surgery for carcinoma: five year results. Dis Colon Rectum 39:S35–S46

Fusco M, Paluzzi M (1993) Abdominal wall recurrence after laparoscopic assisted colectomy for adenocarcinoma of the colon. Dis Colon Rectum 36:858–861

Hewett PJ, Thomas WM, King G, Eaton M (1996) Intraperitoneal cell movement during abdominal carbon dioxide insufflation in laparoscopy. Dis Colon Rectum 39:S62–S66

Jacobs M, Verdeja JC, Goldstei HS (1991) minimally invasive colon resection (laparoscopic colectomy). Surg Laparosc Endosc 1:144–150

Johnstone PAS, Rohde DC, Swartz SE, Fetter JE, Wexner SD (1996) Port-site recurrences after laparoscopic and thoracoscopic procedures in malignancy. J Clin Oncol 14:1950–1956

Jones DB, Guo LW, Reinhard MK, Soper NJ, Philpott GW, Connet J, Fleshman JW (1995) Impact of pneumoperitoneum on trocar site implantation of colon cancer in hamster model. Dis Colon Rectum 38:1182–1188

Mathew G, Watson DI, Ellis T, De Young N, Rofe AM, Jamieson GG (1997) Effect of laparoscopy on the movement of tumor cells and metastases to surgical wounds. Surg Endosc 11:1163–1166

Phillips E, Franklin ME, Carroll B, Fallas M, Ramos R, Rosenthal D (1992) Laparoscopic colectomy. Ann Surg 216:701–702

Plasencia G, Jacobs M, Verdeja J, Viamonte M (1994) Laparoscopic-assisted sigmoid colectomy and low anterior resection. Dis Colon Rectum 37:829–833

Ramos J, Gupta S, Anthone G, Ortega A, Simons A, Beart R (1994) Laparoscopy and colon cancer. Arch Surg 129:897–900

Reymond MA, Kastl S, Schneider C, Hohenberger W, Köckerling F (1997a) Techniques for the prevention of port-site recurrences. Surg Endosc 11:533 (Abstract)

Reymond MA, Schneider C, Hohenberger W, Köckerling F (1997b) Pathogenesis of puncture-site metastasis after laparoscopy (in German). Zbl Chir 122:387–394

Reymond MA, Wittekind C, Jung A, Hohenberger W, Kirchnner T, Köckerling F (1997c) The incidence of port-site recurrences might be reduced. Surg Endosc 11:902–906

Reymond MA, Tannapfel A, Schneider C, Köver S, Jung A, Reck T, Lippert H, Köckerling F (1999) Description of an in-traperitoneal tumor xenograft model in the pig. Eur J Surg Oncol (in press)

Schneider C, Jung A, Reymond MA, Tanapfel A, Balli J, Franklin ME, Hohenberger W, Köckerling F (1999) Efficacy of surgical measures in the prevention of port-site recurrences in a porcine model. Surg Endosc (in press)

Siriwardena A, Samarji WN (1993) Cutaneous tumor seeding from previously undiagnosed pancreatic carcinoma after laparoscopic cholecystectomy. Ann R Coll Surg Engl 75:199–200

Targarona EM, Martinez J, Nadal A, Balague C, Cardesa A, Pascual S, Trias M (1998) Cancer dissemination during laparoscopic surgery: tubes, gas, and cells. World J Surg 22:55–60

Turnbull RB, Kyle K, Watson FR, Spratt J (1967) Cancer: the influence of the no-touch isolation technique on survival rates. Ann Surg 166:420–425

Wexner SD, Cohen SM (1995) Laparoscopic colorectal surgery: are we being honest with our patients ? Dis Colon Rectum 38:723–727

Wu JS, Guo LW, Ruiz MB, Pfister SM, Connett JM, Fleshman JW (1998) Excision of trocar sites reduces tumor implantation in an animal model. Dis Colon Rectum 41:1107–1111

CHAPTER 15

Prevention of Port-Site Recurrences: Chemical Measures

C.A. Jacobi

Introduction

The most important factor influencing tumor cell spillage and growth, as well as development of port-site recurrences in laparoscopic resection of malignant tumors, seems to be the surgeon himself. The large difference (0–25%) in the incidence of port-site recurrences reported after colorectal surgery might also be explained by the experience of the surgical team and, therefore, the intraoperative manipulation of the tumor (Balli et al. 1999; Fleshmann et al. 1996; Franklin et al. 1996; Lacy et al. 1998; Milsom et al. 1998; Pahlman 1997; Reymond et al. 1998; Wexner and Latulippe 1997). The decrease of reported incidence of port-site recurrences in literature over the last 5 years can also be due to the learning curve of the surgeons undertaking laparoscopic cancer resection (Balli et al. 1999; Fleshmann et al. 1996; Franklin et al. 1996; Lacy et al. 1998; Milsom et al. 1998; Pahlman 1997; Wexner and Latulippe 1997). In an overview, Reymond discussed clinical and experimental findings about tumor growth during laparoscopy and found the surgeon to be the most important factor for intraperitoneal tumor cell spillage and the development of abdominal wall metastases (Reymond et al. 1998). Nevertheless, no difference of exfoliated cells in the peritoneal cavity between open and laparoscopic colonic resection could be demonstrated if strict oncologic surgical principles are followed (Kim et al. 1998). Thus, precise laparoscopic techniques and strict oncologic surgical principles can reduce the incidence of intra- and extraperitoneal metastases to a minimum. Reports of a large number of patients undergoing laparoscopic colon cancer resections have shown that the incidence of port-site recurrences is similar or even lower in comparison to conventional open resections (Balli et al. 1999; Fleshmann et al. 1996; Franklin et al. 1996; Milsom et al. 1998; Reymond et al. 1998).

Besides precise oncological surgical techniques, a generally accepted approach to prevent tumor implantation in laparoscopic surgery does not exist. Although the alternative gas helium has been reported to suppress the growth of malignant cells in vitro and in vivo, it has not yet been accepted for routine clinical use (Jacobi et al. 1997b; Neuhaus et al. 1998b). Intraperitoneal instillation of different anti-adherent or cytotoxic agents has been evaluated in animal models in order to avoid port-site recurrences and local tumor recurrence. Irrigation with povidone-iodine caused significant decrease of tumor growth at port-sites and suture material (Jacobi et al. 1999a,b; Neuhaus et al. 1998a; Tsunoda et al. 1997). Furthermore, instillation of taurolidin, a derivative of the amino acid taurine, and heparin has been reported to suppress intra- and extraperitoneal tumor intake and growth in rats (Jacobi et al. 1997a,b; Jacobi et al. 1999a,b). These new therapeutic approaches and their clinical relevance are discussed in the following chapter.

Intraperitoneal Irrigation or Instillation of Cytotoxic or Anti-Adherent Substances

Beside the pathomechanisms of intraoperative tumor cell spillage and attachment, little is known about possible therapeutic interventions to prevent tumor metastases in laparoscopic surgery. In conventional surgery, many surgeons use peritoneal lavage after resection of a malignant tumor in order to remove possible spilled tumor cells from the abdominal cavity. However, since complete irrigation of all peritoneal surfaces does not seem possible, viable cancer cells may remain within the peritoneal cavity causing postoperative metastases. These cells might be able to move to the port-sites and develop metastases after laparoscopic surgery. Thus, tumor cell suspension models in rodents have been used to investigate different therapeutic approaches to inhibit the growth of spilled tumor cells during laparoscopic surgery (Jacobi et al. 1997a,b; Jacobi et al.

1999a,b; Neuhaus et al. 1998a; Paraskeva et al. 1999; Wu et al. 1998b). Although these models can be used to simulate intraoperative tumor spillage during laparoscopy, the number of spilled tumor cells after resection of colon carcinoma in humans is still unknown. Furthermore, the number of injected cells certainly influences the tumor incidence, the total tumor weight and the development of port-site recurrences in these experiments (Wu et al. 1998a).

Heparin and Hyaluronate

A theoretical mechanism for increased tumor cell attachment and implantation might be the injury of the tissue surface mucopolysaccharide layer of the peritoneum and the exposure of extracellular matrix proteins including laminin, fibronectin, and vitronectin to the tumor cells (Castronovo et al. 1991; Ruoslahti and Pierschbacher 1987; Yamada 1983). Tumor cell attachment has been inhibited by binding domains of the extracellular matrix preventing tumor migration and metastases in several animal models (Castronovo et al. 1991; Humphries et al. 1986; Whalen and Ingber 1989). In these studies, adherence of tumor cells, bacteria, and other substances at injured urothelium have been reduced after instillation of heparin into the bladder (Parsons et al. 1979). Furthermore, this approach has been reported to lead to a significant decrease of tumor cell adhesion on injured and noninjured peritoneum in a murine model (Goldstein et al. 1993). It has been suggested that heparin binds to fibronectin and restores the anti-adherence integrity of the peritoneal surface (Gill et al. 1982; Hayman et al. 1985; Parsons et al. 1977).

Results from our department showed a significant decrease of intraperitoneal tumor cell implantation and tumor growth after heparin instillation in a colonic cancer rat model (Jacobi et al. 1997a,c). The animal model used in this study is well established and it is known that rat colonic carcinoma DHD/K12/TRb grows progressively when injected subcutaneously (Reisser et al. 1991) or intraperitoneally (Lagadec et al. 1987) in syngeneic animals. The effects shown in vivo do not appear to be attributable to toxic effects of heparin because heparin did not influence tumor cell viability and growth in vitro (Jacobi et al. 1997a,c). But, in comparison to intraperitoneal tumor growth, development of abdominal wall metastases was not reduced by the intraperitoneal administration of heparin. An explanation for these findings has still to be found. Neuhaus et al. also demonstrated a significant decrease of intraperitoneal tumor growth after heparin instillation in the abdominal cavity during laparoscopy in rats (Neuhaus et al. 1999). Furthermore, increase of tumor growth after additional intraperitoneal instillation of blood during the laparoscopy could be reduced by intraperitoneal heparin.

CD-44, a broadly distributed adhesion molecule, has also been implicated in the spread and adhesion of different tumors. The natural ligand for CD-44 is hyaluronate, which has been used in reduction of postoperative adhesion formations (Paraskeva et al. 1999). These authors investigated the effect of viscous hyaluronate on the invasion of rat colonic cancer cells (cc531 s) in vitro. Tumor cell invasiveness through reconstituted basement membrane (Matrigel) and synthetic filters could significantly be reduced by viscous hyaluronate. Nevertheless, the intraperitoneal or local application of hyaluronate was not performed in this model and in vivo experiments still have to be investigated to confirm the good results in vitro.

Povidone Iodine and Other Cytotoxic Agents

Local application of cytotoxic agents has been discussed in the prevention of tumor metastases by killing spilled tumor cells after laparoscopic interventions. Intraperitoneal instillation of povidone-iodine has been reported to cause significant decrease of port-site recurrences after laparoscopy with carbon dioxide in different cell suspension models (Jacobi et al. 1997a,b; Neuhaus et al. 1998b). In these studies, diluted povidone-iodine, with a concentration of 1% and 0.25%, was able to reduce the incidence of port-site recurrences as well as intraperitoneal tumor growth. These results were also confirmed in a solid tumor model of the spleen in mice undergoing laparoscopic mobilization of the spleen as well as intra-abdominal crushing of the tumor (Lee et al. 1999). In this model, irrigation of the abdominal cavity was performed after tumor manipulation using 5 cc of 8% Betadine solution. Port-site recurrence was significantly reduced after irrigation with Betadine solution when compared to saline irrigation and the control group. In another model, intracaecal application of povidone-iodine at 5% significantly reduced the incidence of tumor growth at transmural sutures of the caecum in rats (Tsunoda et al. 1997). Nevertheless, povidone-iodine is known to be cytotoxic and, therefore, local application of this agent might also cause damage of peritoneal macrophages and other intraperitoneal cells. Growth stimulating cytokines have been significantly increased after povidone-iodine incubation of peritoneal macrophages (Jacobi et al. 1999b). The increase of growth stimulating cytokines was further associated with a significant stimulation of in vivo tumor growth when compared to other anti-adherent or cytotoxic agents in rats (Jacobi et al. 1999b). Additionally, povidone-iodine caused adhesions and fibrin layers on the surface of the liver and the spleen in experimental models (Jacobi et al. 1997a,b, 1999). Therefore, povidone-iodine might not be the best solution in the avoidance of tumor metastases during laparoscopic surgery. Chemotherapeutic agents have also been used in experimental settings of laparoscopic cancer surgery to inhibit port-site recurrences. The intraperitoneal or intravenous application of cyclophosphamide, as described in a murine model, caused significant reduction of tumor growth at the port-sites (Iwanaka et al. 1998). Neuhaus et al. (1998a) investigated the influence of either intraperitoneal or intramuscular injection of 0.125 mg methotrexate on port-site recurrences in rats undergoing laparoscopy and intraperitoneal tumor laceration. In both groups, tumor size and port-site recurrences showed no difference to the control group. Nevertheless, neither local nor systemic chemotherapy can be generally advocated in laparoscopic surgery of gastrointestinal cancer because of major negative side effects.

Immune Modulating Agent Taurolidine

The function of peritoneal macrophages and the local immune response have been suggested to be influenced by carbon dioxide pneumoperitoneum. Thus, Puttick et al. evaluated cancer cell lysis of peritoneal macrophages after gas incubation with 100% helium or 100% carbon dioxide (Puttick et al. 1998). Carbon dioxide led to a significant decrease of cancer cell lysis while helium had no significant influence on cell lysis. Furthermore, it has been demonstrated (Jacobi et al. 1999a,b) that pneumoperitoneum with carbon dioxide caused a significant increase in the production of IL-1β, a strong growth promoting cytokine (Lanfrancone et al. 1992), in peritoneal macrophages. Therefore, intraperitoneal instillation of taurolidine (Taurolin, Hoechst, Germany), a derivative of the amino acid taurine, has been used to inhibit tumor growth during pneumoperitoneum, because it has been demonstrated that taurolidine inhibits the production of IL-1β in pe-

ripheral blood mononuclear cells (PBMC) and has a significant anti-adherence activity on pathogenic microorganisms and tumor cells (Bedrosian et al. 1991; Blenkharn 1988; Jacobi et al. 1997a,c).

A colonic adenocarcinoma of the rat (DHD/K12/ TRb; ECACC – European Collection of all Cultures) and a human colonic adenocarcinoma (CX-1; ECACC) as well as a gallbladder carcinoma of the rat (HV1A3 ; University of Essen, Germany) and a human gallbladder carcinoma (TFK-1; ECACC) were used to investigate the influences of either heparin, povidone-iodine, taurolidine, or taurolidine/heparin on tumor growth in vitro. Furthermore, production of growth stimulating cytokine IL-1β by peritoneal macrophages was investigated after incubation with carbon dioxide and additional incubation with the agents in vitro. Intraperitoneal instillation of either taurolidine, taurolidine/heparin, heparin, and povidone-iodine was then investigated in a colonic tumor cell suspension model of the rat (Jacobi et al. 1999b). All rats underwent pneumoperitoneum with carbon dioxide (8 mm Hg) for 30 min. Laparoscopy was accomplished through three trocars with a diameter of 5 mm. Additionally, the four different agents were instilled intraperitoneally while the control group underwent instillation of culture medium.

In vitro, tumor cell growth decreased after incubation with taurolidine, taurolidine/heparin, and povidone-iodine. Cytokine release was stimulated by incubation with carbon dioxide and could only be suppressed by incubation with taurolidine. Intraperitoneal tumor weight was lower in rats receiving heparin (251 ± 153 mg) and povidone-iodine (134 ± 117 mg) compared to the control group (541 ± 291 mg) but even less when taurolidine (79 ± 82 mg) or taurolidine/heparin (18.3 ± 30 mg) were instilled. Since IL-1β promotes cell growth in vivo it might be that intraperitoneal application of taurolidine indirectly causes decreased tumor growth by inhibiting the IL-1β production of intraperitoneal macrophages, as shown in vitro. Furthermore, it seems that taurolidine acts directly on the tumor cells and inhibits tumor cell growth itself. This suppression is not due to increased cell death but to decreased proliferation which could be shown in earlier experiments (Jacobi et al. 1997a,c). Although it has been reported that taurolidine releases "methylol" groups (hydroxy-methyl groups) are becoming attached to the cell wall of bacteria and causing death of the bacteria (Brodhage et al. 1985), it remains unclear if a similar mechanism is responsible for decreased tumor cell growth. The combination of taurolidine and heparin showed significant synergistic effects on suppression of tumor growth in vivo. It might be that taurolidine is more active on tumor cells and peritoneal macrophages while heparin is active on the peritoneal surface. However, although the pathomechanisms of taurolidine and heparin remain hypothetical, tumor growth could be reduced dramatically by intraperitoneal instillation of both substances without any side effects.

Combination of Chemotherapeutics and Different Gases

Most anti-adherent or cytotoxic agents were used in animals undergoing CO_2 insufflation, although this gas might stimulate tumor growth itself. The combination of anti-adherent or cytotoxic agents with different insufflation gases, like helium or xenon, was evaluated by Jacobi and coworkers in a colonic tumor cell suspension model in rats (Jacobi et al. 1999b). The effect of taurolidine, heparin, and povidone-iodine on growth of colon adenocarcinoma DHD/K12/TRb was measured in rats undergoing laparoscopy with either carbon dioxide ($n = 40$), helium ($n = 40$), or xenon ($n = 40$). 10^4 tumor cells were administered intraperitoneally and pneumoperitoneum was established over 30 min at 8 mm Hg with the different gases. Rats additionally received intraperitoneal instillation of the different agents. A significant decrease of tumor growth was found after intraperitoneal instillation of either taurolidine or taurolidine/heparin compared to controls in all gas groups. While povidone-iodine caused significantly lower tumor growth in the CO_2 group, the combination of helium and xenon with povidone-iodine showed no reduction of tumor growth compared to the control groups (data not shown). Further investigations using the combinations of different gases and the intraperitoneal application of therapeutic agents might lead to new multimodal therapies in cancer patients.

Local Treatment of Port-Sites

Besides additive intraperitoneal instillation, local treatment of port-sites with tumoricidal agents has been reported to reduce metastatic tumor growth in laparoscopic experimental models (Balli et al. 1999; Wu et al. 1998a). Local application of 1% silver sulfadiazine or 10% povidone-iodine at the trocar sites significantly reduced metastatic tumor growth in a hamster model (Wu et al. 1998b). Nevertheless,

tumor incidence was 75% after silver sulfadiazine and 78% after povidone-iodine treatment in comparison to 93% in the control group. The group of Franklin in San Antonio used intraperitoneal and local application of povidone-iodine during laparoscopic colon resection in patients and found no port-site recurrences in over 300 patients (Balli et al. 1999).

The correlation between tumor growth at port-sites and the closure of the peritoneal layer at these sites has been investigated by Farrell and coworkers (Farrell et al. 1999). After closure of the port-sites in a two layer technique (fascia and skin) the incidence of port-site recurrences could be significantly reduced in a colon cancer rat model. The combination of both local tumoricidal treatment and suturing of the peritoneal layer might also lead to prevention of metastatic tumor growth at port-sites.

Conclusion

Laparoscopic procedures in cancer patients and the development of port-site recurrences have brought up some substantial questions which are in general important for oncological surgery. Although the problem of port-site recurrences appears mainly related to the surgeon, the technique, and manipulation of the tumor bearing organ, some other factors, which are related to laparoscopy itself, have been demonstrated to influence tumor growth. The possible stimulation of tumor cell growth and suppression of local immunodefenses by carbon dioxide, as shown in many experimental studies, can be avoided by the alternative use of helium. New therapeutic strategies, including instillation of cytotoxic and immune modulating agents in combination with laparoscopy, were reported to strongly inhibit tumor growth in experimental investigations. Nevertheless, perioperative pathophysiologic and immunologic changes caused by either open or laparoscopic procedures have to be further evaluated to understand the tumor behavior under the conditions of operative intervention and to create new therapeutic strategies including nonsurgical treatments.

References

Balli JE, Franklin ME, Almeida JA, Glass JL, Kazantsev G, Diaz JA (1999) How to prevent port-site recurrence in laparoscopic colorectal surgery. Surg Endosc 13:S4

Bedrosian I, Sofia RD, Wolff SM, Dinarello CA (1991) Taurolidine, an analogue of the amino acid taurine, suppresses interleukin-1 and tumor necrosis factor synthesis in human peripheral blood mononuclear cells. Cytokine 3:568–755

Blenkharn JJ (1988) Sustained anti-adherence activity of taurolidine (Taurolin) and noxythiolin (Noxyflex S). J Pharm Pharmacol 40:509–511

Brodhage H, Pfirrmann RW (1985) Taurolin- Bakteriologe in vitro. In: Brückner WL, Pfirrmann RW (eds) Taurolin. Ein neues Konzept zur antimikrobiellen Chemotherapie chirugischer Infektionen. Urban und Schwarzenberg, Baltimore, pp 38–47

Castronovo V, Tarabolleti G, Sobel ME (1991) Laminin receptor complementary DNA-deduced synthetic peptide inhibits cancer cell attachment to endothelium. Cancer Res 51:5672–5678

Farrell TM, Johnson AB, Metreveli RE, Smith CD, Hunter JG (1999) Fascial closure limits metastasis after pneumoperitoneum. Surg Endosc 13:S33

Fleshmann JW, Nelosn H, Peters WR, Kim HC, Larach S, Boorse R, Ambroze W, Leggett P, Bleday R, Stryker S, Christenson B, Wexner S, Senagore A, Rettner D, Sutton J, Fine A (1996). Early results of laparoscopic surgery for colorectal cancer: retrospective analysis of 372 patients treated by clinical outcomes of surgical therapy (COST) study group. Dis Colon Rectum 39:53–58

Franklin ME, Rosenthal D, Abrego-Medina D, Glass JL, Norem R, Diaz A (1996) Prospective comparison of open versus laparoscopic colon surgery for carcinoma: five year results. Dis Colon Rectum 39:35–46

Gill WB, Jones KW, Ruggiero KJ (1982) Protective effects of heparin and other sulfated glycosaminoglycans on crystal adhesion to injured urothelium. J Urol 127:152–154

Goldstein DS, Lu ML, Hattori T (1993) Inhibition of peritoneal tumor cell implantation: model for laparoscopic cancer surgery. J Endourol 7:237–241

Hayman EG, Pierschbacher D, Ruoslahti E (1985) Detachment of cells from culture substrate by soluble fibronectin peptides. J Cell Biol 100:1948–1954

Humphries MJ, Olden K, Yamada KM (1986) A synthetic peptide from fibronectin inhibits experimental metastasis of murine melanoma cells Science 233:467–470

Iwanaka T, Arya G, Ziegler MM (1998) Mechanism and prevention of port-site tumor recurrence after laparoscopy in a murine model. J Pediatr Surg 33:457–461

Jacobi CA, Ordemann J, Bohm B, Zieren HU, Sabat R, Müller JM (1997a) Inhibition of peritoneal tumor cell growth and implantation in laparoscopic surgery in a rat model. Am J Surg 174:359–363

Jacobi CA, Sabat R, Bohm B, Zieren HU, Volk HD, Müller JM (1997b) Pneumoperitoneum with carbon dioxide stimulates growth of malignant colonic cells. Surgery 121:72–78

Jacobi CA, Sabat R, Ordemann J, Wenger F, Volk HD, Müller JM (1997c) Peritoneal instillation of taurolidine and heparin for preventing intraperitoneal tumor growth and trocar metastases in laparoscopic operations in the rat model. Langenbecks Arch Chir 382:31–36

Jacobi CA, Wildbrett P, Volk T, Müller JM (1999a) Influence of different gases and intraperitoneal instillation of antiadherent or cytotoxic agents on peritoneal tumor cell growth and implantation in laparoscopic surgery in a rat model. Data presented at the Third International Laparoscopic Physiology Conference 1999, New York, USA

Jacobi CA, Peter FJ, Wenger FA, Ordemann J, Müller JM (1999b) New therapeutic strategies to avoid intra- and extraperitoneal metastases during laparoscopy. Results of a tumor model in the rat. Dig Surg (in press)

Kim SH, Milsom JW, Gramlich TL, Toddy SM, Shore GI, Okuda J, Fazio VW (1998) Does laparoscopic vs. conventional surgery increase exfoliated cancer cells in the peritoneal cavity during resection of colorectal cancer ? Dis Colon Rectum 41:971–978

Lacy AM, Delgado S, Garcia-Valdecasas JC, Castells A, Piqué JM, Grande L, Fuster J, Targarona EM, Pera M, Visa J (1998) Port-site recurrences and recurrence after laparoscopic colectomy. A randomized trial. Surg Endosc 12:1039–1042

Lagadec P, Jeannin JF, Reisser D (1987) Treatment with endotoxins of peritoneal carcinomatosis induced by colon tumor cells in rats. Invasion Metastasis 7:83–95

Lanfrancone L, Boraschi D, Ghiara P (1992) Human peritoneal mesothelial cells produce many cytokines (granulocyte colony-stimulating factor, granulocyte-monocyte CSF, macrophage-CSF, interleukin-1 and IL-2) and are activated and stimulated to grow by IL-1. Blood 80:2835–2842

Lee SW, Gleason NR, Chao Zhai BA, Bessler M, Whelan RL (1999) The effects of wound painting and peritoneal irrigation with povidone-iodine solution on port tumor recurrence following laparoscopic splenectomy in a murine model. Data presented at the Third International Laparoscopic Physiology Conference 1999, New York, USA

Milsom JW, Böhm B, Hammerhofer KA, Faszio VW, Steiger E, Elson P (1998) A prospective, randomized trial comparing laparoscopic versus conventional techniques in colorectal cancer surgery: a preliminary report. J Am Coll Surg 187:46–57

Neuhaus SJ, Watson DI, Ellis T, Dodd T, Rofe AM, Jamieson GG (1998a) Efficacy of cytotoxic agents for the prevention of laparoscopic port-site recurrences. Arch Surg 133:762–766

Neuhaus SJ, Watson DI, Ellis T, Rowland R, Rofe AM, Pike GK, Mathey G, Jamieson GG (1998b) Wound metastasis after laparoscopy with different insufflation gases. Surgery 123:579–583

Neuhaus SJ, Ellis T, Jamieson GG, Watson DI (1999) An experimental study of intraperitoneal heparin on tumor implantation following laparoscopy. Data presented at the Third International Laparoscopic Physiology Conference 1999, New York, USA

Pahlman L (1997) The problem of port-site recurrences after laparoscopic cancer surgery. Ann Med 29:477–481

Paraskeva PA, Puttick MI, Rigg A, Lemoine L, Darzi A (1999) Viscous hyaluronate solution: a potential agent for the prevention of post-operative tumor cell invasion following laparoscopic surgery for malignant disease. Data presented at the Third International Laparoscopic Physiology Conference 1999, New York, USA

Parsons CL, Greenspan C, Moore SW, Mulholland SG (1977). Role of surface mucin in primary antibacterial defense of bladder. Urology 9:48–52

Parsons CL, Mulholland SG, Anwar H (1979) Antibacterial activity of bladder surface mucin duplicated by exogenous glycosaminoglycan (heparin). Infect Immun 24:552–557

Puttick MI, Nduka CC, Yong L, Darzi A (1998) Macrophage function is suppressed by a carbon dioxide pneumoperitoneum. Data presented at the Second Workshop of Experimental Laparoscopic Surgery 1998, Rotterdam, Netherlands

Reisser D, Fady C, Lagadec P, Martin F (1991) Influence of the injection site on the tumorigenicity of a cloned colon tumor cell line in the rat. Bull Cancer 78:249–252

Reymond MA, Schneider C, Hohenberger W, Köckerling F (1998) The pneumoperitoneum and its role in tumor seeding. Dig Surg 15:105–109

Ruoslahti E, Pierschbacher D (1987) New perspectives in cell adhesion: RGD and integrins. Science 238:491–497

Tsunoda A, Shinusawa M, Tsunoda Y, Choh H, Takata M, Kusona M (1997) Implantation on suture material and efficacy of povidone-iodine solution. Eur Surg Res 29:473–480

Wexner SD, Latulippe J-F (1997) Laparoscopic colorectal surgery and cancer. Swiss Surg 3:266–273

Whalen GF, Ingber DE (1989) Inhibition of tumor cell attachment to extracellular matrix as a method for preventing tumor recurrence in a surgical wound. Ann Surg 210:758–764

Wu JS, Jones DB, Guo LW, Brasfield EB, Ruiz M, Connet JM, Fleshmann JW (1998a) Effects of pneumoperitoneum on tumor implantation with decreasing tumor inoculum. Dis Colon Rectum 41:141–146

Wu JS, Pfister SM, Ruiz MB, Connett JM, Fleshman JW (1998b) Local treatment of abdominal wound reduces tumor implantation. J Surg Oncol 69:9–14

Yamada KM (1983) Cell surface interactions with extracellular materials. Annu Rev Biochem 52:761–799

CHAPTER 16

Prevention of Port-Site Recurrences: Gasless Laparoscopy and Other Gases

S.J. Neuhaus, D.I. Watson

Introduction

The fundamental difference between open surgical approaches and a resection performed using laparoscopic techniques, other than the size of the wounds, is the need to maintain sufficient space for both vision and operative manipulation. This is usually achieved by the creation of a pneumoperitoneum, by introducing carbon dioxide gas into the peritoneal cavity using positive pressure. It is the pneumoperitoneum which maintains a suitable working space within the abdominal cavity, which when combined with sophisticated fiber optics, permits advanced laparoscopic interventions such as colon resection.

In 1924, Zollikofer first proposed the use of carbon dioxide (CO_2) as an insufflation agent (Zollikofer 1924). Now, CO_2 is almost universally used as the gas to create a laparoscopic pneumoperitoneum, with its role firmly established in the 1960's when Kurt Semm developed the peritoneal insufflator (Lau et al. 1997). CO_2 has properties which make it a very suitable insufflation agent. It is cheap, non combustible and colorless. Furthermore, it is excreted by the lungs during normal respiration, and it is highly soluble in water, which reduces the risk of gas embolism impairing cardiac function. More recently, however, as the physiological effects of laparoscopy have become better understood, debate has arisen about the metabolic and oncologic consequences of insufflating the peritoneal cavity with CO_2. This has resulted in some surgeons re-evaluating the effects of a CO_2 pneumoperitoneum, or perhaps more accurately, capnoperitoneum (Martin and McMahon 1996). Alternatives to CO_2 insufflation are gasless laparoscopy exposure techniques, as well as the use of other insufflation gases such as helium or argon.

Adverse Effects of Carbon Dioxide

Several adverse effects of CO_2 have been documented.

Metabolic

There is now evidence from clinical and experimental studies that CO_2 pneumoperitoneum is associated with adverse physiological effects (Volz et al. 1996a,b), which result in alterations to ventilatory, cellular, hormonal and immunologic parameters. The insufflation of CO_2 into the peritoneal cavity results in hypercarbia and respiratory acidosis due to absorption of CO_2 across the peritoneal membrane. Specific adverse effects which have been identified include acidosis, involving the peritoneal surface and the connective tissue beneath the peritoneal membrane, disturbances in electrical surface charges, and the release of various mediators such as endotoxin (Volz et al. 1996b). In addition, it has been suggested that the use of CO_2 as an insufflating agent promotes the development of postoperative pain (Johnson and Sibert 1997), and that this may occur due to the build-up of carbonic acid at the peritoneal membrane surface.

Cardiovascular and Respiratory

Most pathophysiologic alterations occurring during laparoscopy are secondary to the insufflation of gas under pressure. Significant alterations in central venous pressure, cardiac output, cardiac rhythm and splanchnic and mesenteric blood flow have all been identified (Martin and McMahon 1996). Direct pressure from the use of insufflated gas also results in decreased flow in the inferior vena cava and decreased venous return from the lower limbs and pelvis (Martin and McMahon 1996). Studies which have compared the physiological effects of a pneumoperitoneum using carbon dioxide with helium and argon suggest that whilst hypercapnea is a carbon dioxide-specific effect, the metabolic acidosis observed during pneumoperitoneum is not dependent on the type of gas used, but it is, in fact, a function of impaired tissue perfusion due to pressure in the peritoneal cavity, which results in an accumulation of the end products of hypoxic metabolism (Shuto et al. 1995). Insufflation of CO_2 also causes respiratory acidosis due to absorption of CO_2 into the circulation. This is usually easily managed by the anesthetist increasing the ventilation rate of the mechanical ventilator to maintain a normal end tidal CO_2 partial pressure.

However, in patients with poor cardio-respiratory reserve, this may become clinically important.

Immunological

Recent studies have suggested that minimal access surgery is associated with less overall suppression of the systemic immune system compared to conventional open surgery. This is manifested as decreased surgery-related systemic trauma and stress responses when exposed to a laparoscopic surgical environment (Allendorf et al. 1995; Allendorf et al. 1996; Bouvy et al. 1996; Collet et al. 1995). However, this systemic benefit may not necessarily be acting at the level of the peritoneal membrane interface, as the insufflation of CO_2 under pressure has been shown to adversely modulate the local immune environment (Neuhaus et al. 1998; Volz et al. 1996a; Watson et al. 1995). Volz et al. (1996a,b) proposed that the severe acidosis generated by CO_2 pneumoperitoneum, in combination with elevated intra-abdominal pressure, impairs peritoneal macrophage function. Peritoneal macrophages play an integral role in the primary inflammatory response to infection and cancer within the abdominal cavity.

The insufflation of CO_2 has also been shown to compromise intraperitoneal macrophage activity and depress immunological responses in a range of studies using experimental animals (Jacobi et al. 1998; Watson et al. 1995; West et al. 1997). West et al. (1997) reported a transient inability of peritoneal macrophages to secrete inflammatory cytokines, particularly lipopolysaccharide-stimulated tumor necrosis factor and interleukin-1, following incubation in a CO_2 rich environment. This effect did not occur following either air or helium insufflation. In this study, the depression of macrophage cytokine production by exposure to CO_2 was reversible following incubation for 24 h in a control atmosphere. Recent studies by Jacobi et al. (1998) have suggested that the use of a CO_2 pneumoperitoneum also results in adverse systemic alterations to the experimental immune environment. They demonstrated a decrease in plasma transforming growth factor alpha (TNF-()) levels and an increase in plasma IL-10 in rats undergoing laparoscopy with CO_2 insufflation as compared to control rats and rats undergoing helium laparoscopy. We have recently found a similar in vivo depression of macrophage function occurring within the peritoneal cavity itself in response to CO_2.

In this study, the insufflation of CO_2 was associated with a marked decrease (> 90%) in the ability of peritoneal macrophages to produce TNF-α when harvested 3 days following a 40 min period of pneumoperitoneum in an experimental model. This effect was not seen following helium insufflation or with gasless exposure (unpublished data).

The Role of CO_2 Pneumoperitoneum in the Development of Port-Site Tumors

Factors specific to the CO_2 pneumoperitoneum which may promote the development of port-site recurrences include: mechanical effects of gas under pressure, potential metabolic and immunological effects due to the insufflation gas, alterations in peritoneal humidity, stretching of the abdominal wall and peritoneal lining, and possible electrostatic interactions with trocars and pressure/flow effects related to the use of insufflating gas. Because of these issues, the development of barrier strategies which protect the wounds during laparoscopic surgery may not be sufficient to prevent the development of port-site tumors.

Nduka et al. (1994) suggested that the pneumoperitoneum acts as a closed system through which particulate matter circulates, possibly resulting in "trapping of viable tumor cells by moist peritoneal surfaces". A so-called "chimney phenomenon", whereby the insufflation of CO_2 causes turbulence which displaces tumor cells, has also been proposed (Allardyce et al. 1996). At the port-sites, these cells are concentrated as a result of the leakage of CO_2 alongside trocars leading to high local gas flow at the trocar sites or to tumor cells being wiped off the trocar and deposited within the port-site wound. It is also possible that CO_2 gas under pressure dissects between tissue layers at the port-site, thereby causing additional trauma and allowing tumor cells to lodge between muscle, fascial and peritoneal surfaces.

Experimental Evidence of an Increased Incidence of Wound Recurrences Following Carbon Dioxide Insufflation

Most experimental studies have utilized CO_2 as the only insufflation gas, and have assumed that the physical effects of CO_2 pneumoperitoneum account for the development of subsequent wound recurrences. Experimental studies using small animal models have demonstrated that the incidence of wound recurrences is reduced by eliminating CO_2 insufflation by using gasless laparoscopy (Bouvy et al. 1996; Bouvy et al. 1998; Mathew et al. 1997; Watson et al. 1997), or by replacing CO_2 with the inert gas helium (Neuhaus et al. 1998a,c). Studies both in our department (Mathew et al. 1996; Watson et al. 1997) and by others (Jacobi et al. 1997) suggest that the incidence of wound recurrences when CO_2 is excluded from the peritoneal cavity is similar to that following laparotomy. These studies provide good evidence that either mechanical effects generated by the use of pressurized insufflation or some factor inherent in CO_2 gas per se play a role in the development of metastases in the laparoscopy wounds seen in clinical reports, and that poor surgical technique alone is not sufficient to account for all instances of port-site recurrences.

Alternatives to Carbon Dioxide

Various alternative techniques have been claimed to replace CO_2.

Gasless Laparoscopy

Gasless laparoscopy, which involves the creation of a laparoscopic working space without using positive pressure pneumoperitoneum, is readily achieved and various abdominal wall-lifting devices are commercially available (Luks et al. 1995; Martin and McMahon 1996; Nishii et al. 1997; Yoshida et al. 1997). Gasless laparoscopy may offer some advantages over the use of CO_2 insufflation, including the avoidance of various pneumoperitoneum-specific problems such as: cardiopulmonary compromise, hypothermia due to cold insufflation gas, peripheral

venous stasis, and gas embolism. In addition, the ability to use continuous suction and conventional surgical instruments (there is no requirement to maintain airtight ports) may also be useful. There are two different methods for achieving abdominal wall elevation. This can be achieved by traction of the skin and subcutaneous tissues, e.g., by inserting subcutaneous wires (Hashimoto et al. 1993), or by inserting devices into the peritoneal cavity (Fig. 16.1) which are attached to external retraction frames (Chin et al. 1994; Nishii et al. 1997). In addition; hybrid systems are available which utilize a combination of elevation and low pressure (6–8 mm Hg) gas insufflation (Banting et al. 1993; Martin et al. 1996).

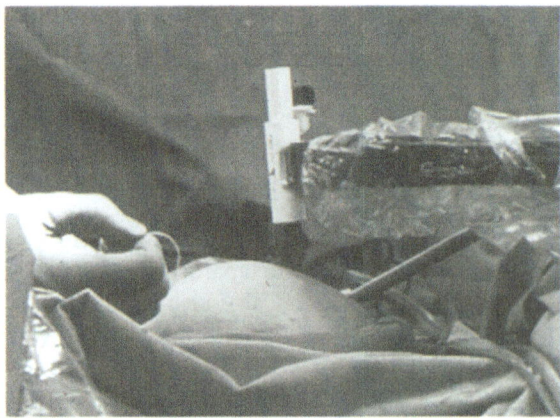

Fig. 16.1. One possible alternative to CO_2-pneumoperitoneum is gasless laparoscopy using, for example, a fan-shaped retractor – which is inserted intraperitoneally – coupled to an external mechanical arm

However, some problems have yet to be overcome with gasless laparoscopy. Principal amongst these is that conventional lifting devices, such as "Laparolift", which involves the use of a fan-shaped retractor which is inserted intraperitoneally and an external mechanical arm, do not uniformly elevate the abdominal wall in the same fashion as a pneumoperitoneum. Therefore, exposure to some areas of the abdomen, particularly the flanks, can be reduced. This may be particularly relevant in laparoscopic colectomy where reduced access to the abdominal flanks may impede colonic mobilization and compromise resection margins by making surgery more difficult. In a randomized trial of gasless versus CO_2 laparoscopy in gynecological surgery, the disadvantages of gasless laparoscopy in terms of impaired exposure, the requirement to convert to conventional pneumoperitoneum, and technical difficulty, outweighed the potential advantages (Johnson and Sibert 1997). In contrast to this, Smith et al. (1993) reported on a series of 58 patients in whom gasless techniques were used without significant technical difficulties. It should be noted, however, that a large percentage of the procedures performed were diagnostic laparoscopies, in which exposure and access may not be as problematic as in colonic mobilization.

Many of the current gasless laparoscopy devices also require complex assembly and additional incisions, which may increase the likelihood of postoperative pain and also offer another potential site for tumor implantation. In theory, compression of the abdominal wall, which can occur when using intraperitoneally sited lifting devices, may also cause local ischemia and/or trauma, which may result in the release of inflammatory mediators. It is possible, but not proven, that a local environment conducive to tumor implantation may even be created (Jones and Rous 1914).

Gasless Laparoscopy and Port-Site Recurrences

On the other hand, the removal of the insufflation gas may eliminate one of the essential environmental components necessary for laparoscopic wound metastasis. Laparoscopy with insufflation gas may transport tumor cells to laparoscopic access wounds and result in the growth of metastases. We reported, using an intraperitoneal suspension of tumor cells in a rat model of laparoscopy, that in gasless laparoscopy tumor, deposits grew largely around the site where tumor was introduced into the peritoneal cavity, rather than evenly throughout the peritoneal cavity, as seen following conventional laparoscopic insufflation (Mathew et al. 1997). A similar study, which involved the laparoscopic laceration of the capsule of an implanted flank tumor, demonstrated a much higher incidence of port-site recurrences following CO_2 laparoscopy compared to gasless laparoscopy (Watson et al. 1997). Gasless laparoscopy was achieved in both studies by suspending the abdominal wall using subcutaneously placed sutures, and no lifting device was inserted into the peritoneal cavity.

In a further study, we introduced viable tumor cells into the upper abdomen of rats undergoing either gasless or conventional laparoscopy (Mathew et al. 1997a), following the introduction of a length of plastic tubing through the anterolateral aspect of the rat's left lower abdominal wall. This tubing was used

to vent the insufflation gas through the abdomen of a further "recipient" rat for 30 min. After 21 days, the peritoneal cavity and surgical wound of the recipient rat were examined, and nodular tumor metastases were found around the site of both the venting port and the inflow tubing site in five out of six of the recipient rats in the group that underwent CO_2 insufflation. However, no tumor was found in any recipient rat in the gasless group. These studies suggest that insufflation (of CO_2) is important for the promotion of wound recurrences.

Other studies utilizing real time imaging of radiolabeled cells instilled into the peritoneal cavity of pigs undergoing laparoscopy demonstrate widespread cell movement throughout the abdominal cavity during CO_2 pneumoperitoneum (Texler et al. 1998), supporting the postulate that CO_2 pneumoperitoneum facilitates tumor cell dispersal throughout the abdominal cavity, thereby bringing cells into contact with potential implantation sites.

Bouvy et al. (1996) have also reported that gasless laparoscopy is associated with decreased tumor implantation and decreased growth of a solid tumor (CC-531 colon adenocarcinoma). In a subsequent study, they confirmed this result by demonstrating decreased tumor growth of an implanted renal subcapsular tumor in rats undergoing laparoscopy using a gasless technique compared to air or CO_2 pneumoperitoneum (ROS-1 osteosarcoma) (Bouvy et al. 1998). As operative trauma and techniques are similar in both the gasless and CO_2 groups in each of these studies, differences in tumor implantation and metastasis may be due to either the mechanical effects of insufflation, a metabolic effect specific to CO_2 gas, or a combination of both. However, tumor growth in their second study was similar in rats undergoing insufflation with air compared to CO_2, suggesting that increased intra-abdominal pressure may be a key factor. Mechanical stretching of the peritoneum secondary to high pressure pneumoperitoneum is associated with an increase in free radical production, and the production of inflammatory mediators in response to local ischemia (Eleftheriadis et al. 1996). Other studies which have compared high and low pressure insufflation, however, have not demonstrated a difference in incidence of tumor metastasis with different insufflation pressures (Neuhaus et al. 1998). Table 16.1 summarizes the experimental studies which have compared CO_2 insufflation with gasless laparoscopy.

Alterations to local peritoneal immune function induced by CO_2 might also contribute to the development of port-site recurrences. The scavenging ac-

Table 16.1. Experimental models: CO_2 insufflation versus gasless laparoscopy

Study	Cell line	Model	Tumors in CO_2 insufflated patients	Tumors in patients of gasless laparoscopy
Watson et al. 1995	Mammary adenocarcinoma	Solid flank tumor	10/12 wounds	3/12 wounds
Mathew et al. 1997b	Mammary adenocarcinoma	Tumor cell suspension	64/72 sectors	37/72 sectors
Mathew et al. 1997a	Mammary adenocarcinoma	Tumor cell suspension	5/6 recipient rats	0/6 recipient rats
Bouvy et al. 1996b	CC-531 colon adenocarcinoma	Solid tumor	Increased tumor growth in CO_2 group; $p < 0.01$	
Bouvy et al. 1996b	CC-531 colon adenocarcinoma	Cell seeding model	Increased tumor seeding in CO_2 group; $p < 0.01$	
Bouvy et al. 1998	ROS-1 osteosarcoma	Solid bolus	Increased subrenal tumor growth in CO_2 group; $p = 0.04$	

tion of peritoneal macrophages is mediated in part by the production of inflammatory cytokines such as TNF-α, which may have a role in the effective killing of tumor cells (Jones and Selby 1980; Rofe et al. 1992). We hypothesize that CO_2-induced depression of macrophage activity, possibly mediated by pH changes, is a contributing factor to the development of port-site recurrences. The depression of peritoneal macrophage function observed with CO_2 insufflation may inhibit effective "scavenging" of viable tumor cells liberated during laparoscopic cancer surgery.

The creation of a capnoperitoneum has also been shown to be associated with structural changes in the peritoneal mesothelial surface layer, which are visible with electron microscopy (Schaeff et al. 1998). This may reflect changes secondary to CO_2 per se or it might be due to desiccation of the peritoneal surface by cold insufflation gas (independent of the gas type). CO_2 is an irritant to the peritoneum, and the subsequent release of inflammatory mediators such as TNF-α, may favor tumor implantation at raw peritoneal surfaces such as those created by laparoscopy access ports (Volz et al. 1996). This effect is eliminated when a gasless exposure technique is used (Bouvy et al. 1996b; Mathew et al. 1997b; Watson et al. 1997).

Helium Pneumoperitoneum

Exclusion of CO_2 can also be achieved by the use of other insufflation gases. Helium and nitrous oxide have been used in clinical practice (Fernandez Cruz et al. 1994; Naude et al. 1996; Neuberger et al. 1996;

Phillips et al. 1987), and argon has been investigated experimentally (Eisenhauer et al. 1994). Helium and argon offer the advantages of a pneumoperitoneum, i.e., exposure and technical access, without the inherent metabolic disadvantages of CO_2. Although neither gas is in common clinical use, helium has been more widely investigated in the laboratory and clinically than argon (Bongard et al. 1991; Fernandez Cruz et al. 1994; Neuberger et al. 1996; Rademaker et al. 1995). Helium has been shown in laboratory studies not to be associated with many of the adverse physiological effects of CO_2 (Naude and Bongard 1995; Neuberger et al. 1996).

However, the use of helium as an insufflation agent requires modifications to the insufflator, as flow regulators in automatic insufflators are gas specific. In addition, helium is more expensive. Nevertheless, initial clinical trials suggest that helium may offer some advantages over CO_2 as an insufflation agent (Neuberger et al. 1996). In particular, patients with borderline cardiorespiratory function, and those undergoing prolonged procedures may benefit from the reduced physiological disturbances associated with helium insufflation (Dorsam et al. 1997; Leighton et al. 1993). In addition, it has been proposed that postoperative shoulder tip pain following laparoscopy may be related to irritation of the peritoneal surface by carbonic acid, which forms as a result of the dissociation of carbon dioxide in water. Theoretically, the use of an inert gas such as helium could achieve a reduction in postoperative pain. This hypothesis has yet to be formally tested in the clinical situation.

Perhaps the most serious possible adverse effect of helium insufflation is the potential for venous gas embolism during insufflation (Wolf et al. 1994). This is because helium is less soluble than CO_2, and therefore a given volume of gas entering the venous system is likely to be eliminated more slowly if it is helium, compared to CO_2, with possibly more serious consequences if a sufficient volume becomes trapped in the right ventricle of the heart, thereby impairing cardiac output. However, gas embolism during laparoscopy is a rare event and there are no reports of helium gas embolism following laparoscopy. Furthermore, it is likely that several hundred milliliters of gas must be introduced into a major vein for cardiac arrest to result. This is only likely to occur if a Verres needle punctures an iliac vein or a vein of similar size, and insufflation occurs directly into the venous lumen, rather than the peritoneal cavity. If this occurs, the choice of insufflation gas is unlikely to make a critical difference to the likely disastrous outcome. Prevention of this scenario is achieved by using an open technique for insertion of the first laparoscopic trocar. Whilst clinical use has been limited, several trials of helium laparoscopy have recently been reported in the international literature (Bongard et al. 1993; McMahon et al. 1994). No complications specific to the use of helium insufflation have been reported.

Helium Insufflation and Port-Site Recurrence

Recent experimental studies using various small animal models have reported that the use of a helium pneumoperitoneum is associated with a reduction in the incidence of port-site recurrences compared to CO_2 insufflation (Jacobi et al. 1997; Neuhaus et al. 1998a,c). Bench top experiments also suggest that helium, unlike CO_2 does not facilitate tumor growth in culture. This effect may have considerable implications for laparoscopic cancer surgery (Jacobi et al. 1997; Neuhaus et al. 1998c). Jacobi et al. (1997) reported a series of in vitro, in vivo and ex vivo experi-

ments using a rat model and a colon cancer cell line in which replacement of CO_2 with helium clearly reduced the likelihood of tumor growth and implantation.

We have also reported (Neuhaus et al. 1998a,c) a reduction in the incidence of port-site recurrences when helium is used as the insufflation agent rather than CO_2, using both a solid tumor and tumor cell suspension model (Table 16.2). This effect was not observed when either medical air or nitrous oxide (N_2O) was used as the insufflation agent.

Because helium is a metabolically inert gas (Neuberger et al. 1996; Rademaker et al. 1995), these studies suggest that the development of port-site recurrences may be dependent, at least in part, on metabolic determinants, and that the physical redistribution of tumor cells alone is insufficient to account for the issue of port-site recurrences. Possible explanations for the reduced rate of tumor metastasis following helium insufflation include this beneficial effect due to the lack of adverse metabolic activity during helium insufflation. Alternatively, but perhaps less likely, is the possibility that helium gas is cytotoxic to cancer cells. Additionally, tumor implantation occurred evenly in all sectors in the study reported by Neuhaus et al. (1998a), suggesting that tumor cells are evenly distributed throughout the peritoneal cavity during laparoscopy, due to the mechanical effect of insufflation, and that the reduced rate of tumor growth in all sectors is a consequence of a metabolic or cytotoxic action of helium insufflation. Gasless laparoscopy, on the other hand, is associated with tumor growth in the area of the abdominal cavity in which tumor cells are placed in experimental models, and the reduction in the likelihood of port-site recurrences and tumor implantation is likely to be due to a reduction in the likelihood of tumor spread to areas in the peritoneal cavity distant from the operative field (Watson et al. 1997b).

It is certainly interesting that the incidence of metastases following helium insufflation is similar to

Table 16.2. Experimental models: CO_2 versus helium laparoscopy

Study	Model	Tumor type	Tumors in CO_2 insufflated patients	Tumors in patients treated with helium laparoscopy
Neuhaus et al. (1998c)	Mammary adenocarcinoma	Solid flank tumor	15/36 sectors	1/36 sectors
Neuhaus et al. (1998a)	Mammary adenocarcinoma	Tumor cell suspension	59/60 sectors, 20/30 port-sites	42/60 sectors, 13/3 port-sites
Jacobi et al. (1997)	DHD/K12/TRb colon adenocarcinoma	Tumor cell suspension	10/15 wounds	6/15 wounds

that following laparotomy and gasless laparoscopy using the similar small animal models (Bouvy et al. 1996b; Mathew et al. 1996), and these findings warrant close evaluation in the clinical setting, as substituting CO_2 with helium insufflation is a potentially a very simple strategy for the prevention of port-site recurrences. Clinical trials investigating the role of helium laparoscopy are now underway in several centers.

Insufflation Using Other Gases

The use of other inert gases may offer similar benefits, and such gases warrant investigation. Nitrogen and argon have both been proposed (Hubens et al. 1996). Argon is the least expensive but may not be entirely physiologically inert and in patients with cardiovascular disease its effects may be clinically important (Eisenhauer et al. 1994). It is also relatively insoluble in blood and therefore carries a theoretical potential for gas embolism (Eisenhauer et al. 1994; Wolf et al. 1994).

The use of N_2O as an insufflation agent has some advantages in terms of improved patient tolerance. However, N_2O supports combustion and is therefore unsuitable for use in therapeutic laparoscopy. The use of N_2O in diagnostic laparoscopy must also be cautioned against, as experimental studies demonstrate no advantage over CO_2 in reducing tumor implantation rates. More recently, nitrogen has been proposed, but there is currently little evidence to support its use. Furthermore, the effects, if any, of N_2O or nitrogen on intraperitoneal immunity are not known.

Conclusions

The weight of experimental evidence suggests that the use of CO_2 as an insufflation agent is associated with facilitation of tumor growth and implantation and that exclusion of CO_2 from the pneumoperitoneum is advantageous. This can be achieved either by the use of gasless exposure techniques or by using an inert gas for insufflation. Which of these options proves to be best will depend on the outcome of further clinical studies. Nevertheless gasless laparoscopy is limited by the fact that poor lateral exposure is achieved, whereas helium insufflation seems to be a more advantageous strategy for further clinical investigation.

References

Allardyce R, Morreau P, Bagshaw P (1996) Tumor cell distribution following laparoscopic colectomy in a porcine model. Dis Colon Rectum 39:S47–S52

Allendorf JD, Bessler M, Kayton ML, Oesterling SD, Treat MR, Nowygrod R, Whelan RL (1995) Increased tumor establishment and growth after laparotomy vs laparoscopy in a murine model. Arch Surg 130:649–653

Allendorf JD, Bessler M, Whelan RL, Trokel M, Laird DA, Terry MB, Treat MR (1996) Better preservation of immune function after laparoscopic-assisted vs. open bowel resection in a murine model. Dis Colon Rectum 39:S67–S72

Banting S, Shimi G, Van der Velpen G, Cushieri A (1993) Abdominal wall lift: low pressure pneumoperitoneum laparoscopic surgery. Surg Endosc 7:57

Bongard FS, Pianim N, Lui SY (1991) Using helium for insufflation during laparoscopy. JAMA 266:3131

Bongard FS, Pianim NA, Leighton TA, Dubecz S, Davis IP, Lippmann M, Klein S, Liu SY (1993) Helium insufflation for laparoscopic operation. Surg Gynecol Obstet 177:140–146

Bouvy ND, Marquet RL, Hamming JF, Jeekel J, Bonjer HJ (1996a) Laparoscopic surgery in the rat. Beneficial effect on body weight and tumor take. Surg Endosc 10:490–494

Bouvy ND, Marquet RL, Jeekel H, Bonjer HJ (1996b) Impact of gas(less) laparoscopy and laparotomy on peritoneal tumor growth and abdominal wall metastases. Ann Surg 224:694–700

Bouvy ND, Giuffrida MC, Tseng LN, Steyerberg EW, Marquet RL, Jeekel H, Bonjer HJ (1998) Effects of carbon dioxide pneumoperitoneum, air pneumoperitoneum, and gasless laparoscopy on body weight and tumor growth. Arch Surg 133:652–656

Chin AK, Eaton J, Tsoi EK, Smith RS, Fry WR, Henderson VJ, McColl MB, Moll FH, Organ CHJ (1994) Gasless laparoscopy using a planar lifting technique. J Am Coll Surg 178:401–403

Collet D, Vitale GC, Reynolds M, Klar E, Cheadle WG (1995) Peritoneal host defenses are less impaired by laparoscopy than by open operation. Surg Endosc 9:1059–1064

Dorsam J, Bucuras CV, Mieck U, Brkovic D, Motsch J, Staehler G (1997) Effects of carbon dioxide pneumoperitoneum in pigs with impaired pulmonary function. J Endourol 11:185–189

Eisenhauer DM, Saunders CJ, Ho HS, Wolfe BM (1994) Hemodynamic effects of argon pneumoperitoneum. Surg Endosc 8:315–320

Eleftheriadis E, Kotzampassi K, Papanotas K, Heliadis N, Sarris K (1996) Gut ischemia, oxidative stress, and bacterial translocation in elevated abdominal pressure in rats. World J Surg 20:11–16

Fernandez Cruz L, Saenz A, Taura P, Benarroch G, Nies C, Astudillo E (1994) Pheochromocytoma: laparoscopic approach with CO2 and helium pneumoperitoneum. Endosc Surg Allied Technol 2:300–304

Hashimoto D, Nayeem SA, Kajiwara S, Hoshino T (1993) Abdominal wall lifting with subcutaneous wiring: an experience of 50 cases of laparoscopic cholesytectomy without pneumoperitoneum. Surg Today 23:786–790

Hubens G, Pauwels M, Hubens A, Vermeulen P, Van Marck E, Eyskens E (1996) The influence of a pneumoperitoneum on the peritoneal implantation of free intraperitoneal colon cancer cells. Surg Endosc 10:809–812

Jacobi CA, Sabat R, Bohm B, Zieren HU, Volk HD, Muller JM (1997) Pneumoperitoneum with carbon dioxide stimulates growth of malignant colonic cells. Surgery 121:72–78

Jacobi CA, Wenger F, Sabat R, Volk T, Ordemann J, Muller JM (1998) The impact of laparoscopy with carbon dioxide versus helium on immunologic function and tumor growth in a rat model. Dig Surg 15:110–116

Johnson PL, Sibert KS (1997) Laparoscopy. Gasless vs. CO2 pneumoperitoneum. J Reprod Med 42:255–259

Jones FS, Rous P (1914) On the cause of the localisation of secondary tumors at points of injury. J Exp Med :404–412

Jones AL, Selby P (1980) Clinical applicati ons of tumor necrosis factor. Prog Growth Factor Res 1:107–122

Lau WY, Leow CK, Li AK (1997) History of endoscopic and laparoscopic surgery. World J Surg 21:444–453

Leighton TA, Liu SY, Bongard FS (1993) Comparative cardiopulmonary effects of carbon dioxide versus helium pneumoperitoneum. Surgery 113:527–531

Luks FI, Peers KH, Deprest JA, Lerut TE (1995) Gasless laparoscopy in infants: the rabbit model. J Pediatr Surg 30:1206–1208

Martin IG, McMahon MJ (1996) Gasless laparoscopy. J R Coll Surg Edinb 41:72–74

Mathew G, Watson DI, Rofe AM, Baigrie CF, Ellis T, Jamieson GG (1996) Wound metastases following laparoscopic and open surgery for abdominal cancer in a rat model. Br J Surg 83:1087–1090

Mathew G, Watson DI, Ellis T, De Young N, Rofe AM, Jamieson GG (1997a) The effect of laparoscopy on the movement of tumor cells and metastasis to surgical wounds. Surg Endosc 11:1163–1166

Mathew G, Watson DI, Rofe AM, Ellis T, Jamieson GG (1997b) Adverse impact of pneumoperitoneum on intraperitoneal implantation and growth of tumor cell suspension in an experimental model. Aust N Z J Surg 67:289–292

McMahon AJ, Baxter JN, Murray W, Imrie CW, Kenny G, O'Dwyer PJ (1994) Helium pneumoperitoneum for laparoscopic cholecystectomy: ventilatory and blood gas changes. Br J Surg 81:1033–1036

Naude GP, Bongard FS (1995) Helium insufflation in laparoscopic surgery. Endosc Surg Allied Technol 3:183–186

Naude GP, Ryan MK, Pianim NA, Klein SR, Lippmann M, Bongard FS (1996) Comparative stress hormone changes during helium versus carbon dioxide laparoscopic cholecystectomy. J Laparoendosc Surg 6:93–98

Nduka CC, Monson JR, Menzies Gow N, Darzi A (1994) Abdominal wall metastases following laparoscopy. Br J Surg 81:648–652

Neuberger TJ, Andrus CH, Wittgen CM, Wade TP, Kaminski DL (1996) Prospective comparison of helium versus carbon dioxide pneumoperitoneum. Gastrointest Endosc 43:38–41

Neuhaus SJ, Ellis T, Pike GK, Rofe AM, Jamieson GG, Watson DI (1998a) tumor implantation following laparoscopy using different insufflation gases. Surg Endosc 12:1300–1302

Neuhaus SJ, Watson DI, Ellis T, Rofe AM, Jamieson GG (1998b) The effect of immune enhancement and suppression of the development of laparoscopic port-site recurrences. Surg Endosc 12:5(abstract)

Neuhaus SJ, Watson DI, Ellis T, Rowland R, Rofe AM, Mathew G, Jamieson GG (1998c) Wound metastasis following different insufflation gases. Surgery 123:579–583

Neuhaus SJ, Watson DI, Ellis T, Dodd T, Jamieson GG (1999) Port-site recurrences are not increased by high pressure insufflation. MITAT (in press)

Nishii H, Hirai T, Ohara H, Maruyama K, Suzuki A, Baba S (1997) Laparoscopic surgery by abdominal wall lifting using original lifting bars. Surg Laparosc Endosc 7:124–128

Phillips RS, Goldberg RI, Watson PW, Marshall JR, Barkin JS (1987) Mechanism of improved patient tolerance to nitrous oxide in diagnostic laparoscopy. Am J Gastroenterol 82:143–144

Rademaker BM, Bannenberg JJ, Kalkman CJ, Meyer DW (1995) Effects of pneumoperitoneum with helium on hemodynamics and oxygen transport: a comparison with carbon dioxide. J Laparoendosc Surg 5:15–20

Rofe AM, Bourgeois CS, Coyle P (1992) Beneficial effects of endotoxin treatment on metabolism in tumor-bearing rats. Immunol Cell Biol 70:1–7

Schaeff B, Paolucci V, Henze A, Encke A (1998) Electron microscopical changes to pneumoperitoneum after laparoscopic operations. Surg Endosc 12:36 (abstract)

Shuto K, Kitano S, Yoshida T, Bandoh T, Mitarai Y, Kobayashi M (1995) Hemodynamic and arterial blood gas changes during carbon dioxide and helium pneumoperitoneum in pigs. Surg Endosc 9:1173–1178

Smith RS, Fry WR, Tsoi EK, Henderson VJ, Hirvela ER, Koehler RH, Brams DM, Morabito DJ, Peskin GW (1993) Gasless laparoscopy and conventional instruments. The next phase of minimally invasive surgery. Arch Surg 128:1102–1107

Texler ML, Luck A, Hewett PJ, King G, Anderson D, Chatterton B (1998) A real time in vivo model of intraperitoneal movement of tumor cells during laparoscopy. Surg Endosc 12:5 (abstract)

Volz J, Koster S, Weiss M, Schmidt R, Urbaschek R, Melchert F, Albrecht M (1996a) Pathophysiologic features of a pneumoperitoneum at laparoscopy: a swine model. Am J Obstet Gynecol 174:132–140

Volz J, Koster S, Melchert F (1996b) The effects of pneumoperitoneum on intraperitoneal tumor implantation in nude mice. Gynaecol Endosc 5:193–196

Watson RW, Redmond HP, McCarthy J, Burke PE, Bouchier Hayes D (1995) Exposure of the peritoneal cavity to air regulates early inflammatory responses to surgery in a murine model. Br J Surg 82:1060–1065

Watson DI, Mathew G, Ellis T, Baigrie CF, Rofe AM, Jamieson GG (1997) Gasless laparoscopy may reduce the risk of port-site recurrences following laparoscopic tumor surgery. Arch Surg 132:166–168

West MA, Hackam DJ, Baker J, Rodriguez JL, Bellingham J, Rotstein OD (1997) Mechanism of decreased in vitro murine macrophage cytokine release after exposure to carbon dioxide: relevance to laparoscopic surgery. Ann Surg 226:179–190

Wolf JS Jr, Carrier S, Stoller ML (1994) Gas embolism: helium is more lethal than carbon dioxide. J Laparoendosc Surg 4:173–177

Yoshida T, Kobayashi E, Suminaga Y, Yamauchi H, Kai T, Toyama N, Kiyozaki H, Fujimura A, Miyata M (1997) Hormone-cytokine response. Pneumoperitoneum vs abdominal wall-lifting in laparoscopic cholecystectomy. Surg Endosc 11:907–910

Zollikofer R (1924) Zur Laparoskopie. Schw Med Wochenschr 54:264

CHAPTER 17

Prevention of Port-Site Recurrences: Role of Therapeutic Pneumoperitoneum

K. Ridwelski, M. Pross, M.A. Reymond

The Problem: CO_2 has Numerous Side-Effects

The automated carbon dioxide (CO_2)-pneumoperitoneum was introduced by Semm in 1980 and is now the accepted standard for exposing the abdominal cavity during laparoscopic procedures (Semm 1980). In the meantime, CO_2-pneumoperitoneum has been demonstrated to have several side effects. In particular, it has recently been documented that CO_2 stimulates tumor growth after laparoscopy for cancer (Jones et al. 1995a), and that it increases bacterial translocation in peritonitis (Bloechle et al. 1998). CO_2 pneumoperitoneum induces a severe acidosis at the peritoneal surface in the animal model (Shah et al., SAGES meeting 1999) and causes morphological changes in mesothelial cells (Bloechle et al. 1999).

The side-effects of CO_2 might be claimed to be a non-issue. In particular, it is possible to operate on hundreds of cancer patients with no port-site recurrence – in the presence of CO_2 (Franklin et al. 1996). Port-site recurrences have been reported – with no CO_2 being used (Fry et al. 1995). In our opinion, the reported side-effects of CO_2 should nevertheless receive special attention. Only such attention will allow further reduction of the physiological and immunological stress for the patient. Further research will permit the desirable evolution from minimally invasive surgery to "minimally disruptive surgery" (Neuhaus 1999).

Gasless laparoscopy has been proposed as an alternative to avoid the side-effects of CO_2 (Paolucci et al. 1995; Bouvy et al. 1996; Watson et al. 1997), but limited exposure might prevent using this technique for advanced laparoscopic procedures such as colonic resections. The occurrence of port-site recurrences after thoracoscopy (Johnstone et al. 1996) also suggests that gasless laparoscopy is not able to prevent such complications.

Alternative types of gas have been proposed for expanding the abdominal cavity without the side-effects of CO_2-pneumoperitoneum (Neuhaus et al. 1998a, Jacobi et al. 1998). In particular, helium has inhibitory effects on tumor growth (Neuhaus et al. 1999). Even though helium appears highly attractive, its acceptance into clinical practice might be limited because this gas is not resorbable and carries therefore a potential risk of lethal gas embolisms in the case of venous lesions (Southern and Mapleson 1993; Bongard et al. 1991). It is important to note, however, that such complications have not been demonstrated so far in clinical practice nor in the animal model (Jacobi, SAGES meeting 1999).

Finally, different drug solutions have been shown to reduce postoperative tumor growth and/or to reduce the incidence of port-site recurrences after CO_2-laparoscopy (Neuhaus et al. 1998b; Jacobi et al. 1997b). Phase III clinical studies are already ongoing that might reproduce in the human patient results obtained in animal models (Jacobi, personal communication), but this demonstration might be difficult in the absence of very large-scaled prospective randomized trials.

Definition of the Therapeutic Pneumoperitoneum

We propose the combination of cytostatic agents with a given carrier gas so that CO_2 might be used not only as an abdominal wall expander, but also as a drug carrier. Arguments for using a drug applied in aerosol form and carried by the insufflation gas rather than as peritoneal washing are: a better distribution of the drug within the abdomen, as well as a better drug diffusion into the tissues – due to the pressurization of the peritoneal cavity. This introduces the novel concept of "therapeutic pneumoperitoneum." Thus, therapeutic pneumoperitoneum might not only prevent the side-effects of CO_2, but it might also improve the results of minimal invasive surgery in selected indications by allowing intraoperative multimodal therapy (Reymond et al. 1999).

Pharmacokinetics Within the Abdominal Cavity

The pharmacokinetic problems i n peritoneal drug administration were recently reviewed (Dedrick and Flessner 1997). Both theory and clinical studies demonstrate that drug concentrations in the peritoneal cavity can greatly exceed concentrations in the plasma following intraperitoneal administration. This regional advantage has been associated with clinical activity (Alberts et al. 1996). Two pharmacokinetic problems appear to limit the effectiveness of intraperitoneal therapy: poor tumor penetration by the drug and incomplete irrigation of serosal surfaces by the drug-containing solution. In both respects, drug aerosolization might have major advantages over conventional irrigation.

Exposure of the Peritoneal Surface

Various observations in experimental animals suggest limited exposure of the peritoneal surface under conditions of peritoneal dialysis. In general, definitive studies have not been conducted on the potential peritoneal surface area of human subjects. The likelihood exists that much of the residual tumor burden after surgery is untreated or undertreated by conventional intraperitoneal irrigation. If the peritoneal surfaces are not exposed to drug-containing solutions or are inadequately exposed, then the rationale for regional administration is compromised (Dedrick and Flessner 1997). Theoretical considerations based on the Laplace law suggest that the pneumoperitoneum should be able to carry microdroplets of active substances to all exposed peritoneal surfaces.

Increasing Drug Penetration

Obtaining large increases in the tissue penetration of a drug might be difficult. Theoretical predictions as well as experimental measurements suggest very limited penetration of drugs into tissues, including tumors, adjacent to the peritoneal cavity. Interestingly, introducing dialysis solution into the peritoneal cavity of rats and raising the intraperitoneal pressure from 0 to 4 cm H_2O caused the extracellular space of the anterior abdominal wall to double. This likely increases the effective diffusivity (Dedrick

and Flessner 1997). However, there are only limited clinical data available to substantiate these preliminary observations (Jacquet et al. 1996).

Reducing First-Pass Hepatic Drug Metabolism

Pneumoperitoneum induces a significant reduction of the portal flow (Gutt et al. 1999). Under those circumstances, diffusion of the drug from the hollow-organ veins to the liver is impaired (Fig. 17.1). Thus, the first-pass liver drug metabolism is expected to be reduced.

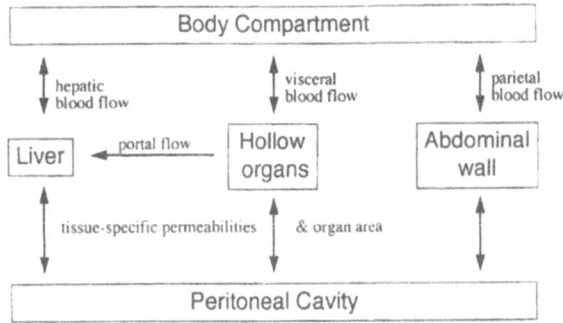

Fig. 17.1. Transfer of drugs from the peritoneal cavity into surrounding tissues. Low-molecular weight drugs move from the peritoneal tissues into the rest of the body primarily via blood flow. Since this flow is reduced during laparoscopy, intraperitoneal concentrations are enhanced (adapted from Flessner and Dedrick 1994)

In summary, therapeutic pneumoperitoneum has many theoretical advantages over irrigation for locoregional, intraperitoneal drug therapy. These advantages might be clinically significance, in particular in the field of multimodal cancer therapy.

Development of a Drug Delivery Device Suitable for Minimally Invasive Surgery

To create such a therapeutic pneumoperitoneum, an intracavitary drug delivery device suitable for minimally invasive surgical procedure is necessary. We developed such an intracavitary drug delivery device suitable for minimally invasive surgery procedures. The device consists of two elements: a micropump and a monitor. The micropump delivers the drug, which is in the form of a liquid substance, as a dispersion of atomized droplets generated by the incorporated monodispersive spray device. The device is located between a gas insufflator and the

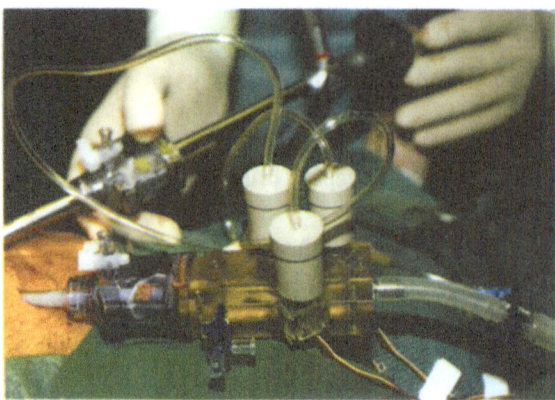

Fig. 17.2. The micropump is inserted between the gas insufflator and the abdominal cavity of the patient

body cavity where surgery is performed, allowing the aerosolization of microdroplets of the therapeutic substance into the pneumoperitoneum. The liquid is aerosolized by excitation of a piezoelectric element. Figure 17.2 shows, in detail, a prototype of the micropump built directly into a 5 mm-trocar, as commercially available (Endopath, Ethicon Endosurgery, Norderstedt, Germany). The monitor is placed in the vicinity of the gas insufflator. Means are provided for regulating the flow rate, concentration and amount of drug delivery according to the gas flow, in a closed loop control system. It is therefore possible to know precisely at each moment of the operation the amount of therapeutic substance that has been administered to the patient.

In Vitro Performance of the Micropump

After designing and manufacturing the prototype, we performed in vitro experiments to determine the behavior of the micropump with various solutions, to assess the flow rate, the influence of viscosity, the optimal delivery rate and the optimal droplet size. To date, we showed that the micropump is able to aerosolize liquids such as water and ethanol, and various solutions including:

- Taurolidine (Taurolin, Geistlich, Wolhusen, Switzerland)
- 5-Fluorouracil (Wyeth-Lederle, Wolfrathshausen, Germany)
- Mitoxantronhydrochlorid (Novantron, Wyeth-Lederle, Wolfrathshausen, Germany)
- Betadine (Betaisodona, Mundipharma, Limburg, Germany), with some limitations due to PVP adhesive characteristics

Application of the Device in a Large Animal Model

We next conducted in vivo experiments to test the intra-abdominal delivery rate and the peritoneal coating uniformity, and to detect possible unexpected events caused by the device during surgical procedures. The decision to use taurolidin in the first animal trial was based on the study of Jacobi et al. that showed that application of taurolidin in the rat model was able to significantly reduce the incidence of port-site recurrences (Jacobi et al. 1997b). Moreover, this drug has been shown to be cytotoxic for colorectal cancer cell lines. Finally, the toxicity of taurolidin in the pig is known to be low (unpublished data, Geistlich, Wolhusen, Switzerland). After obtaining the official authorizations, two German land race pigs were anesthetized using routine protocols. Pneumoperitoneum of 12 mm Hg was established using a Verres needle. At the beginning of the procedure, a second 5-mm commercially available trocar (Endopath, Ethicon Endosurgery, Norderstedt, Germany) was inserted in the left upper quadrant, and then replaced by the micropump. A laparoscopy-assisted resection of the sigmoid colon with transanal double-stapling was performed in both animals, with a four-trocar technique. Operating times were 90 and 97 min. CO_2 volumes were 156 and 195 l (an artificial leak was created by opening a valve on the right lower trocar). During the operation, a solution of taurolidin (2%) was aerosolized into the abdominal cavity. Distribution of the active principle within the abdominal cavity was assessed by aerosolizing 3 ml of a 50% methylene blue solution into a pig cadaver, after installation of a pneumoperitoneum of 12 mm Hg for 30 min. This assay showed a dispersion of the microdroplets within the entire abdominal cavity (Fig. 17.3). It is important to determine that nonexposed surfaces such as the bursa omentalis and the inferior liver aspect were not stained. As expected, the distribution was not homogenous, staining was enhanced in the vicinity and in the axis of the trocar where the micropump had been introduced.

Both surgical procedures, performed by two experienced laparoscopic surgeons, showed no technical difficulties. In particular, vision was not impaired. As soon as a 100% saturation of the humidity of the intraperitoneal space was reached, the micropump was not able to aerosolize anymore. For this reason, we had to create a continuous artificial gas leak through a trocar tap and an usual gas line. This allowed the device to continue functioning throughout the procedure.

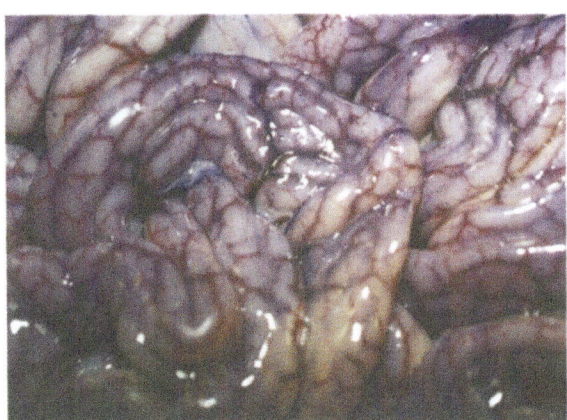

Fig. 17.3. Distribution of 3 ml of 50% methylene blue solution after 30 min pneumoperitoneum, showing a diffuse staining of the bowel loops

Clinical Applications

Prevention of Local Recurrence

The main causes of local recurrence are inadequate excision of the primary tumor, or the draining lymph nodes, and intraoperative tumor cell implantation (Abulafi and Williams 1994). Because they break the natural barrier formed by mesothelium and hyaluronic acid, peritoneal wounds (van den Tol et al. 1998) such as trocar sites (Jones et al. 1995a) or anastomoses are major sites of recurrence. The presence of growth factors and other cytokines in surgical wounds following cancer resections might stimulate growth of minimal residual disease. Avoidance of unnecessary surgical trauma by using gentle techniques, control of spilled cells by intraoperative locoregional cytostatic drug delivery, and treatment of peritoneal wounds by the aerosolization of coating agents could therefore reduce the local recurrence rate.

Prevention of Port-Site Recurrences

Jacobi et al. have shown that intraperitoneal lavage with taurolidine in cancer laparoscopy was able to markedly reduce the incidence of port-site recurrences in the rat model (Jacobi et al. 1997b). At this step, the micropump has been shown to aerosolize a 2% taurolidine solution, and since the therapeutic substance reaches the anterior and lateral abdominal walls in the present animal model, it can be hypothesized that a preventive effect will be achieved. Therapeutic pneumoperitoneum might also be introduced in thoracoscopy. Since port-site recurrences have also been described during such proce-

dures (Downey et al. 1996), aerosolization of taurolidine (Jacobi et al. 1997b) or other hyaluronates might also be indicated.

Intraperitoneal and Intrapleural Chemotherapy

The response of established carcinoma or sarcoma implants to intraperitoneal and intrapleural chemotherapy is multifactorial. Three of these factors that influence pharmacokinetics of intraperitoneal drugs are contact area, pressure (Jacquet et al. 1996) and heath (Sugarbaker 1998). Contact area is limited in conventional intraperitoneal chemotherapy (Fig. 17.4). Application of an intraperitoneal hyperpressure – such as pneumoperitoneum in laparoscopy – and heated CO_2 might be a promising approach to increase the drug diffusion into the tumor and to enhance the efficiency of intraperitoneal chemotherapy. These points deserve further research since, in the case of colorectal adenocarcinoma, there are insufficient data on which to make a clearcut conclusion of the real benefits (Penna and Nordlinger 1996).

In summary, we introduce the novel concept of "therapeutic pneumoperitoneum" in laparoscopic and thoracoscopic surgery to prevent some side effects of CO_2-pneumoperitoneum without increasing the difficulty of the surgical procedures nor the risks

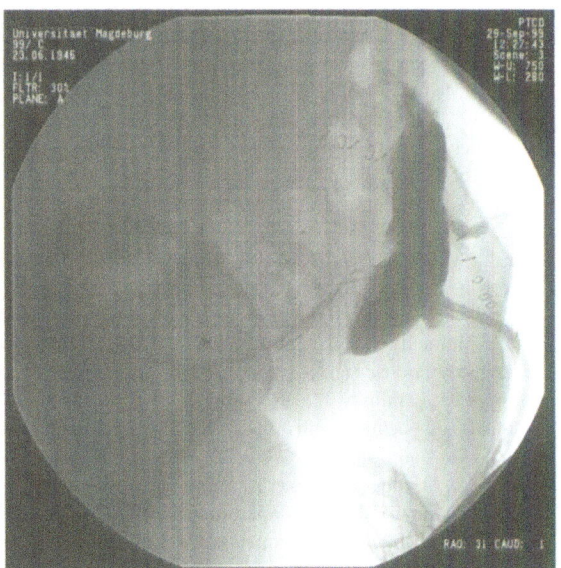

Fig. 17.4. Postoperative distribution of a contrast-enhanced intraperitoneal lavage at postoperative day 2 after debulking for ovarian carcinoma: the contact area between the solution and the peritoneum is limited to one flank and to a small subhepatic space

for the patient. Our results show that it is possible to create such a therapeutic pneumoperitoneum – associating of a carrier gas with an aerosolized therapeutic substance – using the present drug delivery device. It was simultaneously possible to perform resections of the sigmoid colon with no special surgical difficulty. So far, the data were only in a preclinical model, and positive and negative target effects of drugs have not been assessed at this stage of development. Thus, major work is still necessary before the micropump can be applied routinely to the human patient.

Therapeutic pneumoperitoneum has numerous theoretical advantages over peritoneal irrigation or even direct spraying: in particular, it might allow better tissue penetration and distribution of the drug to all exposed serosal surfaces. Expected and unexpected effects of various drugs have yet to be assessed in appropriate animal and clinical studies, taking into account the specific pharmacokinetic problems associated with peritoneal drug administration. These might be exciting fields of research for engineers, pharmaceutical companies, oncologists and laparoscopic surgeons.

References

Abulafi AM, Williams NS (1994) Local recurrence of colorectal cancer: the problem, mechanisms, management and adjuvant therapy. Br J Surg 81:7–19

Alberts DS, Liu PY, Hannigan EV, O'Toole R, Williams SD, Young JA (1996) Intraperitoneal cisplatin plus intravenous cyclophosphamide versus intravenous cisplatin plus intravenous cyclophosphamide for stage III ovarian cancer. N Engl J Med 335:1950–1955

Bloechle C, Emmermann A, State T, Scheurlen UJ, Schneider C, Achilles E, Wolf M, Mack D, Zornig C, Broelsch CE (1998) Laparoscopic vs open repair of gastric perforation and abdominal lavage of associated peritonitis in pigs. Surg Endosc 12:212–218

Bloechle C, Kluth D, Holstein AF, Emmermann A, Strate T, Zornig C, Izbicki JR (1999) A pneumoperitoneum perpetuates severe damage to the ultrastructural integrity of parietal peritoneum in gastric perforation-induced peritonitis in rats. Surg Endosc 13:683–8

Bongard FS, Pianim N, Liu SY, Lippmann M, Davis I, Klein S (1991) Using helium for insufflation during laparoscopy (letter). JAMA 266:3131

Bouvy ND, Marquet RL, Jeekel H, Bonjer HJ (1996) Impact of gas(less) laparoscopy and laparotomy on peritoneal tumor growth and abdominal wall metastases. Surg Endosc 10:1618 (abstract)

Dedrick RL, Flessner MF (1997) Pharmacokinetic problems in peritoneal drug administration: tissue penetration and surface exposure. J Natl Cancer Inst 89:480–487

Downey RJ, McCormack P, LoCicero III J, the Video-Assisted Thoracic Surgery Study Group (1996) Dissemination of ma-

lignancies following video-assisted thoracic surgery. J Cardiovasc Thor Surg 111:954–960

Flessner MF, Dedrick RL (1994) Role of the liver in small-solute transport during peritoneal dialysis. J Am Soc Nephrol 5:116–120

Franklin ME, Rosenthal D, Abrego-Medina D, Dorman JP, Glass JL, Norem R, Diaz A (1996) Prospective comparison of open vs. laparoscopic colon surgery for carcinoma. Dis Colon Rectum 39:S35–S46

Fry WA, Siddiqui A, Pensler JM, Mostafavi H (1995) Thoracoscopic implantation of cancer with a fatal outcome (see comments). Ann Thorac Surg 59:42–45

Gutt CN, Schmandra TC (1999) Portal flow during CO_2 pneumoperitoneum in the rat. Surg Endosc 13:902.

Jacobi CA, Ordemann J, Bohm M, Zieren HU, Sabat R, Muller JM (1997a) Inhibition of peritoneal tumor cell growth and implantation in laparoscopic surgery in a rat model. Am J Surg 174:359–363

Jacobi CA, Sabat R, Ordemann J, Wenger F, Volk HD, Müller JM (1997b) [Peritoneal instillation of taurolidin and heparin for preventing intraperitoneal tumor growth and trocar metastases in laparoscopic operations in the rat model]. Langenbecks Arch Chir 382:S31–S36

Jacobi CA, Sabat R, Ordemann J, Müller JM (1998) The impact of laparoscopy with carbon dioxide versus helium on immunologic function and tumor growth in a rat model. Dig Surg 15: 110–6

Jacobi CA, Junghans T, Peter F, Ordemann J, Müller JM. Gas embolism during laparoscopy with CO_2 or helium. SAGES Annual Meeting, San Antonio, 24–27.3.1999

Jacquet P, Stuart OA, Chang D, Sugarbaker PH (1996) Effects of intraabdominal pressure on pharmacokinetics and tissue distribution of doxorubicin after intraperitoneal administration. Anticancer Drugs 7:596–603

Johnstone PAS, Rohde DC, Swartz SE, Fetter JE, Wexner SD (1996) Port-site recurrences after laparoscopic and thoracoscopic procedures in malignancy. J Clin Oncol 14:1950–1956

Jones DB, Guo LW, Reinhard MK, Soper NJ, Philpott GW, Connet J, Fleshman JW (1995a) Impact of pneumoperitoneum on trocar site implantation of colon cancer in hamster model. Dis Colon Rectum 38:1182–1188

Jones LM, Gardner MJ, Catterall JB, Turner GA (1995b) Hyaluronic acid secreted by mesothelial cells: a natural barrier to ovarian cancer cell adhesion. Clin Exp Metastasis 13:373–380

Neuhaus S, 3rd International Conference in Basic Science in Laparoscopy, Columbia University, New York, 29–30.3.1999

Neuhaus SJ, Ellis T, Rofe AM, Pike GK, Jamieson GG, Watson DI (1998a) Tumor implantation following laparoscopy using different insufflation gases. Surg Endosc 12:1300–1302

Neuhaus SJ, Watson DJ, Ellis T, Rofe AM, Mathew G, Jamieson CG (1998b) Efficacy of cytotoxic agents for the prevention of laparoscopic port-site recurrences. Surg Endosc 12:515 (abstract)

Neuhaus SJ, Ellis TS, Barret MW, Rofe AM, Jamieson GG, Watson DI (1999) In vitro inhibition of tumor growth in a helium-rich environment : implications for laparoscopic surgery. Aust N Z J Surg 69:52–55

Paolucci V, Gutt CN, Schaeff B, Encke A (1995) Gasless laparoscopy in abdominal surgery. Surg Endosc 9:497–500

Penna C, Nordlinger B (1996) Locoregional therapy for adjuvant treatment of colorectal adenocarcinoma. Eur J Cancer 32A:1117–1122

Reymond MA, Hu B, Garcia A, Reck T, Köckerling F, Hess J, Morel P (1999) Feasibility of therapeutic pneumoperitoneum in a large animal model using a microvaporisator. Surg Endosc (in press)

Semm K (1980) Die Automatisierung des Pneumoperitoneums für die endoskopische Abdominalchirurgie. Arch Gynäkol 232:738

Southern DA, Mapleson WW (1993) Which insufflation gas for laparoscopy (letter). BMJ 307:1424

Sugarbaker PH (1998) Intraperitoneal chemotherapy and cytoreductive surgery for the prevention and treatment of peritoneal carcinomatosis and sarcomatosis. Semin Surg Oncol 14:254–261

Tol PM van den, van Rossen EE, van Eijck CH, Bonthuis F, Marquet RL, Jeekel H (1998) Reduction of peritoneal trauma by using nonsurgical gauze leads to less implantation metastasis of spilled tumor cells. Ann Surg 227:242–248

Watson DI, Mathew G, Ellis T, Baigrie CF, Rofe AM, Jamieson GG (1997) Gasless laparoscopy may reduce the risk of port-site recurrences following laparoscopic tumor surgery. Arch Surg 132:166–168

CHAPTER 18

Treatment of Port-Site Recurrences

F. Köckerling, C. Schug

Introduction

In addition to abdominal and thoracic surgeons, those specialized in gynecology and urology are also well aware of the possibility of implantation metastases. These occur in patients with carcinoma who have undergone laparoscopic or open procedures, including needle biopsy, diagnostic laparoscopy, laparoscopic resection for expected as well as unexpected tumors, and laparotomy.

Reported incidences differ depending on tumor type: recurrence of colorectal cancer in abdominal wounds after conventional surgery is about 0.6%/0.69%, according to the studies by Hohenberger et al. (1995) and Hughes et al. (1983). Reilly et al. (1996) found a wound recurrence of 1.5%, but only 0.2% had isolated scar recurrence with no other sites of metastatic lesions. Gunderson and Sosin (1974) reported a rate of 3.3% in abdominal surgical scars at a routine relaparotomy at 3 months after resection. Two thirds of these lesions escaped detection during physical examination. In a review article, Fortner and Lawrence (1960) reported an overall rate of 1.9% for incisional tumors following resection of gastric cancer, with most of the cases (1.5%) undergoing "curative" gastrectomy. Surgical wound recurrences have also been described after biopsy and resection of hepatocellular carcinoma (Koffi et al. 1996), as well as pancreatic cancer (Jorgensen et al. 1995).

Initially, port-site recurrences have been reported with a rate of more than 20% after laparoscopic surgery for cancer (Wexner and Cohen 1995). In the meantime, on the basis of current studies (Lacy et al. 1998), the rate of port-site recurrences after laparoscopic resection is about 2%, with a lower incidence being found in laparoscopically resected colonic carcinoma (about 0.7%) (Nduka et al. 1994). A higher incidence was reported after gallbladder and bile duct surgery, namely 6.7% (Schaeff et al. 1998). In unexpected gallbladder carcinoma Z'graggen et al. (1998) noted a recurrence rate of 14%.

The rate of tumor seeding into the thoracic wall after biopsies for pleural mesothelioma is approximately 19% (Boutin et al. 1995) as compared with minimal (about 0.1%) implantation of tumor cells of other histological types (Downey et al. 1996). Incisional recurrences following mediastinoscopy occur with a similar, low frequency (Hoyer et al. 1992).

Following laparoscopic procedures for gynecologic tumors, about 1% (Childers et al. 1994) of the patients develop port-site recurrences. The rate of all soft-tissue metastases including port-site recurrences in renal and bladder carcinoma is reported to be 0.1–0.2%. Autopsy figures of 6%, 9% and 1% for soft-tissue recurrences have been reported in carcinoma of the bladder, kidneys and prostate, respectively (Hohenberger et al. 1995). Thus, on the basis of current data, the incidence of port-site recurrences in laparoscopic surgery appears to be similar to that associated with open surgery (Franklin et al. 1996; Stage et al. 1997).

Although optimal therapy aims to prevent port-site recurrences, we are unable to avoid them in every case. This means that a small number of abdominal and thoracic wall metastases must always be expected after both open and laparoscopic surgery. Treatment of these recurrences is the subject of the present chapter.

Clinical Presentation

The period of time elapsing between surgical procedure and occurrence of port-site recurrences ranges from 1 week to several years, with a mean of between 3 and 9 months (Nduka et al. 1994; Wexner and Cohen 1995). It is postulated that the development of port-site recurrences correlates with the aggressiveness and the stage of the tumor. While we hope that such lesions remain a solitary occurrence, they are unfortunately often signs of general progression of tumor disease. For this reason, close surveillance of the patient's general clinical status, including incision sites, is necessary.

Suspicious changes in subcutaneous tissue might be early recurrences. These metastases typically present as hard, painful or indolent nodules at one or several sites. In some cases they are easily confused with inflammatory infiltration. Tumor growth may be rapid, and more than one port-site may be affected. Among the ports, those used for extraction are more often involved, but this relative difference is not striking.

Diagnosis

Our awareness of possible wound or port-site recurrence underscores the need for further diagnostic procedures, including ultrasound, X-rays, CT/NMR-scans, and biopsy of the tumor if its biological significance is unknown. Before surgery, data on tumor extension and infiltration, as well as possible local recurrence of primary cancer, additional metastases, pleural/peritoneal carcinomatosis or systemic involvement should be obtained. Only a small subgroup of patients have isolated, solitary met astases.

In most cases, recurrent lesions are a sign of general tumor involvement, and manifestation of port-site recurrence worsens the chance of survival. Data collected by Hughes et al. (1983) in patients undergoing open surgery for large bowel cancer showed that more than half of the patients died within 6 months, and all had died within 4 years.

Treatment – Review of the Literature

Since recurrences are rare for all types of carcinoma, we still have no standardized recommended treatment for these lesions. It is well known that different carcinomas differ in their susceptibility to surgery alone versus a combination of resection with radiotherapy and/or chemotherapy. Also, a distinction must be made between an isolated recurrence located in the abdominal or thoracic wall, and recurrence as a symptom of peritoneal/pleural carcinomatosis or systemic tumor progression.

By definition, a curative treatment removes the tumor completely (R0), with no microscopic (R1) nor macroscopic (R2) residual disease. In the light of these data we have to ask ourselves whether there is a real chance of achieving curative treatment or whether all our efforts are merely palliative? A brief review of the literature with regard to treatment may

help us to make decisions on how to manage port-site recurrences.

Abdominal Malignancies

Most cases of port-site recurrences are reported in gastrointestinal surgery (Hohenberger et al. 1995): soft-tissue metastases occur in about 1% of all patients treated for a solid malignant tumor. In almost all cases, this implies generalized disease. Pearlstone et al. (1999) showed that three (0.61%) out of four (0.8%) patients with port-site recurrences, from a total number of 533 patients undergoing laparoscopy for abdominal malignancy, had carcinomatosis or positive peritoneal washing at the time of laparoscopy. Organ-specific data are available for the following cancers:

Gastric Cancer

Gastric cancer (0.3%): one third of the metastases were isolated lesions that were treated by local excision, but the majority were associated with other metastases at various sites and treatment comprised chemotherapy, irradiation and analgesia; the median survival of all the patients reported was 3 months. Fortner and Lawrence (1960) reported only minimal regression of gastric tumor metastases following local radiotherapy over a 21-day period in patients undergoing open resection for gastric cancer.

Colorectal Cancer

In general, metastases are treated by local excision, sometimes in combination with radio-/chemotherapy. For local excision of a wound recurrence after curative (R0) resection for colorectal cancer, the 5-year survival rate is about 31%, which is comparable with that seen after curative resection of lung and liver metastases, as well as after resection of local recurrent lesions.

In colorectal carcinoma, one third of soft-tissue metastases have reportedly been resected curatively – in two cases in combination with radiotherapy. Reilly et al. (1996) published data on wound recurrences in patients undergoing conventional surgical treatment for colorectal carcinoma: mean time of presentation was about 1.5 years after adjuvant chemotherapy. The rate of recurrence involving surgical wounds was 0.64%. Most of the patients had peritoneal carcinomatosis or metastases at other sites, and some underwent local excision, with or without radiotherapy. Similar results were already reported by Hughes et al. in 1983: despite local excision or deep radiotherapy after conventional resection for colonic cancer, all of the patients with recurrences had died of disseminated cancer within 4 years. Ledesma et al. (1982) reported on 22 patients with incision-site recurrences after conventional resection for colorectal cancer (Dukes B/C), 9 of whom had been treated with radio-/chemotherapy prior to admission. After a diagnostic work-up for further signs of disease, the recurrences were treated by local excision that included adherent structures. Mesh was used to close the fascial defect, and a few cases required secondary skin grafting, while other defects were treated with delayed primary closure. The 5-year survival rate was 45%. All the patients who died had generalized carcinomatosis.

In the case of laparoscopy, similar data are to be found in the review by Schaeff et al. (1998), showing that excision of port-site recurrences developing after laparoscopic resection of colorectal cancer is followed by peritoneal carcinomatosis, secondary metastases or further metastases in more than half of the patients. Fusco and Paluzzi (1993) reported on the recurrence of well-differentiated adenocarcinoma following laparoscopic right hemicolectomy (T3N1M0), treated by wide excision and reconstruction with synthetic mesh, but no data were provided on the long-term results. Encouraging results were reported with two patients undergoing laparoscopic resection for a colon carcinoma who developed port-site recurrences. They both had peritoneal carcinomatosis with no lymph node or liver metastases. After resection they received chemotherapy with heated intraperitoneal mitomycin C and early postoperative intraperitoneal 5-fluorouracil for 5 days. Eighteen months after therapy they were clinically free of disease (Jacquet et al. 1995). In addition, there is a comparable case report on chemotherapy with 5-fluorouracil and folate prior to excision of abdominal wall metastases from an adenocarcinoma treated by laparoscopic colectomy, including reconstruction with polypropylene mesh. Histology revealed almost complete necrosis of the tumor. Six months later the patient was still alive and recurrence-free (Montorsi 1995).

Carcinoma of the Gallbladder

Port-site recurrences in carcinoma of the gallbladder are more frequent than in other malignant abdominal tumors, especially when the malignant nature of disease was unknown at the time of cholecys-

tectomy. Jacobi et al. (1995) described the local resection of unexpected recurrences after laparoscopic cholecystectomy. In two other patients, wide excision of the abdominal wall for such a recurrent lesion after laparoscopic resection of an undetected gallbladder carcinoma, with no signs of further metastases, appeared to be curative after 11 months of follow-up (Sandor et al. 1995). In a large multicenter study, Z'graggen et al. (1998) reported that resection was possible in about two thirds of port-site recurrences from unexpected gallbladder carcinoma. After extirpation more than 85% again developed one or more incision-site recurrences or other metastases and subsequent peritoneal carcinomatosis. In this study, all patients with port-site recurrences after laparoscopic resection of an unexpected gallbladder carcinoma presented with early distant metastases after local excision.

Pleural Mesothelioma, Lung Cancer and Metastases Found After Thoracoscopy and Mediastinoscopy

Quite different types of malignant cells may be responsible for incision-site metastases following thoracic surgery and they are associated with different treatments and outcome. Fry et al. (1995) described a chest wall recurrence after video-assisted biopsy of a well-differentiated adenocarcinoma of the lung, subsequently treated with lobectomy. This recurrent lesion was managed by a full-thickness resection and a 4 cm margin, followed by reconstruction with a Goretex patch, a latissimus dorsi muscle flap and a skin graft. The patient developed a second recurrence that failed to respond to chemotherapy and radiation therapy. In a few case reports, Wille et al. (1997) showed that chest-wall recurrences developing after video-assisted thoracoscopic resection of pulmonary metastases may be resected curatively without radiotherapy, but may also recur despite adjuvant radiotherapy. Sullivan and Passamonte (1982) and Hoyer et al. (1992) reported on several incision-site recurrences developing after diagnostic mediastinoscopy that were successfully treated with local radiotherapy. The tumor mass decreased in all cases, but recurred in one case a few months later.

In diagnostic procedures for malignant mesothelioma, there is no comparable alternative to percutaneous approaches, including thoracoscopy. In the literature, the mean incidence of malignant seeding in this particular tumor is reported to be about 19%. A randomized prospective study confirmed the efficacy of local radiotherapy after thoracoscopy (3–7 Gy, over 10–15 days) in minimizing the risk of recurrence (Boutin et al. 1995). None of the patients who received radiotherapy developed subcutaneous metastases, as compared with 40% of those not so treated. Low et al. (1995) presented similar data showing no recurrences after immediate irradiation. These results were supported by those reported by Emri et al. (1996), who described the successful prevention of metastases by a combination of local or systemic chemotherapy and local radiotherapy after thoracoscopy for pleural mesothelioma.

Gynecological Malignancies

A negative outcome for gynecological tumors was reported by Kadar (1997): in metastatic cervical or endometrial carcinoma, extended-field or pelvic radiation, as well as chemotherapy (taxol, cis-platinum), after laparoscopy failed to prevent port-site recurrences. Solitary recurrences were excised and electron beam radiation was applied, while metastatic disease was treated conservatively; all patients died within 4 months. Positive results were found by Kohler et al. (1991) in two patients developing port-site recurrences after intraperitoneal radioactive chromic phosphate therapy for resected ovarian carcinoma. After undergoing resection of wound recurrences, the patients were treated with combination chemotherapy comprising cisplatin, doxorubicin and cyclophosphamide, and remained free of recurrence for at least 5 years.

On the basis of the above mentioned results reported in the literature, a few conclusions may be drawn with regard to the therapy of port-site recurrences. Most of the time, curative treatment by local excision of incision- or port-site recurrences is not possible. This is due to dissemination of malignant cells before surgical therapy is applied. Nevertheless, abdominal and chest-wall metastases may be resected in curative as well as palliative intent.

Surgical Treatment

Most recurrences can be managed surgically with good results. To confirm the indication for an extended resection, a frozen section evaluation may be requested. For surgery in curative intent, en-bloc resection with a margin of about 4–5 cm, if possible including adjacent organs, is performed (Fig. 18.1). If small bowel, colon, lung or further organs are in-

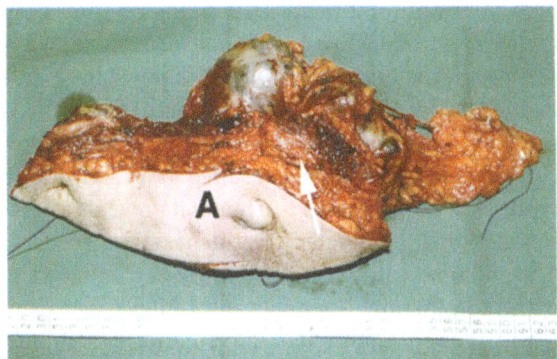

Fig. 18.1. Port-site recurrences should be treated with a wide en-bloc excision of the tumor together with the complete abdominal wall. Note that the recurrence occurred at the extraction port. *A*, umbilicus. (Courtesy of Prof. H. Lippert, Department of Surgery, University Hospital Magdeburg, Germany)

volved, they have to be removed en-bloc with no attempt made to separate adherent organs.

Management of the surgical defect is a secondary problem. Primary closure is desirable, but not always possible. A large fascial defect that does not permit primary closure, or extreme suture line tension after extended resection requires the use of graft materials. Today, synthetic materials are preferentially used to close large fascial defects: they are immediately available, totally inert with no antigenic properties, and are of high tensile strength. Subcutaneous tissue defects may be closed immediately with the aid of musculo-cutaneous flaps. A mesh graft is necessary to replace missing cutaneous layers.

Adjuvant Therapy

In patients with solitary port-site recurrences, surgical therapy as a possible curative procedure remains the treatment of choice. In patients with progressive carcinoma in whom excision will probably be only palliative, systemic chemotherapy oriented to the biological type of the tumor, might be a useful adjuvant capable of halting further progress of the disease, as illustrated below.

Adjuvant Therapy in Gastrointestinal Tumors

The results reported in the literature suggest that neither radio- nor chemotherapy can be generally recommended as adjuvant therapy of port-site recurrences in gastrointestinal cancer surgery, since both fail to prevent them. Depending on their biological type, many tumors are not susceptible to radiation or chemotherapy, while the port-site is not involved in initial local irradiation of the tumor bed. As already mentioned, radiation of incision-site recurrences prior to surgery resulted in no significant regression of the tumor. Current data reveals no rationale for differentiated treatment of recurrences. The outcome with surgery alone or in combination with radiotherapy is similar and rather discouraging. Although reports by Sullivan and Passamonte (1982) and Hoyer et al. (1992) suggest some effect of adjuvant radiotherapy in recurrent lesions arising from tumor cell implantation during mediastinoscopy, which achieved a certain degree of regression, long-term results with radiotherapy alone are not impressive.

On the other hand, a case report by Montorsi et al. (1995) showed that systemic chemotherapy with 5-fluorouracil and folate, prior to excision of the recurrence together with adherent bowel, was effective (based on histology showing tumor necrosis, and disease-free survival). This might well be relevant therapy for large, possibly unresectable, tumors susceptible to chemotherapy and/or radiotherapy. A few years ago, Sugarbaker et al. (1989) came out in favor of early postoperative intraperitoneal chemotherapy after surgical treatment of gastrointestinal cancer. In view of the fact that laparoscopy for primary tumor or recurrences is often associated with positive peritoneal cytology, there is a rational basis for local intraperitoneal chemotherapy after resection of port-site recurrence. Even in peritoneal carcinomatosis, treatment with heated intraperitoneal mitomycin C followed by intraperitoneal 5-fluorouracil led to disease-free survival of at least 1.5 years. In the light of these results, further therapeutic trials are necessary to investigate the value of adjuvant chemotherapy.

Adjuvant Therapy in Gynecological Tumors

Adjuvant systemic chemotherapy in combination with local resection of port-site recurrences proved effective curative treatment in women undergoing resection for ovarian carcinoma followed by intraperitoneal treatment with radioactive chromic phosphate (Kadar 1997).

These results certainly cannot form a basis for general recommendations for the treatment of gynecological tumors, since some authors failed to find any benefit of adjuvant therapy, especially irra-

diation. In most of the cases, peritoneal tumor spread is already present and is not curable. Again, local resection should be adequate treatment for localized recurrence. Only a small number of patients might benefit from adjuvant therapy in the event of highly susceptible malignant cells.

Adjuvant Treatment of Thoracic Tumors

The potential role of adjuvant therapy is underscored by the good results achieved with local radiotherapy after thoracoscopy for a special kind of tumor, namely pleural mesothelioma, which is extremely susceptible to preventive local radiotherapy, as reported by Boutin et al. (1995) and Emri et al. (1996).

Laparotomy and laparoscopy, as well as thoracotomy, thoracoscopy and mediastinoscopy, are associated with comparable rates of port-site recurrences from various types of primary malignant tumor. In general, the results of treatment, whether surgery alone or combined treatment, are discouraging. This is due in particular to generalized malignant tumor spread, which is found in more than two thirds of patients with port-site recurrences – presumably already prior to the primary surgical intervention, or as a result of incurable secondary spread from the incision-site lesion. Owing to the rarity of the port-site/incision-site recurrences, which, it is to be hoped, may be reduced even further by measures aimed at preventing tumor cell implantation, we still have no generally recommended treatment for this entity. Further experience still needs to be gained.

References

Boutin C, Rey F, Viallat JR (1995) Prevention of malignant seeding after invasive diagnostic procedures in patients with pleural mesothelioma. Chest 108:754–758
Childers JM, Aqua KA, Surwit AE, Hallum AV, Hatch KD (1994) Abdominal-wall tumor implantation after laparoscopy for malignant conditions. Obstet Gynecol 84:765–769
Downey RJ, McCormack P, LoCicero III J (1996) Dissemination of malignant tumors after video-assisted thoracic surgery: a report of twenty-one cases. J Thorac Cardiovasc Surg 111:954–960
Emri S, Karakoca Y, Baris YI, Zorlu F, Akyol F, Akay H (1996) Preventive irradiation after invasive diagnostic and therapeutic procedures in malignant pleural mesothelioma. Chest 109:1665–1666
Fortner JG, Lawrence W (1960) Implantation of gastric cancer in abdominal wounds. Ann Surg 152:789–794
Franklin ME, Rosenthal D, Abrego-Medina D, Dorman JP,

Glass JL, Norem R, Diaz A (1996) Prospective comparison of open vs. laparoscopic surgery for carcinoma. Dis Colon Rectum 39:S35–S46

Fry WA, Siddiqui A, Pensler JM, Mostafavi H (1995) Thoracoscopic implantation of cancer with a fatal outcome. Ann Thorac Surg 59:42–45

Fusco MA, Paluzzi MW (1993) Abdominal wall recurrence after laparoscopic-assisted colectomy for adenocarcinoma of the colon. Dis Colon Rectum 36:858–861

Gunderson LL, Sosin H (1974) Areas of failure found at reoperation (second symtomatic look) following "curative surgery" for adenocarcinoma of the rectum. Cancer 34:1278–1292

Hohenberger W, Altendorf-Hofmann A, Schmidt O (1995) Surgical therapy for metastases of the soft tissue. Langenbecks Arch Chir [Suppl II]:288–294

Hoyer ER, Leonard CE, Hazuka MB, Wechsler-Jentzsch K (1992) Mediastinoscopy incisional metastasis. Cancer 70:1612–1615

Hughes ESR, McDermott FT, Polglase AL, Johnson WR (1983) Tumor recurrence in the abdominal wall scar tissue after large-bowel cancer surgery. Dis Colon Rectum 26:571–572

Jacobi CA, Keller H, Monig S, Said S (1995) Implantation metastasis of unexpected gallbladder carcinoma after laparoscopy. Surg Endosc 9:351–352

Jacquet P, Averbach AM, Stephens AD, Sugarbaker PH (1995) Cancer recurrence following laparoscopic colectomy. Dis Colon Rectum 38:1110–1114

Jorgensen JO, McCall JL, Morris DL (1995) Port-site seeding after laparoscopic ultrasonographic staging of pancreatic carcinoma. Surgery 117:118–119

Kadar N (1997) Port-site recurrences following laparoscopic operations for gynaecological malignancies. Br J Obst Gyn 104:1308–1313

Koffi E, Moutardier V, Sauvanat A, Noun R, Flejou JF, Belghiti J (1996) Wound recurrence after resection of hepatocellular carcinoma. Liver Transpl Surg 2:301–303

Kohler MF, Soper JT, Tucker JA, Clarke-Pearson DL (1991) Isolated incisional metastases after intraperitoneal radioactive chromic phosphate therapy for ovarian carcinoma. Cancer 68:1380–1383

Lacy AM, Delgado S, Garcia-Valdecasas JC, Castells A, Piqué JM, Grande L, Fuster J, Targarona EM, Pera M, Visa J (1998) Port-site recurrences and recurrence after laparoscopic colectomy. Surg Endosc 12:1039–1042

Ledesma EJ, Tseng M, Mittelman A (1982) Surgical treatment of isolated abdominal wall metastasis in colorectal cancer. Cancer 50:1884–1887

Low EM, Khoury GG, Matthews AW, Neville E (1995) Prevention of tumor seeding following thoracoscopy in mesothelioma by prophylactic radiotherapy. Clin Oncol (R Coll Radiol) 7:317–318

Montorsi M, Fumagalli U, Rosati R, Bona S, Chella B, Huscher C (1995) Early parietal recurrence of adenocarcinoma of the colon after laparoscopic colectomy. Br J Surg 82:1036–1037

Nduka CC, Monson JRT, Menzies-Gow N, Darzi A (1994) Abdominal wall metastases following laparoscopy. Br J Surg 81:648–652

Pearlstone DB, Mansfield PF, Curley SA, Kumparatana M, Cook P, Feig BW (1999) Laparoscopy in 533 patients with abdominal malignancy. Surgery 125:67–72

Reilly WT, Nelson H, Schroeder G, Wieand HS, Bolton J, O'Connell MJ (1996) Wound recurrence following conventional treatment of colorectal cancer. Dis Colon Rectum 39:200–207

Sandor J, Ihasz M, Fazekas T, Regoly-Mérei J, Batorfi J (1995) Unexpected gallbladder cancer and laparoscopic surgery. Surg Endosc 9:1207–1210

Schaeff B, Paolucci V, Thomopoulos J (1998) Port-site recurrences after laparoscopic surgery. Dig Surg 15:124–134

Stage JG, Schulze S, Moller P, Overgaard H, Andersen M, Rebsdorf-Pedersen VB, Nielsen HJ (1997) Prospective randomized study of laparoscopic versus open colonic resection for adenocarcinoma. Br J Surg 84:391–396

Sugarbaker PH, Cunliffe WJ, Belliveau J, Bruijn EA de, Graves T, Mullins RE, Schlag P (1989) Rationale for integrating early postoperative intraperitoneal chemotherapy into the surgical treatment of gastrointestinal cancer. Semin Oncol 16:83–97

Sullivan WD, Passamonte PM (1982) Mediastinoscopy incision site metastasis: response to radiation therapy. South Med J 75:1428

Wexner SD, Cohen SM (1995) Port-site recurrences after laparoscopic colorectal surgery for cure of malignancy. Br J Surg 82:295–298

Wille GA, Gregory R, Guernsey JM (1997) Tumor implantation at port-site of video-assisted thoracoscopic resection of pulmonary metastasis. West J Med 166:65–66

Z'graggen K, Birrer S, Maurer CA, Wehrli H, Klaiber C, Baer HU (1998) Incidence of port-site recurrence after laparoscopic cholecystectomy for preoperatively unsuspected gallbladder carcinoma. Surgery 124:831–838

CHAPTER 19

Illustrated Practical Notes for the Surgeon

C. Schneider, C. Schug, F. Köckerling

Introduction

The significance of port-site recurrences has already been discussed in detail in earlier chapters of this book. Every port-site recurrence represents a problematical situation for the patient, since recurrence tumor, at whatever localization, has a considerable influence on the prognosis. The first reports in the early days of laparoscopic colorectal surgery performed in curative intent noted port-site recurrence rates of between 4% and 20% (Berends et al. 1994; Wexner and Cohen 1995), figures that differed considerably from those reported for open surgery, namely less than 1% (Hoffman et al. 1996; Hohenberger et al. 1995).

As a general rule, port-site recurrences occur very early on, usually after 3–6 months (Johnstone et al. 1996; Reymond et al. 1998; Wexner and Cohen 1995), and it must be concluded from this that there is a direct, massive seeding of cells into the incision wounds. This means that tumor cells must have been present within the abdominal cavity which, in one way or another, were able to gain access to the incision wounds. In a certain percentage of the cases, in particular in locally advanced tumors, it has been shown that tumor cells are present in the peritoneal cavity prior to the start of surgery (Horattas et al. 1997; Solomon et al. 1997). In many cases, however, traumatization of the tumor, resulting in the liberation of tumor cells, must be presum ed.

Against this background, all the individual steps in the surgical procedure need to be investigated for their potential for the implantation of tumor cells present in the abdominal cavity, and, on the basis of the contamination pathways identified, consequences should be drawn for possible prophylactic measures.

Tumor Cell Seeding and Ways of Preventing It

Patient Selection

Tumors of the colon, in particular, are often of large diameter. Furthermore, about 10% of all colorectal carcinomas show infiltration into adjacent structures (Hermanek 1992; Lopez and Montafo 1993). This means that these tumors are difficult to manipulate laparoscopically in the abdominal cavity. As a result, such situations are associated with a considerably increased danger of iatrogenic traumatization to the tumor. Furthermore, in tumors that have already invaded other organs, multivisceral resection – where applicable, with dissection also of the lymphatics associated with the organs – is indicated. Not only does this make greater demands on the laparoscopic surgeon, it is also associated with a considerable risk of tearing the tumor during surgery (Köckerling et al. 1997).

On the basis of these factors, all patients in whom, preoperatively, an inordinately large tumor or involvement of adjacent structures is known to be present should not be operated on using the laparoscopic modality. All patients operated on laparoscopically for a colorectal cancer should be staged preoperatively with a computerized tomography, and additionally for rectal tumors by endosonography. Equally, planned laparoscopic interventions, during which an overdimensioned tumor or an infiltrating carcinoma is discovered, should be converted to open surgery.

Trocar Placement

Errors during the placement, introduction and movement of trocars are a major factor in possible tumor implantation. Placement of a trocar, for example, in a position that is unfavorable for the task intended, or which is located too far from the oper-

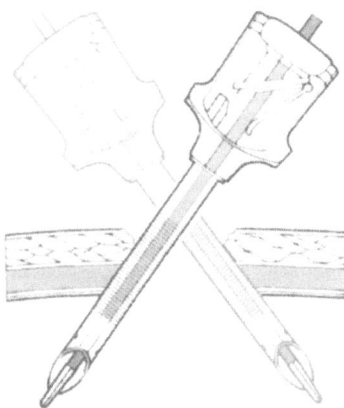

Fig. 19.1. The effect of levering forces in the case of a poorly placed trocar, with resultant enlargement of the incision, extensive peritoneal tearing and risk of gas and liquids leakage

ating site, will make it difficult for the surgeon to manipulate the tumor-bearing tissue and, in this way alone, can promote direct traumatization of the tumor. A trocar inserted in the wrong direction (blunt angle to the area of dissection) results in massive leverage at the port-site and thus leads to enlargement of the port wound with extensive tearing of the peritoneum. In this way, as well as with a primarily overdimensioned incision, leakage of gas can occur at the wound (Fig. 19.1). The resulting "chimney effect" (Hewett et al. 1996; Reymond et al. 1998) leads to a movement of cell material out of the peritoneal cavity together with the escaping pneumoperitoneum gas, and increases the risk of inoculation of the port wound. This fluid and gas escape can be prevented by using blunt balloon trocars.

There is thus clearly a need, when planning the position of the trocar incisions, to consider the tasks to be carried out via the respective ports. Each trocar should be placed at the most favorable site for the task for which it is intended. Also, the incision should be as small as possible to ensure optimal sealing of the trocar. Furthermore, the angle of the incision for the trocar must be selected such that levering forces at the port wound are avoided when using the instruments (avoidance of abdominal wall trauma).

Instruments

The laparoscopic instruments themselves have been found to be often highly contaminated with intra-abdominal tumor cells; that is, they have a considerable role to play in the dissemination or inoculation of such cells (Allardyce et al. 1997; Hewett et al. 1996).

For this reason, it would appear to make good sense, to eliminate the tumor cells likely to be adhering to the instruments. For this purpose, placement of the instruments that are not presently in use in a bath on the instrument table containing a cytotoxic solution (e.g., Betadine, taurolidine) is recommended.

Tumor Handling

When dissecting in close proximity to the tumor and manipulating the latter during this work, tension or pressure has to be applied to the lesion. The use of unsuitable instruments (e.g., sharp forceps such as Babcock), and the excessive tension/pressure applied with a 5 mm instrument, are associated with a very real risk of traumatizing the tumor (Köckerling et al. 1997).

For this reason, all manipulations involving the bowel wall should be effected either with blunt hooks (Endo-Langenbeck) or atraumatic (non-crushing) forceps or swabs, in order to avoid injuring the tumor and thus causing dissemination of tumor cells (Fig. 19.2). Indirect tumor handling is much better than direct manipulation.

If tumor localization is not apparent from the peritoneal side, there is a risk of inaccurate tumor manipulation. Thus, preoperative tatooing with India ink or perioperative coloscopy, combined or not with ultrasonosgraphy, is indicated. If indicated, it is advisable to clamp the proximal colon to prevent insufflation of the small bowel.

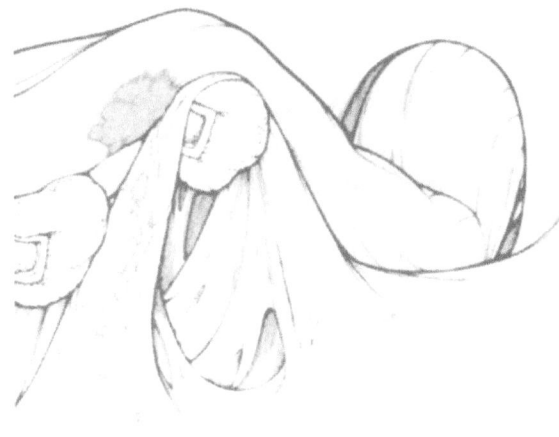

Fig. 19.2. An important principle for avoiding intraoperative seeding of tumor cells resulting from injury to the tumor is the atraumatic handling of the tumor-bearing bowel using suitable instruments

Minilaparotomy

In order, after dissection and freeing of the tumor-bearing segment, to recover the surgical specimen through the abdominal wall, a minilaparotomy is always needed – an exception being amputation of the rectum in which recovery via the perineal wound is possible. The minilaparotomy should also be kept as small as possible, so as to minimize abdominal wall trauma, but size is dictated by the size of the surgical specimen. Specimen recovery is a complex problem and will be discussed separately below. Furthermore, if prior to carrying out the minilaparotomy the pneumoperitoneum has not been vented via a trocar, the "chimney effect" (Hewett et al. 1996; Reymond et al. 1998b) will come into play when liquids, including tumor cells are projected into the minilaparotomy wound. Here too cell inoculation is highly likely. When the peritoneum is not closed, tumor cell seeding to the abdominal wall at the end of the operation is an additional possibility for the initiation of port-site recurrences, since the integrity of the peritoneum is a major immunological and cellular barrier (Murthy et al. 1989).

For all of these reasons, we propose the following procedure: prior to minilaparotomy, the peritoneum should always be desufflated. Thereafter, a minilaparotomy should be performed. After recovering the surgical specimen and preparing the anastomosis by inserting the anvil, the wound is closed layer by layer. This means, in particular, closing the peritoneum. Before closure of the abdominal wall, the surgical wound should be washed out with a cytotoxic solution (e.g., Betadine, taurolidine) (Schneider et al. 1999).

Specimen Recovery

The minilaparotomy will, of course, be relatively small. This means that the specimen can only just be withdrawn through the wound. During this procedure, shearing and also compressive forces will act on the tumor. Either is capable of resulting in tearing of the tumor and, thus, if the specimen is unprotected, tumor inoculation can occur (Köckerling et al. 1997; Schlag et al. 1994; Treat et al. 1995).

There are two possibilities for recovering the specimen: firstly, it can be divided with the cutter/stapler at both proximal and distal ends, and freed from the central supplying vessels. In this case, it can be recovered in toto in an appropriately dimensioned cell- and water-tight recovery bag (Fig. 19.3).

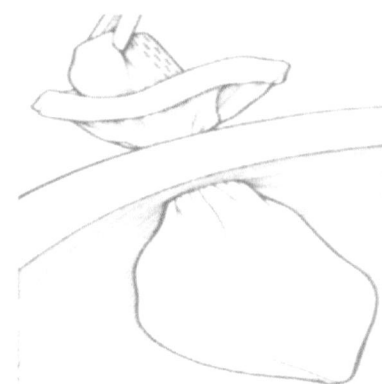

Fig. 19.3. The important measure for avoiding tumor cell implantation during retrieval of the surgical specimen from the abdominal cavity is protection of the recovery incision using cell- and watertight recovery bags or sleeves

A disadvantage of this option is that the oral arm of the bowel has to be drawn, unprotected, through the abdominal wall in order to be able to insert the anvil of the stapler. In a second option, a self-expanding protective sleeve is introduced through the minilaparotomy. The specimen divided distally with the stapler is then drawn through the protected abdominal wound and oral division and the introduction of the anvil is then effected outside the abdominal cavity.

Irrigation of the Abdominal Cavity

In the case of locally advanced tumors, a certain percentage of tumor cells can be found in the peritoneal irrigation fluid already at the time the operation is started (Horattas et al. 1997; Solomon et al. 1997). In addition, tumor cells can be liberated by inappropriate manouvers during dissection and recovery of the tumor. These cells circulating within the peritoneal cavity can thus enter the open wounds at any time or, after the conclusion of surgery, may migrate into a wound that has not been meticulously closed.

For these reasons, we recommend reducing the intra-abdominal cell load by irrigating the abdominal cavity with a cytotoxic solution (e.g, Betadine, taurolidine) (Jacobi et al. 1997; Reymond et al. 1997, Schneider et al. 1999).

Closure of the Trocar Incisions

In addition to the above mentioned measures that should be employed at the beginning and end of the procedure to protect the trocar wound (planning of trocar placement, small incisions made in the direction of working, fixation of the trocars), and which take account of the problems of placement and instrument use, additional aspects are involved when the trocars are removed. At the end of the operation, as has been shown, the trocars are contaminated with tumor cells (Allardyce et al. 1997; Hewett et al. 1996; Reymond et al. 1997, 1998a,b), and can thus inoculate the port wound on being withdrawn. Again, intra-abdominal cells can be "sucked" through the port wound when the peritoneum is vented via the ports (Schneider et al. 1999). Finally, the same concerns apply to the small peritoneal wounds as to the minilaparotomy, which represents a sizable peritoneal defect in which seeding of tumor cells is readily possible during the concluding phase of the operation (Murthy et al. 1989).

For all of the above reasons, we consider the following approach to be indicated: prior to the removal of the trocars, the intra-abdominal parts of all trocars should be washed with a cytotoxic solution in order to remove, as far as possible, all the cells adhering to them and thus prevent implantation in the incisions (Fig. 19.4). For all incisions of more than 5 mm in length, a suture should be prepared for the peritoneum (e.g., using the Berci suturing instrument). After suturing, the pneumoperitoneum should be vented via the trocars and only when the CO_2 has been completely vented should the trocars be removed. Thereafter, all the incisions should be washed with cytotoxic solution, in the same way as with the minilaparotomies, before the externalized suture is knotted (Fig. 19.5).

The Experience of the Surgeon

It is a known fact that the experience of the surgeon correlates directly with his/her results. This means that an oncological intervention, in particular when performed in curative intent, should not be carried out by a surgeon with little experience with the laparoscopic modality (Johnstone et al. 1996).

We recommend that any surgeon wishing to perform a laparoscopic intervention on the colorectum in curative intent, in addition to extensive experience with other and simpler laparoscopic interventions (cholecystectomy, hernia, appendectomy, etc.), should also have appropriate experience with laparoscopic colorectal procedures for benign diseases.

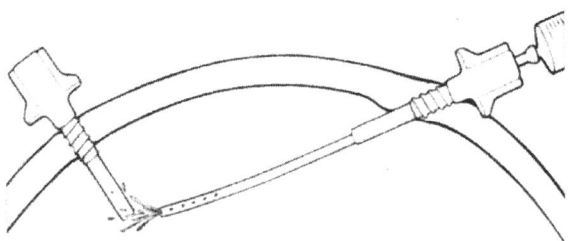

Fig. 19.4. Since cell contamination is known to be a major factor in port-site recurrences, the trocars should be washed with a cytotoxic solution prior to removal

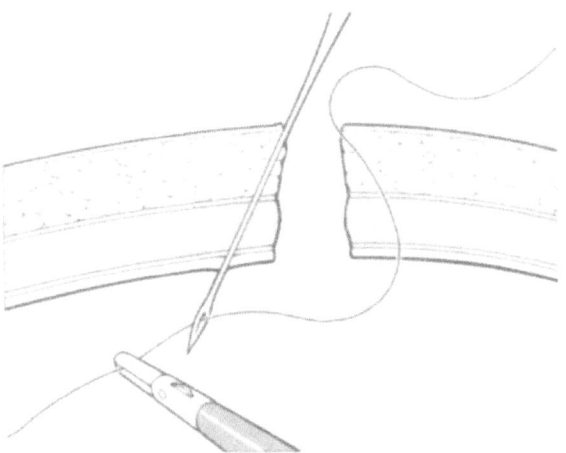

Fig. 19.5. To preserve the barrier function of the peritoneum, closure of the peritoneum should be done in all incisions longer than 5 mm

Summary

Laparoscopic procedures on the colorectum make great demands on the surgeon. They are technically complex and require extensive practical training and experience. To this may be added the responsibility for the oncological fate of the patient – in particular in the case of a potentially curative intervention – which may be radically changed by a recurrence at another site. In this connection, a recurrent lesion in the port-site wound is certainly a major problem in comparison with op en surgery, for which recurrence in the laparotomy wound is reported to occur in less than 1% of the cases. Since, however, early publications considering such complications following procedures done in curative intent reported considerably higher incidences (4–21%) (Berends et al. 1994; Wexner and Cohen 1995), the avoidance of a recurrent tumor at the trocar site should be an overriding concern for all laparoscopic surgeons.

For an appreciation of the pathogenesis of port-site metasization, it is important to understand that the problem results from a seeding of tumor cells to the port wound. The tumor cells subsequently inoculated may either have been present in the peritoneal cavity already at the start of the operation, or may have been liberated by the manipulations of the surgeon. Whatever the cause in the individual case, however, the recurrence is always a result of inadequate surgical performance, and may thus be regarded as a surgical failure.

The sources of error during surgery have been discussed above, and the possible contamination pathways to the port wounds and minilaparotomy at the various stages of the procedure, identified. For each of these stages, possible ways of avoiding tumor cell contamination were proposed. Although the effect of each individual measure has not been investigated for all of the above mentioned steps (Schneider et al. 1999), nevertheless, a large measure of efficacy in avoiding port-site metastases with a high level of significance has been attained by combining these measures. Against this background, we urgently recommend that careful consideration should be given to all the above mentioned suggestions aimed at reducing port-site recurrences when oncological laparoscopic procedures are carried out in curative intent.

References

Allardyce RA, Morreau P, Bagshaw PF (1997) Operative factors affecting tumor cell distribution following laparoscopic colectomy in a porcine model. Dis Colon Rectum 40:939–945

Berends FJ, Kazemier G, Bonjer HJ, Lange JF (1994) Subcutaneous metastases after laparoscopic colectomy. Lancet 344:58

Hermanek P (1992) Multiviscerale Resektion beim kolorektalen Karzinom – Erfahrungen der SGKRK-Studie. Langenbecks Arch Chir Suppl Kongressbd:95–100

Hewett PJ, Thomas WM, King G, Eaton M (1996) Intraperitoneal cell movement during abdominal carbon dioxide insufflation and laparoscopy. Dis Colon Rectum 39:S62–S66

Hoffman GC, Baker JW, Doxey JB, Hubbard GW, Ruffin WK, Wishner JA (1996) Minimally invasive surgery for colorectal cancer. Ann Surg 223:790–796

Hohenberger W, Altendorf-Hofmann A, Schmidt O (1995) Chirurgische Therapie von Weichteilmetastasen. Langenbecks Arch Chir Suppl Kongressbd:288

Horattas MC, Evasovich MR, Topham N (1997) Colorectal carcinoma and the relationship of peritoneal cytology. Am J Surg 174:334–337

Jacobi CA, Ordemann J, Bohm M, Zieren HU, Sabat R, Juller JM (1997) Inhibition of peritoneal tumor cell growth and implantation in laparoscopic surgery in a rat model. Am J Surg 174:359–363

Johnstone PA, Rohde DC, Swartz SE, Fetter JE, Wexner SD (1996) Port-site recurrences after laparoscopic and thoracoscopic procedures in malignancy. J Clin Oncol 14:1950–1956

Köckerling F, Reymond MA, Schneider C, Hohenberger W (1997) [Mistakes and hazards in oncological laparoscopic surgery.] Chirurg 68:215–224

Lopez MJ, Montafo WW (1993) Role of extended resection in the initial treatment of locally advanced colorectal carcinoma. Surgery 113:365–372

Murthy SM, Goldschmidt RA, Rao LN, Ammirati M, Buchmann T, Scanlon EF (1989) The influence of surgical trauma on experimental metastasis. Cancer 64:2035–2044

Reymond MA, Schneider C, Hohenberger W, Köckerling F (1998a) The pneumoperitoneum and its role in tumor seeding. Dig Surg 15:105–109

Reymond MA, Wittekind Ch, Jung A, Hohenberger W, Kirchner T, Köckerling F (1997) The incidence of port-site recurrences might be reduced. Surg Endosc 11:902–906

Reymond MA, Schneider C, Kastl S, Hohenberger W, Köckerling F (1998b) The pathogenesis of port-site recurrences. J Gastrointest Surg 2:406–414

Schlag PM, Hünerbein M, Rau B (1994) Diagnostic and operative laparoscopy in oncology. Onkologie 17:226

Schneider C, Jung A, Reymond MA, Tannapfel A, Balli J, Franklin ME, Hohenberger W, Köckerling F (1999) Efficacy of surgical measures in the prevention of port-site recurrences in a porcine model. Surg Endosc (in press)

Solomon MJ, Egan M, Robert RA, Philips J, Russell P (1997) Incidence of free colorectal cancer cells on the peritoneal surface. Dis Colon Rectum 40:1294–1298

Treat MR, Bessler M, Whelan RL (1995) Mechanisms to reduce incidence of tumor implantation during minimal access procedures for colon cancer. Semin Laparosc Surg 2:176

Watson DI, Mathew G, Ellis T, Baigrie CF, Rofe AM, Jamieson GG (1997) gasless laparoscopy may reduce the risk of port-site recurrences following laparoscopic tumor surgery. Arch Surg 132:166–168

Wexner SD, Cohen SM (1995) Port-site recurrences after laparoscopic colorectal surgery for cure of malignancy. Br J Surg 82:295–298

CHAPTER 20

Conclusions and Perspectives

M.A. Reymond, J.H. Bonjer, F. Köckerling

Introduction

The application of laparoscopic surgery to cancer has been associated with an increased number of secondary tumors implanted into the abdominal wall, termed "port-site recurrences." Since it was first described after colorectal surgery (Alexander et al. 1993), this complication has been reported for hundreds of patients in the literature. In a famous paper, based on a series of anecdotes, Wexner et al. estimated the incidence of port-site recurrences in laparoscopic cancer surgery around 4% (Wexner and Cohen 1995), whereas the incidence in open surgery had generally been accepted to lie between 0.6% and 1.6% (Hugues et al. 1983; Hohenberger et al. 1995).

At the same time, numerous observations in the small animal model showed a clear-cut adjuvant effect of carbon dioxide pneumoperitoneum on intra-abdominal tumor growth (Jones et al. 1995; Jacobi et al. 1996a,b; Bouvy et al. 1996; Dorrance et al. 1996; Hubens et al. 1996; Mathew et al. 1996). Thus, it appeared that application of laparoscopy to cancer patients was inappropriate (Wexner et al. 1995; Wexner and Reissman 1994) so that most surgeons were discouraged to apply minimally invasive methods to cancer treatment.

Quality of Surgery Is a Major Outcome Criteria in Laparoscopic and Open Surgery

However, large differences in the incidence of port-site recurrences (between 0 and 21%) and in the quality of laparoscopic colorectal cancer resections (Köckerling et al. 1998) were soon reported. These differences stressed the role of the surgeon as a prognostic factor in laparoscopic surgery. In fact, this was all but a surprise, since major differences had already been documented after conventional colorectal cancer surgery (Hermanek et al. 1995).

Soon thereafter, Wexner and colleagues suggested that port-site recurrences might be mainly due to technical factors related to the expertise of the operator (Johnstone et al. 1996). Other authors claimed the incidence of port-site recurrence might be reduced (Reymond et al. 1997) if efficient preventive strategies could be developed (Franklin et al. 1996). In the meantime, publication of large consecutive, prospective series with low incidences of port-site recurrences (Franklin et al. 1996; Vukasin et al. 1996) confirmed that the importance of local wound recurrences following laparoscopy had been overestimated. A milestone publication by Heidi Nelson and colleagues concluded that the incidence of wound recurrences in open surgery is low, but also that this incidence might have been underestimated (Reilly et al. 1996).

To ensure high quality treatment in laparoscopic surgery, surgeons could consider following recommendations:

- Better training
  Residents should receive advanced laparoscopic training in cancer surgery, in particular during staging procedures and palliative cases. They could be trained to avoid surgical mistakes and to apply preventive measures against local wound recurrence that have been described in the literature (Köckerling et al. 1997). This opportunity should be integrated into formal surgical training.
- Accreditation of surgeons
  After having received corresponding training, laparoscopic surgeons should be awarded with an accreditation of the SAGES, the EAES and/or the ELSA.
- Quality control
  Surgeons performing laparoscopic surgery in curative intent should be open to a quality control. For example, they can enter their patients prospectively and consecutively into an independent database.

As long as the long-term outcome of cancer patients operated on using the laparoscope has not been determined by prospective randomized trials, we consider it unethical to operate on those patients outside the boundaries of prospective, independent registries or randomized trials.

The Incidence of Port-Site Recurrences Is Low Using Careful Operating Technique

It is now reasonable to state that both incidences of port-site recurrences in laparoscopic surgery and wound recurrences in open surgery are low (around 1% when careful technique is used). For statistical reasons related to the rarity of the outcome event, it is questionable if significant differences might ever be demonstrated in the incidence of wound recurrences between open and laparoscopic surgery.

Studies on port-site recurrences have focused surgeons again on the presence and liberation of free viable cancer cells during surgery. Even if it is true that the historical publication by Turnbull, promoting a "no-touch", atraumatic operating technique (Turnbull et al. 1967), was not confirmed by enough high-level evidence studies, atraumatic surgery and dissection within anatomic planes are back in the forefront. Zirngibl and colleagues clearly demonstrated that intraoperative perforations during open curative rectal surgery are associated with an increased rate of local recurrence (Zirngibl et al. 1989). In contrast, Heald et al. presented evidence that total mesorectal excision – in the anatomic, "holy" plane – is the clue to pelvic recurrence (Heald et al. 1982). The outcome of cancer surgery – open or laparoscopic – might benefit from a better method of dealing with free and spilled cells.

A few typical situations are associated with port-site recurrences. Examples are unsuspected gallbladder carcinoma and multiple colon tumors, which represent a significant number of port-site recurrences in the literature. In those cases, the surgeon begins the procedure with an inaccurate idea of the disease, so that the kind of operating procedure and the corresponding technique might be inadequate. Thus, unexpected complications such as port-site recurrences might occur. There is no simple solution to this problem. For example, pre- or intra-operative diagnosis of gallbladder carcinoma might be very difficult, and second or third colorectal tumors might be missed during endoscopic procedures. Thus, careful operating and bagging techniques should always been used in all laparoscopic

procedures, which is possible at low cost. Small and multiple colon cancers require detailed preoperative localization including inking, or laparoscopic procedures combined with coloscopy.

Most port-site recurrences have been documented in advanced stages of cancer. Such recurrences are, in a majority of cases, the expression of disseminated disease, for example, when disseminated tumor cells can be found within the abdominal cavity during the primary operation. Thus, it is difficult to conclude much about the prognostic significance of port-site recurrences.

Evidently, our main concern is patients suffering from early stages of disease (Dukes A or B) who have developed port-site recurrences. In such cases, port-site recurrences might not express advanced disease: they are rather caused by iatrogenic inoculation of tumor cells into the trocar wound during the procedure. Thus, poor laparoscopic technique represents an additional risk for these patients. If an isolated recurrence is observed at a port-site, it appears that radical excision of the port-site is associated with a good chance of cure.

Pathogenesis of Port-Site and Wound Recurrences

Animal studies have helped to reveal some of the mysteries of port-site and wound recurrences, notably as to the origin of the cells from which the secondary tumor arises, the means by which they are dispersed, and how local effects in the port-site wound can favor implantation. It is difficult to relate all of the published experimental animal protocols to the clinical setting.

Several problems are linked to the use of animal models. Most studies used suspension models reflecting disseminated disease. We still lack a solid tumor model that would reproduce the clinical practice. The type and length of surgical procedures performed in small animal studies are different from those in human patients.

Only if we can evaluate the models critically can we evaluate the conclusions drawn from the experiments presented in the literature. Only if we can determine the part that each model plays, by knowing the behavior of the tumor cell lines, can we reliably identify those features of laparoscopy which have fostered implantation of cancer in small wounds.

The available studies suggest that possibly poor operative technique and not the type of surgery may lead to tumor cell exfoliation. The surgeon needs to breach the tumor, liberating cells into the peritoneal cavity and onto laparoscopic instruments. In advanced tumor stages, large amounts of tumor cells can present in the abdominal cavity at the beginning of the procedure and represent a major risk factor, since the development of port-site recurrences appears to be dose-dependent in various intraperitoneal seeding models.

Tumor cells are carried across the peritoneal cavity by peritoneal fluid currents. These fluid currents are influenced by physical factors. Laparoscopic instruments and trocars act as the major mode of tumor cell transport. Circumstances where the port-site is brought into prolonged contact with free cells (such as during exsufflation) will facilitate port-site contamination. Aerosolization of tumor cells only occurs during grossly contaminated and prolonged surgery, and does not act as a major mode of tumor cell transport.

CO_2 Pneumoperitoneum Has Adverse Effects

Although the problem of port-site recurrences is mainly related to the surgeon, the technique, and manipulation of the tumor bearing organ, some other factors, which are related to laparoscopy itself, have been demonstrated to influence tumor growth.

There are many indications that CO_2 pneumoperitoneum might have adverse effects that could cancel some of the advantages of the minimal access approach due to the unfavorable modification of the intracavitary environment. The possible stimulation of tumor cell growth and suppression of local immune defense by CO_2 has been shown in many experimental studies. This can be prevented either by the use of gasless exposure techniques or by using an inert gas for insufflation. Which of these options proves to be best will depend on the outcome of further clinical studies. Nevertheless, gasless laparoscopy is limited by the fact that poor lateral exposure is achieved, whereas helium insufflation seems to be a more advantageous strategy for further clinical investigation. Therefore, helium should be evaluated in prospective randomized clinical trials.

New therapeutic strategies, including instillation of cytotoxic and immune modulating agents in combination with laparoscopy and different gases, were reported to strongly inhibit tumor growth in experimental investigations. Adding various agents (cytotoxic, immunomodulating, adhesion blocking agents, etc.) to the gas (local) or intravenously (systemic) during the operation might further improve the outcome of curative cancer surgery.

Minimally Invasive Surgery Reduces the Immunological Trauma

Experimental data document that minimally invasive surgery reduces immunological trauma and might reduce postoperative tumor growth. There also seems to be a protective effect overall of a minimally invasive approach which reduces systemic immunodepression. Nevertheless, there is no simple pat answer to the question: "Is laparoscopy better for the immune system than open surgery?" There are a multitude of different effects at numerous levels of the immune system which can be interpreted in numerous ways.

Further studies will be needed in order to better work out the import of subtle differences in immune parameters and to better explain just where along the complex intertwined immune system pathways surgical trauma exerts itself. Despite these limitations, evaluation of the impact of surgery of all types on immune function remains a promising field of study. Armed with a better understanding, it may prove possible, via alterations in our surgical methods or via pharmacological means, to limit the detrimental immune system changes that occur after both open and laparoscopic surgery.

Perspectives

In the meantime, port-site recurrences are no longer considered as a major problem by most experienced laparoscopic surgeons, since they obviously can be prevented by careful technique and preventive measures. Nevertheless, in our opinion, the demonstrated benefits of diminished pain, shortened hospitalization, and preserved perioperative pulmonary function after laparoscopic surgery are still not sufficient to choose this technique for curative cancer treatment. To date, the proof that stage for stage, disease-free, and overall survival are identical or better than that achieved with more traditional open surgical techniques is still not available.

This situation will change in the next few years. Multicenter prospective data obtained for colorectal surgery have already documented that accurate oncological resection is possible using the laparoscope (Köckerling et al. 1998). Preliminary data from limited, prospective, randomized trials show that the laparoscopic approach achieves short-term oncologic results similar to those observed after open procedures for colon cancer (Lacy et al. 1998; Milsom et al. 1998). Large prospective randomized trials are under way that will provide surgeons with sufficient long-term oncologic data in a few years (Nelson et al. 1995; Wittich et al. 1997).

This worldwide clinical research effort is supported by active laboratory research focusing on:

- Surgical tumor seeding
- Influence of surgical trauma on postoperative tumor growth
- Relationship between wound healing, inflammation and carcinogenesis
- Better control of the operating environment

If we are able to deal with these issues, we will create new therapeutic strategies, including nonsurgical treatments. Patient outcome after curative cancer surgery will be further improved. This might be the most unexpected effect of the laparoscopic revolution.

References

Alexander RJ, Jaques BC, Mitchell KG (1993) Laparoscopically assisted colectomy and wound recurrence (letter; comment). Lancet 341:249–250

Bouvy ND, Marquet RL, Lambert SWJ, Jeekel J, Bonjer HJ (1996) Laparoscopic bowel resection in the rat: earlier restoration of IGF-1 and less tumor growth. Surg Endosc 10:567 (abstract)

Dorrance HR, Oein K, O'Dwyer PJ (1996) Laparoscopy promotes tumor growth in an animal model. Surg Endosc 10:559 (abstract)

Franklin ME, Rosenthal D, Abrego-Medina D, Dorman JP, Glass JL, Norem R, Diaz A (1996) Prospective comparison of open vs. laparoscopic colon surgery for carcinoma. Dis Colon Rectum 39:S35–S46

Heald RJ, Husband EM, Ryall RDH (1982) The mesorectum in rectal cancer surgery: the clue to pelvic recurrence ? Br J Surg 82:613–616

Hermanek P, Wiebelt H, Staimmer D, Riedel S, The German Study Group Colo-Rectal Carcinoma (SGCRC) (1995) Prognostic factors of rectum carcinoma. Experience of the German multicenter study SGCRC. Tumori 81[S1]:60–64

Hohenberger W, Altendorf-Hofmann A, Schmidt O (1995) [Surgical therapy for metastases of the soft tissue.] Langenbecks Arch Chir Suppl II:288–294

Hubens G, Pauwels M, Hubens A, Vermeulen P, Van Marck E, Eyskens E (1996) The influence of pneumoperitoneum on the peritoneal implantation of free intraperitoneal colon cancer cells. Surg Endosc 10:181 (abstract)

Hugues ESR, McDermott FT, Polgase A (1983) Tumor recurrence in the abdominal wall scar after large-bowel cancer surgery. Dis Colon Rectum 26:571–572

Jacobi CA, Sabat R, Ordemann J, Müller JM (1996a) [Influence of different gases on the tumor cell growth in laparoscopic surgery. Preliminary results of an experimental study in a rat model.] Langenbecks. Arch Chir 381[Suppl 1]: 127–130

Jacobi CA, Sabat R, Böhm B, Zieren HU, Volk HD, Müller JM (1996b) Pneumoperitoneum with CO_2 stimulates malignant tumor growth. Surg Endosc 10:551 (abstract)

Johnstone PAS, Rohde DC, Swartz SE, Fetter JE, Wexner SD (1996) Port-site recurrences after laparoscopic and thoracoscopic procedures in malignancy. J Clin Oncol 14:1950–1956

Jones DB, Guo LW, Reinhard MK, Soper NJ, Philpott GW, Connet J, Fleshman JW (1995) Impact of pneumoperitoneum on trocar site implantation of colon cancer in hamster model. Dis Colon Rectum 38:1182–1188

Köckerling F, Reymond MA, Schneider C, Hohenberger W (1997) [Mistakes and hazards in oncological laparoscopic surgery.] Chirurg 68:215–224

Köckerling F, Reymond MA, Schneider C, Wittekind C, Scheidbach H, Konradt J, Köhler L, Börlehner E, Kuthe A, Bruch HP, Hohenberger W (1998) Prospective multicenter study of the quality of oncological resection in patients undergoing laparoscopic colorectal surgery for cancer. The laparoscopic colorectal surgery study group. Dis Colon Rectum 41:963–970

Lacy AM, Delgado S, Garcia-Valdecasas JC, Castells A, Pique JM, Grande L, Fuster J, Targarona EM, Pera M, Visa J (1998) Port-site recurrences and recurrence after laparoscopic colectomy. Surg Endosc 12:1039–1042

Mathew G, Watson DI, Rofe AM, Baigrie CF, Ellis T, Jamieson GG (1996) Wound metastases following laparoscopic and open surgery for abdominal cancer in a rat model. Br J Surg 83:1087–1090

Milsom JW, Bohm B, Hammerhofer KA, Fazio V, Steiger E, Elson P (1998) A prospective, randomized trial comparing laparoscopic versus conventional techniques in colorectal cancer surgery: a preliminary report. J Am Coll Surg 187:46–54

Nelson H, Weeks JC, Wieand HS (1995) Proposed Phase III trial comparing laparoscopic-assisted colectomy versus open colectomy. J Natl Cancer Inst Monogr 19:51–56

Reilly WT, Nelson H, Schroeder G, Wieand HS, Bolton J, O'Connell MJ (1996) Wound recurrence following conventional treatment of colorectal cancer. Dis Colon Rectum 39:200–207

Reymond MA, Wittekind C, Jung A, Hohenberger W, Kirchner T, Köckerling F (1997) The incidence of port-site recurrences might be reduced. Surg Endosc 11:902–906

Turnbull RB, Kyle K, Watson FR, Spratt J (1967) Cancer: the influence of the no-touch isolation technique on survival rates. Ann Surg 166:420–425

Vukasin P, Ortega AE, Greene FL, Steele GD, Simons AJ, Anthone GJ, Weston LA, Beart RW (1996) wound recurrence following laparoscopic colon cancer resection. Results of The American Society of Colon and Rectal Surgeons Laparoscopic Registry. Dis Colon Rectum 39:S20–S23

Wexner SD, Cohen SM (1995) Port-site recurrences after laparoscopic colorectal surgery for cure of malignancy. Br J Surg 82:295–298

Wexner SD, Reissman P (1994) Laparoscopic colorectal surgery. A provocative critique. Int Surg 79:235–239

Wexner SD, Cohen SM, Ulrich A, Reissman P (1995) Laparoscopic colorectal surgery – are we being honest with our patients? Dis Colon Rectum 38:723–727

Wittich P, Kazemier G, Schouten WR, Jeekel J, Lange JF, Bonjer HJ (1997) [The 'colon cancer laparoscopic or open resection' (COLOR) trial.] Ned Tijdschr Geneeskd 141:1870–1871

Zirngibl H, Husemann B, Hermanek P (1989) Intra-operative spillage of tumor cells in surgery for rectal cancer. Dis Colon Rectum 33:610

Subject Index

The manufacturer's authorised representative in the EU is Springer
Nature Customer Service Centre GmbH, Europaplatz 3, 69115 Heidelberg,
Germany. If you have any concerns regarding our products, please
contact ProductSafety@springernature.com

Printed and bound by CPI Group (UK) Ltd, Croydon, CR0 4YY
06/05/2026
02103785-0001